The Clinical Interview and Physical Examination

The Clinical Interview and Physical Examination

EDITED BY
James C. Guckian, M.D.
Professor of Internal Medicine
Vice President for Medical Professional Affairs
The University of Texas Medical Branch
Galveston, Texas

Nine Contributors

J. B. Lippincott Company
Philadelphia London Mexico City New York St. Louis São Paulo Sydney

Acquisitions Editor: David A. Barnes
Sponsoring Editor: Richard Winters
Manuscript Editor: Lee Henderson
Indexer: Angela Holt
Design Coordinator: Caren Erlichman
Production Manager: Carol A. Florence
Compositor: Digitype
Printer/Binder: R. R. Donnelley & Sons Co.
Cover Printer: Philips Offset

 Printed in the United States of America. For information write J. B. Lippincott Company, East Washington Square, Philadelphia, Pennsylvania 19105.

6 5 4 3 2

Library of Congress Cataloging-in-Publication Data
The clinical interview and physical examination.

Includes index.
1. Medical history taking. 2. Physical diagnosis.
I. Guckian, James C., DATE. [DNLM: 1. Interviews
— methods. 2. Physical Examination — methods.
WB 205 C641]
RC65.C58 1987 616.07′51 87-3180
ISBN 0-397-50853-0

Contributors

John C. Barber, M.D.
Associate Professor and Chairman of Ophthalmology
The University of Texas Medical Branch
Galveston, Texas

James C. Guckian, M.D.
Professor of Internal Medicine
Vice President for Medical Professional Affairs
The University of Texas Medical Branch
Galveston, Texas

Joan R. Hebeler, M.D., F.A.A.P.
Formerly Associate Professor of Pediatrics
The University of Texas Medical Branch
Galveston, Texas

Alvin L. LeBlanc, M.D.
Professor of Obstetrics and Gynecology
Vice President for Hospital Affairs
The University of Texas Medical Branch
Galveston, Texas

Donald McDonald, M.D.
Professor Emeritus of Surgery (Urology)
The University of Texas Medical Branch
Galveston, Texas

Roger McNeil, M.D.
Clinical Assistant Professor of Otolaryngology
The University of Texas Medical Branch
Galveston, Texas

Harold H. Morris III, M.D.
Staff Physician
Department of Neurology
Section of Epilepsy and Clinical Neurophysiology
The Cleveland Clinic Foundation
Cleveland, Ohio

Murphy T. Scurry, M.D.
Clinical Professor of Internal Medicine
The University of Texas Medical Branch
Galveston, Texas

J. Marc Shabot, M.D.
Associate Professor of Internal Medicine
The University of Texas Medical Branch
Galveston, Texas

Preface

The Clinical Interview and Physical Examination includes discussions of the medical interview, how to perform a physical examination, normal physical findings, the contents of a general screening physical examination, and elementary physical diagnosis. It attempts to integrate data collection (interviewing skills, the content of a medical interview, and the general physical examination).

For a number of years, committees at the University of Texas Medical Branch have identified what is believed to be the "core" for a beginning clinical student. This book presents this core in a format that categorizes, interrelates, sequences, and graphically presents information for learning and reference. The format has been derived from a synthesis of research on learning modes, instructional strategies, information processing, and graphic design.

The objectives of the textbook are to facilitate the following goals:

- *Instilling in students professional attitudes toward their future roles as physicians. Students should*
  - Recognize their professional capabilities and limitations
  - Accept the necessity of maintaining professional competence by

    Being willing to learn from each patient

    Accepting responsibility to learn from reading

    Learning to evaluate critically the information received from faculty, house officers, and other students

    Learning to evaluate the reliability of information obtained from resources, using knowledge of the scientific method and normal and abnormal physiology

    Recognizing the need for all physicians to be teachers of other physicians, students, nurses, patients, and the public

    Being aware that their position as educated professionals requires certain commitments to professional associations and to the community, especially in regard to their special expertise as physicians
  - Relate effectively to patients and family by

    Being concerned about the welfare of the patient and the patient's family

    Being willing to devote the time and effort necessary to understand and solve the patient's problems

    Recognizing the patient's need to accept responsibility for his own health program

Recognizing the special needs of dying patients, those with incurable diseases, and their families, while becoming aware of how one's own attitudes toward death may affect the relationship with the patient

- Develop awareness and knowledge of religious, moral, and ethical issues as they relate to medicine and patient care, and develop a willingness to make their own convictions known while maintaining sensitivity and respect for the attitudes of others

- *Developing students' skill in solving clinical problems. Students should be able to*
  - Elicit appropriate historical information from the patient
  - Obtain information by means of an appropriate physical examination
  - Obtain information by laboratory examination or procedures by

    Asking for appropriate information

    Considering appropriate timing and sequencing of laboratory examinations

    Interpreting the significance of laboratory results with awareness of the finite limits of reliability and inherent sources of error in diagnostic tests
  - Skillfully record, maintain, and report clinical data, using the problem-oriented method
  - Develop adequate pathophysiologic and psychosocial knowledge so that they can begin to translate problems into diagnoses and to organize plans to solve problems
  - Organize and use resource material (books, etc.) to solve problems
  - Be willing to reexamine data bases (historical, physical, and laboratory) and their own decision-making process, and to alter decisions as new information is uncovered
  - Begin to recognize when consultation is necessary and how to integrate the information obtained
  - "Test" their assessments of problems
  - Learn to review problem lists to be certain that all problems have been considered and priorities established
  - Begin to learn how to react appropriately to emergency and nonemergency situations, to evaluate the seriousness of problems, and to establish appropriate priorities

The Clinical Interview and Physical Examination was designed to introduce students to the practice of medicine and to prepare them for additional training in clinical medicine. It presupposes that students entering clinical clerkships must have the ability *to interview and examine a patient, to interpret the data obtained, and to begin problem-solving.*

- The major part of the text involves teaching approaches to *adult* patients and strategies for interview and examination. A basic general interview and examination must be mastered; more detailed examinations can then be done as indicated by the history and general examination.

- A special chapter deals with a special problem in both interviewing and examination—the pediatric patient.

Finally, this textbook has the limitations of all textbooks: it does not contain adequate illustrations of the subject matter. Slide–tape or videotape programs illustrating examination techniques, skin lesions, lesions of the head and neck, heart sounds and murmurs, lung sounds, and so forth can be used in conjunction with the text.

I wish to acknowledge the following persons:

- My colleagues, Emil Petrusa, Ph.D., and Paul Horvatich, Ph.D.
- Peter Bowman, Ph.D., Division of Biomedical Communications, University of Texas Medical Branch, who rewrote the first draft into the format that is used in this text
- The Photography Section of the Division of Biomedical Communications
- Reneé Robillard, who rewrote many of the chapters
- And especially Bonnie Rhew, who not only kept the editor and authors on track but did all of the typing

James C. Guckian, M.D.

Contents

The Clinical Interview and Physical Examination

Patients' Bill of Rights

- Patients have the right to considerate and respectful care.
- Patients have the right to obtain from their physician complete current information concerning their diagnosis, treatment, and prognosis in terms patients can be reasonably expected to understand. When it is not medically advisable to give such information to patients, the information should be made available to an appropriate person in their behalf. Patients have the right to know, by name, the physician responsible for coordinating their care.
- Patients have the right to receive from their physician information necessary to give informed consent prior to the start of any procedure and/or treatment. Except in emergencies, such information for informed consent should include, but not necessarily be limited to, the specific procedures and/or treatment, the medically significant risks involved, and the probable duration of incapacitation. Where medically significant alternatives for care or treatment exist, or when patients request information concerning medical alternatives, they have the right to such information. Patients also have the right to know the name of the person responsible for the procedures and/or treatment.
- Patients have the right to refuse treatment to the extent permitted by law and to be informed of the medical consequences of their action.
- Patients have the right to every consideration of privacy concerning their own medical care program. Case discussion, consultation, examination, and treatment are confidential and should be conducted discreetly. Those not directly involved in patients' care must have their permission to be present.
- Patients have the right to expect that all communications and records pertaining to their care should be treated as confidential.
- Patients have the right to expect that within its capacity a hospital must make reasonable response to the request of a patient for services. The hospital must provide evaluation, service, and/or referral as indicated by the urgency of the case. When medically permissible patients may be transferred to another facility only after they have received a complete explanation concerning the needs for and alternatives to such a transfer. The institution to which patients are to be transferred must first have accepted them for transfer.
- Patients have the right to obtain information as to any relationship of their hospital to other health care and educational institutions insofar as their care is concerned. Patients have the right to obtain information as to the existence of any professional relationships among individuals, by name, who are treating them.
- Patients have the right to be advised if the hospital proposes to engage in or perform human experimentation affecting their care or treatment. The patients have the right to refuse to participate in such research projects.
- Patients have the right to expect reasonable continuity of care. They have the right to know in advance what appointment times and physicians are available and where. Patients have the right to expect that the hospital will provide a mechanism whereby they are informed by their physician or a delegate of the physician of their continuing health care requirements following discharge.
- Patients have the right to examine and receive an explanation of their bill regardless of source of payment.
- Patients have the right to know what hospital rules and regulations apply to their conduct as a patient.

PART ONE

The Medical Interview

CHAPTER ONE

Establishing an Effective Patient–Physician Relationship

James C. Guckian, M.D.

GENERAL OVERVIEW

Purposes

The purposes of the medical interview are to:

- collect information about patients and illnesses
- establish a therapeutic contract
- understand patients' environments
- establish lists of problems that should be solved
- develop problem-solving plans that encompass
  - diagnostic studies
  - therapy (the interview itself may initiate therapy)
  - education of the person and the person's family

Collection of Information

Diagnosis and treatment in medicine begin with the interview. The more skilled the interviewer, the more complete and reliable the data on which diagnoses and treatment are based. In addition, skilled interviewers can explain findings and treatment plans to patients without creating anxiety and can get patients to trust them and to feel confident of their abilities to deal with their problems. Proper collection of information from patients requries:

- precision and specificity
- quantitative evaluation
- completeness

Precision

Assessment of patients in an interview is a "scientific" evaluation. Thus, the information that is gathered about dates, times, and particular circumstances must be precise and specific.

Quantitation

Measurements that are more quantitative than "mild" or "severe" should be attempted.

EXAMPLES:

- shortness of breath after walking two blocks at a regular pace
- severe pain in the mid-chest lasting 15 minutes
- ten to 12 loose watery brown bowel movements per day

Completeness

Enough data must be gathered for the physician to feel comfortable with the accuracy of the diagnosis.

COMMUNICATION SKILLS

The Most Important Factor	The physician's skill in communicating with the patient is an important factor in determining how much the physician can help the patient. NOTE: Also important, of course, are such factors as professional and technical competence, fees, and courtesy of office staff. A good interview will allow the physician to understand the patient's illness and the social, psychological, ethnic, and economic influences on the patient's health.
NOTE! The Pediatric Patient	The first eight chapters of this textbook address interviewing and the principles of interviewing generally. Interviewing under special circumstances is covered later. Specifically, Chapter 17 deals with interviewing parents of infants and children and interviewing children themselves.
Frank Discussion	Young physicians have a tendency to revert to techniques that people usually use to handle questions that make them uncomfortable; they change the topic, talk about a neutral topic (such as the weather), or become evasive. In a patient-physician relationship, however, it is inappropriate to avoid discussing unpleasant matters. Physicians should never fall back on social small talk to avoid discussing topics that make them uncomfortable.
Patients' Concern	Patients are concerned about such things as: • the severity of their symptoms • the possibility of their recovery or death • the effect of their illness on personal activities • the embarrassment of having to disrobe for a physical examination
Patients' Strong Feelings	Patients may develop feelings of anger over waiting to see physicians or feelings of confusion over the use of medical jargon. These strong feelings are not communicated directly to their physicians, but if they are allowed to build up, they may disrupt the patient-physician relationship.

(Continued)

COMMUNICATION SKILLS, Continued

Sensitivity

To free patients to express their fears, anger, and confusion openly, physicians must be sensitive to feelings that patients express indirectly and make it possible for patients to discuss these feelings in the interview.

EXAMPLES:

- When a patient looks apprehensive after a physician states that an injection must be given, the physician might respond:
  - "Come now, this isn't going to hurt that much!"

  OR
  - "Injections are unpleasant and frightening, aren't they?"
- After a physican explains to a patient that he has high blood pressure and must take medication, the patient mentions that he had a close friend who died from high blood pressure. The physician might respond:
  - "Your friend probably didn't take care of himself."

  OR
  - "Yes, high blood pressure is dangerous, and you're right to be concerned. With proper treatment, however, high blood pressure can be controlled, and you can live a normal life."
- The physician should consider which of these responses is likely to promote cooperation and a beneficial relationship between physician and patient. Such consideration necessitates recognition of the patient's feelings.

TRUST AND CONFIDENCE

Introduction

Symptoms that bring people to physicians often promote anxiety, feelings of helplessness, disruption of personal relationships, and loss of income. Thus, patients come to physicians with both hope and fear. They hope that the cause of their symptoms will be discovered and appropriate steps taken to correct them. At the same time, they fear that the physicians will not be able to help them. These fears may be accompanied by anxiety over the cost of care and fear of diagnostic or therapeutic procedures.

Trust in Professional Skill

Trust in the professional skill of physicians is usually created by the confidence physicians display and by patients' perceptions of the professionalism of physicians' offices (patients notice diplomas on the walls).

Most Important Factor

The relationship that is formed between the patient and physician is the most important factor in the development of trust and confidence. Patients cannot usually judge a physician's medical skills and knowledge.

Personal Trust

Trust and confidence are created when physicians maintain a friendly but dignified demeanor that is becoming to a professional and when they treat their patients with interest, respect, and competence.

NOTE: Previous successful treatment of the patient, the patient's family, or friends also creates trust.

PATIENTS' EXPECTATIONS

What Patients Expect	Patients' expectations are influenced by their pain and fear, but almost all patients do expect: • to have the cause of their symptoms located and corrected • to get some reassurance from their physician • to have a feeling of well-being after treatment NOTE: Patients (except for those who achieve satifaction from being sick) have trouble accepting the fact that they cannot always return to being their "same old selves" again.
IMPORTANT!	Physicians should deal with all of their patients' expectations realistically.

INDEPENDENCE

Types of Relationships

Three types of interview relationships are possible.

IF THE PHYSICIAN	THEN THE PATIENT	COMMENT
is completely authoritarian	• may lose independence • tries to please the physician • may not take an active part in treatment	This relationship is usually necessary in emergencies, but is not useful in usual interviewing and data-gathering.
exercises some authority	has a greater feeling of independence and participates more actively in the treatment	In this relationship, a desire to please the physician may still cause the patient to provide information that he or she thinks the physician wants to hear. Alertness and skill in phrasing questions can neutralize this tendency, however, and the interview can be successful.
moderates the use of authority and encourages the patient to collaborate actively with the physician	• feels more independence • feels responsible for the accuracy of the diagnosis • feels responsible for the outcome of treatment • participates actively in treatment	This mutual-participation relationship greatly facilitates the collection of accurate, complete information.

Allowance for Changing Conditions

The physician-patient relationship should be continuous, but it should allow for changing conditions. Physicians must be able to provide a wide range of services to their patients --from routine immunizations to treatment of emergencies to counseling for emotional problems. The ability of the relationship to accommodate these changing conditions depends upon the patterns established in early interviews.

THE THERAPEUTIC CONTRACT

Introduction

An unwritten, implicit contract must be formed between a patient and physician. The patient expects the physician to make an accurate diagnosis and provide appropriate treatment. The physician expects the patient to provide accurate information and to follow the treatment regimen. This implicit therapeutic contract is influenced a great deal by the relationship established through interviews. Unless a sound contract is formed, diagnosis and treatment are seldom successful.

Importance of the Patient's Environment

Understanding a patient's personality and life situation is essential to the development of therapeutic plans. The patient's job and family situation should be explored, and sometimes other social relationships as well. Such exploration often requires several interviews so that the patient can learn to trust the physician and not feel that the physician is making value judgments about his or her life-style.

Establishing a Problem List

During an interview, the interviewer receives and categorizes a large amount of information. A problem list is a way to organize the physical, emotional, or situational difficulties the patient or physician feels are affecting the patient's health. The list helps the physician to develop hypotheses about the causes of these difficulties.

Developing a Plan for Solving Problems

During the interview, tentative plans are also developed for solving the problems. The interviewer seeks specific information on how the patient or other physicians have attempted to solve the problems in the past. The patient and the family of the patient receive information about the problems and the plans that are being developed to solve them, which includes information about the nature of the illness and ways in which health can be maintained.

CHAPTER TWO

Interview Strategies

James C. Guckian, M.D.

THE INTERVIEW COMPONENTS

Opening of Interview	When seeing a new patient for the first ime, interviewers should introduce themselves. EXAMPLE: "I am student physician, ____(name)____." If it is not clear how the patient's name should be pronounced, the pronunciation should be checked with the patient at this time. Some interviewers feel that some social talk at the outset of interview will set the patient at ease, but since most patients come to physicians with specific problems, they expect those problems to be addressed immediately. Thus, the interview should begin with an open-ended question. EXAMPLES: • "What problems have you been having?" • "What has brought you to see me today?"
Middle of Interview	Most of an interview involves collection of information on the patient and his or her problems. The interviewer moves from open-ended questions to more specific questions as the interview progresses.
Closing of Interview	Closing an interview is often a difficult time for the inexperienced interviewer, who may not be aware that the closing does not usually take place until after the physical examination has been completed. Before the examination, experienced interviewers frequently ask two questions: • "Is there anything that hasn't been covered and needs to be brought up?" • "Do you have any questions?" Once these questions are answered, the interviewer can say, "Now we will proceed with the physical examination."
End of Visit	After the physical examination is completed, the patient returns to the interview room. At this time, the physician: • answers the patient's questions • tells the patient what he or she thinks is wrong or thinks the problems represent • outlines a diagnostic and treatment plan EXAMPLE: "Mr. Jones, I am not sure what is causing the pain and diarrhea you've been having for the past 3 weeks, so we need to do some tests to find out. As you indicated, these symptoms may be related to a personal problem you have, that is, your impending divorce.

(Continued)

THE INTERVIEW COMPONENTS, Continued

Plan Outline

The plan may include:

- diagnostic tests
- medications
- obtaining information from other sources
- a follow-up interview

EXAMPLE "Mr. Jones, I think there are a number of things that we should do. First, I would like to obtain the reports of the x-rays you had done in the other hospital. I then want to schedule a procto-scopic exam and collect a stool specimen for culture. My secretary will schedule these for you and a return appointment in 3 days. Do you have any questions?"

A beginning student should probably not speak in such definitive terms. A more proper response may include a reference to the supervising physician.

EXAMPLE: "Mr. Jones, I think there are a number of things that we might do. I would like to discuss your problems with Dr. Smith. We will return in a few minutes to discuss our plans with you. Do you have any questions?"

TYPES OF INTERVIEWS

Introduction	There are two main types of interviews: the open-ended interview and the direct-question interview.
Direct-Question Interview	In the direct-question interview, the interviewer asks questions about a list of items and expects the patient to answer only those questions. When the patient provides information about a general topic, the physician asks specific questions about the topic. The patient responds passively and limits his or her responses to short, direct answers to the interviewer's questions. Sometimes the patient may not even understand the interviewer's vocabulary, jargon or diction. This type of interview does not produce an effective patient-physician relationship and does not give the interviewer access to psychological and social factors that may be affecting the patient's health.
Open-Ended Interview	The open-ended interview involves both data-collection and establishment of rapport between patient and interviewer. In this type of interview, the interviewer initially uses the minimal amount of prompting of the patient to obtain the maximal amount of information.
Conditions	To be successful, the open-ended interview requires four conditions: • The interview should be conducted in a setting that encourages spontaneous behavior on the part of patients. • The manner of the interviewer should encourage the patient to speak freely. • The interviewer should be alert to the patient's nonverbal, as well as verbal, communication. • The interviewer should begin by providing little direction to the interview and should increase the direction as the interview progresses.
Setting	Comfort and privacy should be provided, and the interviewer should arrange for the fewest possible interruptions.

(Continued)

TYPES OF INTERVIEWS, Continued

Encourage Communication	In general, the patient will respond more freely if the interviewer says little other than to encourage the patient to describe his or her problems, especially in the earlier part of the interview.
Attention to Nonverbal Behavior	Nonverbal communication, which often indicates more about patients' inner feelings than verbal messages, may occur through patients' behavior, manner, and appearance. Interviewers may call patients' attention to the non-verbal messages to facilitate verbal communication.
Information-Seeking	The interview should begin with a broad, open-ended question. EXAMPLE: "What kind of difficulties are you having?" As the patient begins to answer, the interviewer should encourage elaboration of the story through words and gestures.

IF	THEN
the interviewer sees that the patient is having trouble describing his or her problems OR if the interviewer cannot follow the patient's account	the interviewer should point this out to the patient
the interviewer sees contradictions between the patient's behavior and the account	the patient's attention should be drawn to the behavior
the interviewer feels that not enough specific information is being provided where it is needed	the interviewer may ask more direct questions

(Continued)

TYPES OF INTERVIEWS, Continued

Directing the Interview

Although the interviewer will usually learn most about patients by letting them tell their stories in their own ways, the interviewer is still in charge of the interview, which must usually be conducted within a certain period. Some patients may wander from the main topic to avoid discussing problems that they fear may be serious. In these situations, the interviewer must interrupt and redirect the interview. Sometimes only a simple statement is required.

> EXAMPLE: "Mrs. Brown, I want to get back to your chest pains."

At other times, a direct question may be necessary.

Medical Jargon

It is sometimes tempting for beginning students (and even for some experienced physicians) to use some of their newly discovered medical vocabulary. Though some sophisticated persons will understand some medical terms, most persons do not. Beware of using medical terminology unless it is appropriate for the person being interviewed.

REMEMBER!

Above all else, a good interviewer MUST GIVE THE PATIENT UNDIVIDED ATTENTION.

EXAMPLE OF THE DIRECT-QUESTION INTERVIEW

Introduction	In this example of the direct-question approach, the physician often interrupts the patient's sequence of thought and directs the patient to one question after another, thus preventing the patient from telling the story in his or her own way.

Example

Physician: "What brings you in today?"

Patient: "Last night I had a terrible pain in my stomach -- right here" (the patient points to his lower abdomen).

Physician: "Have you ever had it before?"

Patient: "No, not that I can remember."

Physician: "Have you ever had a pain like this before?"

Patient: "Well, no, not exactly. I have had slight stomachaches before, but I've never had anything like this."

Physician: "Do you have any other symptoms?"

Patient: "No, doctor."

Physician: "Ever been troubled with constipation or diarrhea?"

Patient: "No."

Physician: "Have you had any vomiting?"

Patient: "No."

Physician: "Have you ever had diabetes or tuberculosis or kidney difficulties or any sort of liver disease or asthma or hay fever or allergies?"

Patient: "No."

Physician: "How are your teeth?"

Patient: "O.K."

Physician: "Have you ever had any operations or serious illnesses or accidents?"

Patient: "I had my tonsils taken out some time ago."

Physician: "How long ago?"

Patient: "Oh, a long time ago. I was about 4 -- or 5 -- years old."

(Continued)

EXAMPLE OF THE DIRECT-QUESTION INTERVIEW, Continued

Analysis

This interview revealed only the kind of information that is obtained by asking patients to fill out questionnaires. By using an interview method that limited the patient's responses chiefly to "yes" or "no," the physician did not obtain data that the patient might have revealed if more open-ended questions had been asked.

Use of Specific Questions

Sometimes, of course, questions must be asked about times, places, dates, and events. The interviewer, however, should wait to ask such questions until the patient stops talking or until near the end of the interview so as not to interfere with patients' telling their own story.

> EXAMPLE: A 42-year-old man was arguing with his 16-year-old son. The boy demanded that he listen to what he was about to say. And, to comply, the father leaned out from the ladder that he was on. He fell off the ladder and sustained a serious back injury, which brought him to the hospital. When asked what caused his injury, the father launched into an angry description of the argument with his son, including a description of his smoking, drinking, and carousing.

Although it is important to know how far the patient fell and when he fell, the interviewer should not interrupt this patient's display of anger with specific questions. The relationship with his son may be a more important problem in his life than the injury he received from his fall. Thus, the flow of spontaneous information should not be interrupted unless necessary.

> NOTE: Information gathered in this fashion does not emerge in a precise order that fits record-keeping forms. Organizing historical information into a systematic history is a different process from that used to gather information during an interview.

EXAMPLE OF THE OPEN-ENDED INTERVIEW

Introduction

An open-ended interview begins with broad questions that invite an unrestricted response.

EXAMPLE: "When you called me, you said you felt bad. Could you tell me more about that?"

When patients begin to tell why they came to the physician, they should be allowed to continue without interruption. Any pauses or points of hesitation should be used _not_ to change the course of the interview, but to encourage continuation.

EXAMPLE: If a patient pauses briefly, it is better to simply encourage conversation by a simple comment such as "Go ahead," "Can you tell me more?" or "Un-huh."

Attention to Patient's Story

The physician should pay attention to how patients:

- describe their complaints
- express concern about their complaints
- relate their complaints to events in their lives
- describe the sequence of the events

EXAMPLE: A 32-year-old man describes headaches. If the physician interrupts with questions about past treatment and dates, the physician diverts the patient from the next topic he might have discussed. For instance, the patient might have gone from talking about his headaches to describing a stressful relationship with his wife, and the physician would have obtained important information about the cause of the headaches.

Example

An example of an interview conducted in the open-ended fashion follows. The kind of information that is obtained with this method should be compared with that obtained with the direct-question type of interview.

(Continued)

EXAMPLE OF THE OPEN-ENDED INTERVIEW, Continued

Physician: "Could you tell what brought you to see me?"

Patient: "Well, like I told you over the telephone, I've been having these pains in my stomach. They started about a month ago and they are getting worse...to the point sometimes that I find it hard to continue work and I just have to go home. Like last week, it was so bad that I stayed home every day. My stomach is really bothering me."

Physician: "Go on."

Patient: "You see, I am the chief accountant at the Interstate Bank, and it is audit time. We are already behind. I am not sure if we will be able to make the federal deadlines. We just have to get these things out in time. I just can't have the board and the feds on me all at once."

Physician: "Yes, I can see that."

Patient: "I suppose, well, I should get this out right away. I should tell you I have been really worried about stomach cancer. You see, my uncle died of stomach cancer 2 years ago, and, well, his wife moved in with my folks. My folks have been pretty busy taking care of his wife, and she is feeling pretty bad. Then my father died of a heart attack a month ago. I have only been married a short time, and I just got to thinking that I wouldn't want to leave my wife and my new baby in that position. Well, you know how someone can get when it hits this close to home."

Physician: "I can see you are pretty worried about that."

Patient: "You can say that again, doctor. This stomachache began just after I got married; and the job...I don't know...maybe it's just the tension. Sometimes I wonder if all of these are connected in some way."

Physician: "You see some connection between your pain, your job, and your recent marriage?"

Patient: "Well, I've thought about it. I have had stomachaches before in my life. You know, the usual kind that go away. They came on after I had eaten too much. But nothing like this. Rolaids won't even touch this. I just feel scared."

Physician: (Silence)

Patient: "I'm beginning to wonder about that cancer stuff. My God, if it is cancer.... I don't know, I'm just scared."

(Continued)

EXAMPLE OF THE OPEN-ENDED INTERVIEW, Continued

Analysis	Abdominal pain is a common complaint. After this patient mentioned such pain, the physician could have: • attempted to localize the pain, to get a more accurate description of it, and to concentrate on developing a diagnosis • inquired about other symptoms • begun to take a more complete history If the physician had made one of these choices, however, the circumstances of the patient's life situation that seem to relate directly to the pain (particularly his concern about stomach cancer) would not have been revealed. Yet, all these circumstances have a powerful influence on the nature of the relationship the patient may develop with this physician.
Information Revealed	After asking only five open-ended questions, the physician in this case already knows: • the duration of the patient's symptoms • the patient's occupation • the patient's marital status • information about the patient's father's death • information about the patient's uncle's death • the patient's feelings about the two deaths in his family • the possible connection between the symptoms and the patient's life stress If the physician continues in this fashion, he or she will be able to formulate some questions that are worthy of diagnostic exploration. • Is the abdominal pain associated with anger or fear of failure in both his job <u>and</u> his marriage? • Since his uncle died just 2 years ago, is it possible that the symptoms represent a reaction to that event? • Is the pain related to the father's death? NOTE: Of course, we still know nothing about the patient's relationship with his uncle or his father.

(Continued)

EXAMPLE OF THE OPEN-ENDED INTERVIEW, Continued

Encouraging Elaboration	Not every patient will speak as freely, without prompting, as this one. If patients seem to want to continue but hestitates, the interviewer can facilitate continuation. EXAMPLE: "I'm not quite sure I understand; can you explain a little more?" or "I can see that this is important to you, please continue if you would like." Statements of this sort will encourage patients to elaborate on matters that they have introduced, without feeling that they are being pushed.

SPECIFIC QUESTIONS

Introduction

At some point in any interview, more specific information will be needed, and direct questions must be asked. If the interview has not been limited to questions that require only brief answers or "yes" or "no" answers up to this point, however, the specific questions will clarify matters without stifling free communication.

Guidelines

The following guidelines should help to ensure that direct questions are used appropriately:

- Questions should progress from the general to the specific.
- Questions should progress from the less personal to the more personal.
- Questions should be worded so that answers of a sentence or more are required rather than just a "yes" or "no."
- Questions should be worded in such a way that the interviewer's bias is not injected into the interview.

General to Specific

The physician should start with relatively broad questions and move to progressively more specific, focused questions.

> EXAMPLE: The first question might be something like, "You say you think the headaches might be connected with your job. Can you tell me why you feel that way?"

At this time, the patient might express more concern about his new job responsibilities. The physician could then ask a question about the stresses in the patient's life that will allow the patient to feel free to talk about his fears. As the discussion becomes more specific, the foundation will be laid for open and unbiased responses.

Less Personal to More Personal

Most people cherish and protect their privacy, even when speaking to their physicians. If physicians show consideration and develop a sound professional relationship with their patients from the beginning of their interviews, however, and if they begin the interview with questions that do not threaten patients' privacy, patients will be relaxed, trusting, and cooperative when questions that are more personal must be asked.

(Continued)

SPECIFIC QUESTIONS, Continued

Avoiding "Yes" and "No" Responses

Even when specific questions must be asked, patients should be allowed to continue to talk freely. Questions that require only a "yes" or "no" answer interrupt the spontaneity of the patients' thoughts and conversation and invites them only to wait for another question after their short response.

> EXAMPLE: The physician could say to a patient, "Tell me something about your marriage," as opposed to asking, "Are you happily married?"
> OR
> "Tell me what your headache is like," rather than "Is the pain sharp?"

Avoiding Interviewer Bias

Patients' responses depend largely on the wording of the questions. Therefore, interviewers can introduce bias into the interview in several ways. For instance, questions can be loaded; that is, a question can be asked in such a way that it is much easier for a patient to give a certain answer.

> EXAMPLE: If the physician says, during a physical examination, "It hurts here, doesn't it?" the patient will assume that the doctor expects a "yes" answer and is more likely to answer "yes" than "no."

Another way to load a question is to use words that elict strong emotions.

> EXAMPLE: "Do you have to spank your children often?" will produce more emotion than "How do you discipline your children?"

The interviewer's tone of voice, manner, and body language can also introduce bias.

(Continued)

SPECIFIC QUESTIONS, Continued

Speaking the Patient's Language

Sometimes the vocabulary or cultural background of physician and patient are vastly different, and this may lead to confusion during the interview. Sometimes patients will reply "yes" or "no" to questions to cover their embarrassment at not knowing the meaning of the physician's words. Since physicians must use language understandable to patients to ensure communication, they must assess, in their first interaction with their patients, the level of communication that is appropriate.

IF	THEN
patients do not understand the words used	physicians should use language that the patients _do_ understand
patients do understand some medical vocabulary	physicians should _not_ oversimplify

Misinterpretation

Sometimes a physician will interpret an answer according to his or her own bias.

> _EXAMPLE_: If the physican asks, "Have you had the usual childhood immunizations?" and the patient replies "Yes," the physician might assume that the patient has had mumps, measles, rubella, DPT, and polio immunizations. The patient, however, might be referring to only DPT, and the physician would then have missed an important therapeutic point.

SELF-ASSESSMENT

Mark the Single Correct Answer, or Answer as Indicated

1. A 25-year-old woman complains of recurrent headaches. She says, "I've had this headache for so long, and no doctor has ever been able to find the cause. What do you think it could be?" Which of the following is the best response? What is wrong with the others?

   a. You seem upset. Is there a problem at home that's bothering you?
   b. Could you tell me more about the headaches, so that I can understand more about them?
   c. Don't worry. I'm sure we can find the cause.
   d. You shouldn't expect someone to understand and diagnose your problem immediately. Give me some more information.

2. Your nurse gives you a paper with the patient's name and age on it. You know nothing about the patient's problem.

   A. When you walk into the examining room where the patient is seated, what is the first thing you should do?

   ____

   B. The patient may present his/her chief complaint in a few words or a short sentence. Your response to this may facilitate or hinder communication. Place a plus sign (+) in the space in front of the response that would facilitate communication and a minus sign (-) in the space in front of the response that would hinder communication if the patient states, "This persistent diarrhea just has me baffled."

_____(1) "Uh humm."
_____(2) "Yes?"
_____(3) "Can you tell me a little more about that?"
_____(4) "Have you been traveling abroad?"

   C. As you pursue a chronological history of the patient's chief complaint, you also want to be aware of responses that facilitate communication. Place a plus sign (+) in the space in front of the open-ended questions and a minus sign (-) in the space in front of the closed questions.

_____(1) "How many times have you had this before?"
_____(2) "Is the pain sharp?"
_____(3) "What is the pain like?"
_____(4) "Do you have nausea with the pain?"
_____(5) "Where is the pain located?"

(Continued)

SELF-ASSESSMENT, Continued

Questions 3 through 6 contain statements by a patient and a series of possible responses by a physician. Select the response that is most appropriate. Explain why the others may not be as appropriate.

3. Man-- Age 40: "It's not that I don't want to do something about my nerves ... I just ... well ... I know what I ought to do ... but for some reason or other, I just can't do a thing."

    a. I am sure that if we talk over what you've thought of doing, we can figure out what is best to do.
    b. Obviously this is a complicated problem or else you could have decided what to do about it. Tell me more about it.
    c. Are you sure you know what you ought to do? It seems to me that if you really had a clear idea of what you ought to do, you'd be able to go ahead and do it.
    d. I think that doing something--anything--would help you overcome your inertia.

4. Woman-- Age 54: "I couldn't let my daughter help me now that I'm down and out. I've got that shred of pride left ... because you see I remember when she was a kid I didn't provide any care or support for her. I worked 50 hours a week ... her father died when the kid was born ... and I let the relatives push her around ... and now ... it certainly was like a knife stuck in me when she visited me the other day and said, "We can make a go of it Mom." No! No! I won't let her do it. It'll be hard...."

    a. Have you investigated the possibility of social security pension? Possiblysomething could be worked out there that wouldn't make it necessary for you to impose on your daughter.
    b. What was your married life like? Had you and your husband planned for a child?
    c. You seem to feel that your behavior in the past makes you unworthy of the help your daughter wants to give you now. Is that what you mean?
    d. Have you thought about what it will mean to your daughter if you don't let her do this thing for you?
    e. Well, you certainly have no right to expect to ruin her life any further.

    (Continued)

SELF-ASSESSMENT, Continued

5. Woman-- Age 22: "I can't decide what to do without help. Please tell me what you think I should do. It's like at the lab.... I can't go ahead on my own. I just can't. I want to be told, ... then it's not my fault if things go wrong. And they would go wrong. I feel so helpless."

   a. You say it's not your fault if things go wrong even after you've been told what to do. Can you tell me what you mean?
   b. You feel that you just aren't capable of doing things unaided, but you know that's not true. You are capable.
   c. It's not really that you can't go ahead on your own. It's just that you think you can't.
   d. You've really got a system. If things go wrong, it's not your fault, and if they go well, I expect you take the credit for it.

6. Man-- Age 46: "Well, this new young guy came into the group. He's a big shot, has all the answers. Thinks he's going places. But-- my God-- he doesn't know me! I'll get ahead of him, if I have a stroke trying."

   a. I don't care how you run your business life, but I wish you'd quit trying to be such a big shot here on the ward.
   b. It's a fine thing to try to get ahead, but do you think that by starting out with such an attitude toward him you're going at it right?
   c. And that will probably take a lot of careful planning and thinking. You'll want to go carefully.
   d. You're really determined that he won't beat you out. Can you tell me more about that?
   e. Let's wait a minute there. Why is it so important to you to want to get ahead of this man?

7. Which opening will allow the greatest independence for the patient?

   a. I am Dr. Foster. The nurse tells me that you have high blood pressure. Have a seat and tell me about it.
   b. Good morning, Mrs. Jones. I am Dr. Foster. I understand that you may have a problem with your blood pressure. Won't you have a seat and tell me what you can about it?
   c. Mrs. Jones, the nurse tells me that you are hypertensive. Be seated and tell me how long your blood pressure has been high.

(Continued)

SELF-ASSESSMENT, Continued

8. Which response would most reasonably fulfill the patient's expectations?

Patient: "Doctor, these headaches are killing me. I can't sleep, I can't drive, I can't even find a comfortable position."

Physician:
a. Miss Adams, I am sure that we can find the cause and relieve the pain.
b. Miss Adams, you are very upset. If you can calm down, we can deal with the matter.
c. I can understand your discomfort, Miss Adams. When we know more about the cause of your headaches, I think we can design a plan that will help.

9. Name the four characteristics of open-ended interviewing.

1. ______________________________
2. ______________________________
3. ______________________________
4. ______________________________

Answer the following questions either TRUE or FALSE.

10. An interview should be opened with a series of direct questions, to obtain as much factual information as rapidly as possible.

11. When specific questions are asked, relatively broad questions should be followed by more narrowly focused ones, and giving advice should be avoided before the patient's complete history is elicted.

Choose the best response. Explain why the other choices are not as appropriate.

12. In beginning an interview, which type of questions should be asked first?

a. Questions that offer a choice of topics but can be answered with one word.
b. Questions that offer a choice of topics but cannot be answered with one word.
c. Questions that offer direct suggestions of a topic and can be answered with one word.
d. Questions that ask for information in specific terms, thus specifying the topic to be discussed.

13. A young woman comes to you and says that her mother has recently died from cancer of the ovary. She begins to cry. Which one of the following is the best response?

a. Lean forward, listen intently, and remain silent for a few moments.
b. Immediately reassure her that this is a natural grief reaction and that she will begin feeling better soon.
c. Ask her to describe in detail her mother's death.
d. Immediately suggest to her that she go see her minister.

(Continued)

SELF-ASSESSMENT, Continued

14. In closing an office visit, following the interview and physical examination, the physician should:

    a. get as much additional information as possible in the remaining alloted time
    b. make a final summary statement, present the patient with a plan, and ask if the patient has questions
    c. reassure the patient that his/her problem can be corrected
    d. tell the patient the visit is over

15. A 17-year-old girl comes to you concerned that she might be pregnant. You have not seen her before, but her concern is written on her chart. Of the ways to open the interview, which one of the following is best?

    a. I see you think you're pregnant. What does your husband think about this?
    b. What problem brings you to see my today?
    c. I see you think you're pregnant. Is there anything else that's bothering you?
    d. I see you think you're pregnant. Can you tell me about that?

16. While talking to the girl (Question 15), she tells you she is considering an abortion, but is concerned because her family doesn't know about the pregnancy. Of the responses listed below, which one is best?

    a. I understand you feel abortion is one of your choices, but it is difficult because your parents don't know, is that right?
    b. Don't you think you should consider alternatives other than abortion?
    c. It's a difficult situation, but you are young and this will just be a small crisis when you consider your total lifetime.
    d. Why don't you sit down with your parents and tell them all about it tonight?

17. As the interview continues, the girl (Questions 15 and 16) asks you what she should do. Of the responses listed below, which one is best?

    a. I can't help you. You're on your own.
    b. If I were you, I'd let my parents in on the whole thing.
    c. In the long run, an abortion will cause you to have numerous guilt feelings.
    d. This is a difficult decision for you to make. Let's think of the alternatives and the disadvantages and advantages of each.

(Continued)

SELF-ASSESSMENT, Continued

18. A 60-year-old man comes to you complaining of shortness of breath and cough. At this point in the interview, you are trying to get more specific information. You ask when he first began to notice the shortness of breath. He answers, "Some time ago." Of the responses listed below, which one is best?

    a. "Tell me a little about the cough."
    b. "Some time ago?"
    c. "Do you smoke?"
    d. "Have you had blood in the sputum?"

ANSWERS TO THE SELF-ASSESSMENT

1. b
2. A. See text.
   B. 1. + 2. + 3. + 4. -
   C. 1. - 2. - 3. + 4. - 5. -
3. b
4. c
5. a
6. d
7. b
8. c
9. a. setting that encourages spontaneous behavior
   b. interviewer encourages communication
   c. interviewer gives attention to nonverbal behavior
   d. interviewer exercises least direction first and most direction last
10. F
11. T
12. b
13. a
14. b
15. b
16. a
17. d
18. b

CHAPTER THREE

Recording and Reporting the Medical History

James C. Guckian, M.D.

OVERVIEW

Introduction

Recording a medical history is the final stage of a three-stage, data-gathering process that constitutes the medical interview. The three stages are:

STAGE	DESCRIPTION
1	Interviewing the patient in order to obtain data
2	Ordering the data chronologically
3	Putting the data into written form according to categories

Interview and Notes

Since a large body of information with:

- dates
- relationships
- times
- numbers

is obtained, interviewers may not be able to remember the data. Thus, they must jot down brief notes, dates, names, etc.; that is, sufficient information to write the history after the interview is concluded. Note-taking during the interview must be done unobtrusively, without distracting the patient or interviewer and without detracting from the flow of the interview.

Chronologic Sequencing

Chronologic sequencing is the first step in ordering interview data. Data are to be put in precise chronological order after the interview is completed. In this fashion one arranges the exact date or time of significant events and symptoms.

Written History

Once the data are ordered chronologically, the history is easy to write. Each category of the history should be properly labeled and put in the following sequence (the abbreviations are acceptable):

- identifying data
- chief complaint (CC)
- present illness (PI)
- past medical history (PMH)
- family history (FH)
- patient profile (PP)
- problem list (PL)

DATA CATEGORIES

Identifying Data	The interviewer should collect identifying data, including: • name • age • sex • race • place of residence • marital status • occupation • if an informant (person knowledgeable about the history) was used and, if so, his or her relationship to the patient The date of the interview should also be recorded. An example of the written interview appears at the end of this chapter, before the self-assessment questions.
Chief Complaint (CC)	The chief complaint is the difficulty that brings the patient to the physician. It should be recorded in the patient's own words.
Present Illness (PI)	The <u>most important</u> part of the interview is the PI One must <u>always</u> include in the description of the present problem(s): • when it began, i.e., the exact time and date • what brought it on, i.e., the precipitating event • where it was, i.e., the anatomical location • mode of onset (sudden, gradual, unknown) • severity • number of times or frequency • method of relief or worsening • character or quality, e.g., the type of pain or disturbed function The PI is a chronological prose-style account of the patient's symptoms with dates and should include: • presence or absence of all symptoms related to the organ system involved in the illness • other physicians' diagnoses • medications (if known) • patient's diagnosis of and reaction to the illness NOTE: Diagnoses should <u>not</u> be used unless they are given by the patient or by another physician (and then so designate)

(Continued)

DATA CATEGORIES, Continued

Past Medical History (PMH)

Having allowed the patient to "tell his own story" and filled in the story with more questions, one now can turn to the past medical history. Once again an open-ended question is a good opener; for example, "How was your health before this problem began?" If necessary, one can increase the specificity of the questions until all of the data in the past medical history are obtained.

Identifying Diagnosis

The patient's report of a given diagnosis should <u>not</u> be accepted at face value. It is better to try to identify it from the account of:

- onset
- course
- duration
- type of treatment
- symptoms or functional limitation following the illness

This part of the interview will usually make it possible to place the present illness in the context of general health and previous illnesses and injuries.

PMH Data

The past medical history must include inquiry about and data on:

- illness history
  - major illnesses
  - hospitalizations and operations
  - medications and other treatments
  - allergies
- health maintenance
  - past physician contact
  - what the patient does to maintain "good" health
  - immunizations
- health-related habits
  - tobacco
  - medications
  - alcohol
  - illicit drugs

(Continued)

DATA CATEGORIES, Continued

In conjunction with PMH data, the following should also be recorded:

- dates
- adequate description
- name of physician(s)
- name of hospital(s) or clinic(s)

The recorder must quantify the amount and kind of:

- tobacco
- drugs
- alcohol

Family History (FH)

Once again an open-ended question may be most useful; for example, "Tell me about your family." This section should list the members of the patient's:

- family of origin (mother, father, siblings)
- family of marriage (spouse, children-- also called family of procreation)

Family Member Data

For each member, the following data should be recorded:

- age (or age of death and cause of death if deceased)
- state of health or significant past health problems

Important!

The interviewer should specifically inquire whether there are any diseases that occur in the family. Even if the answer is no, ask whether family members have had:

- cancer
- diabetes
- hypertension
- heart disease
- bleeding disorders

COMMON SYMPTOMS

Introduction	Interviewing will almost always elicit symptoms referable to an organ or a group of organs. The apprentice physician will learn that when a patient complains of a symptom, it frequently means disease of an organ system or possibly a group of organ systems. The following information on such symptoms may indicate the origin of the problems and serve as a guide in facilitating the interview. The beginning physician should learn these symptoms and the organ system(s) with which they are associated.
General	General or constitutional symptoms include: • weight change • weakness • fatigue • fever • malaise (lack of energy) • chills
Head and Neck	• eyes loss of vision diplopia (double vision) eye pain or discharge (drainage of fluid) scotomata (spots, flashes, or blind spots in visual field) • ears discharge vertigo (feeling of whirling or spinning) pain hearing loss tinnitus (sensation of ringing or buzzing in the ears) • nose rhinorrhea (nasal discharge) postnasal discharge (drainage of fluid into nasopharynx) epistaxis (nose bleed) stuffiness loss of smell • throat sore throat hoarseness abnormal speech • mouth sores bleeding • neck swollen glands (lymph nodes) pain masses or swelling

(Continued)

COMMON SYMPTOMS, Continued

Skin	• rashes • pruritus (itching) • alterations in pigment • moles • brittleness or other alterations in nails • loss of hair or changes in its color or texture

Cardiorespiratory System	• cough
	• sputum (exudate coughed from the lower respiratory tract)
	• character of sputum
	• hemoptysis (coughing of blood)
	• wheezing
	• dyspnea (sensation of breathlessness or shortness of breath)
	• orthopnea (dyspnea when assuming supine position)
	• chest pain
	• pleurisy (sharp chest pain on inspiration or coughing)
	• palpitations (conscious awareness of the heartbeat)
	• edema (swelling) of:
	  • hands
	  • feet
	  • face
	• syncope (fainting)

Gastrointestinal System	• dysphagia (difficulty in swallowing or sensation of food lodging in the esophagus) • loss of appetite (anorexia) • pyrosis (substernal or epigastric burning; heartburn) • abdominal pain • nausea • vomiting • diarrhea • constipation • eructation (belching) • food intolerances • hematemesis (vomiting of blood) • blood in feces (hematochezia) • coffee-ground appearance of vomitus (often partially digested blood) • melena (tarry, black, loose feces) • jaundice • hemorrhoids (dilated perianal veins) • rectal pain • tenesmus (painful straining with diarrhea)

(Continued)

COMMON SYMPTOMS, Continued

Urinary Tract	• dysuria (painful urination) • stranguria (difficulty or straining to start stream) • hematuria (blood in the urine) • suprapubic pain • pain in the costovertebral angle or flank • incontinence (involuntary loss of urine) • hernia (swelling in the groin)

Genital Tract	• female
	  • difficulties or irregularities in menstrual cycle
	  • sexual dissatisfaction
	  • dyspareunia (pelvic pain on sexual intercourse)
	  • excessive vaginal bleeding
	  • sexually transmitted disease
	  • vaginal discharge
	  • lower abdominal or genital pain
	• male
	  • swelling or pain in the scrotum
	  • penile discharge or sores
	  • inability to achieve and maintain an erection satisfactorily (impotence)
	  • unsatisfactory sexual activity
	  • sexually transmitted disease

Musculoskeletal System	• arthralgia (pain in joints) • arthritis (inflammation with pain, swelling, tenderness, and increased heat in the joints) • back or neck pain • myalgia (pain in muscles) • joint stiffness (limitation of motion with respect to usual range) • weakness of a group of muscles • general muscle weakness • swelling on a bone • pain in a bone

(Continued)

COMMON SYMPTOMS, Continued

Neurologic	• headaches • change in personality or memory • paralysis • poor coordination • tremors • anesthesia (loss of sensation) • hypesthesia (diminished sensation) • paresthesia (strange sensations; tingling, burning sensation) • loss of consciousness • disturbance of equilibrium

Psychiatric	• change in key biological functions
	  • sleep patterns
	  • appetite
	  • sexual activity
	  • energy and physical stamina
	• disturbance of mood
	• unusual ideas and experiences
	  • delusions (unusual thoughts or ideas that other people consider strange or untrue)
	  • hallucinations (seeing or hearing things that are not there)
	  • phobias (unusual fears of some situation or object; e.g., being afraid of high places or of particular animals)
	  • obsessions (thoughts that the subject dislikes but cannot get rid of)
	  • compulsions (being compelled to do things aginst one's will; e.g., washing hands repeatedly)

PATIENT PROFILE: OVERVIEW

Introduction

A detailed patient profile will help the physician understand the patient as a person. Much of this information is obtained in the open interview. What is not must be obtained by more specific questions.

THESE PATIENT DATA	WILL INFLUENCE
• the kind of background from which the patient comes	• how the patient responds to the stress of illness
• the personality pattern he or she has developed	• how well he or she tolerates pain
• current factors in the patient's life situation	• how well he or she cooperates in the treatment • how he or she relates to the physician

Current Life Factors

Categories of current life factors include:

- personal
- social
- economic
- religious
- ethnic
- cultural
- psychological

Variations of Importance

The importance of obtaining information about these factors will vary greatly from one case to another.

IF	THEN
a patient has an acute, easily treated, and brief illness	these factors are less important to know in great detail
a patient has a prolonged, debilitating condition	these factors become more important

(Continued)

PATIENT PROFILE: OVERVIEW, Continued

Illustration

Current personal factors are relatively insignificant in the treatment of appendicitis in a previously well-adjusted, 25-year-old man who has a good job, stable work history, happy marriage, and adequate backup support from good health insurance.

> NOTE: Of course, unless this information is acquired, the physician does not know that there are not significant problems.

On the other hand, if the physician is evaluating a 25-year-old man with chronic renal failure, careful consideration of these factors is essential in deciding whether or not the patient will derive a net benefit from an artificial kidney machine that he uses in his own home. The decision to place such a patient on a chronic home dialysis program may well mean the difference between life and death for that patient.

Categories of Data

Much of the data needed to write an adequate patient profile will come out spontaneously in the course of an open-ended interview. To obtain other data the physician must make specific inquiries. A patient profile must cover the following categories:

- personal data
  - appearance
  - behavior
  - education
  - occupation
- interpersonal relationships
  - familial
  - social
  - sexual
- stress response

PATIENT PROFILE: PERSONAL DATA

Appearance and Behavior	The interviewer should observe the patient and make subjective assessments of the patient's: • mood • appearance • dress • mannerisms that help or hinder the interview • nonverbal and verbal communications • attitude toward and cooperation with the interviewer • ability for self-expression The interviewer should record his or her subjective assessment of the patient and the objective observations that support the assessment.
Occupation	How effectively and consistently a person works or runs a family and household is an important index of personal maturity and emotional competence. It is said that if a person loses the ability to work productively, he or she loses dignity. Illnesses that impair work ability are frequently devastating to the patient's entire outlook on life.
Indication of Cooperation	One can accurately predict how effectively a person will work with the physician to regain health if one knows how that person has worked at jobs. Difficulties or successes in working with others and the capacity to stick with a task will often indicate how well or how poorly one can expect a patient to cooperate in the treatment.
Consideration of Work Factors	A patient's work and economic situation profoundly affects medical decisions, length of hospitalization, and adequacy of follow-up care. Some illnesses will necessitate changes in work habits and type of job in order to avoid physical and emotional stress beyond the patient's capabilities. Working conditions, length of workday, and other such factors may sometimes have to be changed in the interest of the patient's health.

(Continued)

PATIENT PROFILE: PERSONAL DATA, Continued

Education	One's education is a good indicator of basic familiarity with and sophistication about health matters. For young patients who have not yet worked full time, how well they coped with academic work and extracurricular activities in school is a good indicator of personality and adjustments, ability to tolerate stress, and ability to stick with a task and cope with adversity.

PERSONAL DATA: INTERPERSONAL RELATIONSHIPS

Family Relationships

The history of medical problems, serious illness, causes of death, and ages of family members is recorded in a separate category, the Family History. This portion of the Patient Profile emphasizes relationships, support structures, conflicts, and changes. The physician needs to know the quality of relationships the patient has with:

- father
- mother
- spouse
- children
- siblings
- significant other persons

Four key questions are:

- "Tell me about your family."
- "Where do (the family members) live?"
- "What type of work do they do?"
- "With whom do you live?"

Changes in relationships with persons emotionally important to the patient are of special note. These changes may come about owing to:

- death
- divorce
- angry disagreements
- moves to distant cities
- children growing up and leaving home

Example

The following is an example of the Family Relationship portion of the Patient Profile:

"Father is a college graduate and works as a chemist. He is described as a 'pleasant, hardworking, affectionate man.' Since the death of his wife he has maintained the house. He visits the patient often.

"Mother died in 1976 at age 40 of breast cancer. She was a 'warm and loving person.' She was a college graduate and school teacher.

"Husband is a high school graduate and works as a repairman for the telephone company. He and patient have a warm, affectionate relationship.

"Son suffers from asthma. He is described as a 'cuddly child who clings to his mother.' Asthma attacks often occur if mother leaves him with a sitter."

(Continued)

PERSONAL DATA: INTERPERSONAL RELATIONSHIPS, Continued

Social Relationships

Any ill person is under stress. The most effective protection against stress of illness and life events is relationships with people whom the patient knows, trusts, and respects; people who can show concern for the patient and who are willing to support him or her emotionally. A careful survey to determine the presence or absence of such relationships may profoundly influence the physician's treatment plan. A patient with a loyal and loving family may do well, even through he or she suffers from a debilitating illness. Another patient who has exactly the same illness, but no family or close friends, may do poorly for want of emotional support.

Religion

Religious faith--including a relationship with a minister, priest, or rabbi--is another source of support for some people. For others it is *not* a source of support.

Physician and Others

A relationship of trust and confidence between patient and physician is a *sine qua non* for optimal medical care. Frequently, the physician must also enlist the assistance of other people in the patient's life. When additional help is needed, it is important for the physician to know to whom the patient will listen.

Sexual Relationships

An important part of marital and social adjustment is sexual satisfaction. Thus, the physician should determine whether the patient:

- is satisfied sexually if married
- is involved in a sexual relationship if unmarried and, if so, whether the relationship is satisfactory

---

Caution!

Despite the so-called "sexual revolution" and the popularity of encounter and other groups (noted for their frank discussion of personal matters), sexual relationships are still regarded as strictly private matters by many people. Questions about them may be offensive, and are best raised in the context of clarifying interpersonal relationships.

PERSONAL DATA: STRESS RESPONSE

Stress Reactions	Illness of any significant degree is a stress to which each patient will react in a characteristic fashion. • Some patients are mature and confident and will have a positive attitude toward their physician and their treatment. • Some will feel terribly threatened and will tend to deny that there is very much wrong with them, even in the face of serious symptoms. • Others will seem resigned to their fate, become depressed, or resort to drugs or alcohol to lessen their apprehension.
Personality, Stress, and Cooperation	Beyond the adolescent years, people change little in their usual pattern or response to stress and adversities in life. It is important for the physician to know the patient's ability to tolerate frustration, endure physical discomfort, and face anxiety-producing situations. • A conscientious, emotionally mature, and intelligent person will cooperate with his or her physician effectively and faithfully, even if illness and health care impose major discomforts, limitations, and stress. • An immature person who tolerates pain poorly and who easily becomes impatient and frustrated often does not cooperate with his or her physician.
Amount and Variety of Stress	It is equally important to know the amount and variety of stress a patient is currently experiencing. Too much stress in too short a time overwhelms any person's physical and emotional capacity to adapt. Such varied physical illnesses as myocardial infarction (heart attack) and tuberculosis often occur in the context of an accumulation of life stresses over a year or two.

(Continued)

PERSONAL DATA: STRESS RESPONSE, Continued

Loss and Change

Two kinds of life events are especially stressful--loss and change.

- LOSS-- the loss of any person, thing, or situation that is emotionally important is very stressful.
  EXAMPLES: The loss of:
  - a spouse through death
  - an important possession (such as a house) from fire
  - prestige or status (such as that attendant on a job) through discharge or retirement
  - financial security from bankruptcy
  - self-esteem from indictment for a crime
- CHANGE-- any event that necessitates considerable readjustment imposes stress. The greater the readjustment that is required, the greater the stress associated with that event.
  EXAMPLES: Stressful events due to readjustment are:
  - marriage
  - birth of a child
  - promotion to an important new job

Obtaining the Data

Most stressful circumstances will be obvious from the open interview and from responses to earlier questions. One may reasonably ask, "Do you recognize any stresses?" if the interviewer cannot determine whether the patient is experiencing any stressful circumstances.

PROBLEM LIST

Definition of Problem

A problem is any physical, emotional, or situational difficulty that disturbs the patient's health and that is bothersome to either the patient or the physician. It is something that requires diagnostic evaluation or a management decision.

CATEGORIES

A problem can be a:

- symptom
  - shortness of breath
  - chest pain
  - dizziness
- physical sign
  - coma
  - fractured femur
  - hallucinations
- social problem
  - inadequate housing
  - rats
- economic situation
  - inadequate diet
  - inability to buy drugs
- psychological sign
  - depression
  - crying spells
  - loss of interest
- established diagnosis
  - diabetes mellitus
  - coronary artery disease
  - schizophrenia
- pathophysiologic syndrome
  - heart failure
  - metabolic acidosis

CONFIDENTIALITY OF MEDICAL RECORDS

Access

What the physician writes concerning a patient is as confidential as the content of the interview. A written document may be scrutinized by colleagues and other medical personnel, but it cannot be obtained for public record except by legal process. While care should be taken to preserve the confidentiality of records, a patient does sometimes see his or her own record when it is inadvertently left out, and, in fact, has a right to review the record in the presence of his/her physician. Because the written document is subject to scrutiny by colleagues, the patient, and the judicial system, the physician must be certain that the record is accurate, unbiased, and nonjudgmental.

Rule

A good rule is to write the history in such a fashion that one would be comfortable in reading the document in a court of law (before a jury of lay persons), before one's peers, or before the patient.

STRUCTURE OF THE INTERVIEW

Example

The open-ended interview and more specific questions related to the present illness are followed by rather direct questions concerning:

- past medical history
- family history
- the patient profile

A sequence of questions is depicted below.

NO.	QUESTION	TOPIC
1	"Tell me what brings you to the clinic today."	chief complaint
2	"Could you tell me more about that?"	present illness, open-ended question
3	"When did it begin?"	present illness, more direct question to obtain details about complaint
4	"You have described the pain in your chest. Does it ever go elsewhere?"	present illness, specific question to obtain data
5	"Do you ever get short of breath?"	direct question concerning symptoms of system involved in PI
6	"Can you think of anything else that might help us?"	reflection on data obtained in PI
7	• "Have you ever been hospitalized?" • "Have you had any serious accidents or injuries?" • "Do you take any medications or other treatments?" • "Do you have any allergies?" • "Do you smoke? How much?" • "Do you drink alcohol? How much?" • "Do you have a regular physician?" • "What do you do to stay in good health?" • "What immunizations have you had?"	past medical history

(Continued)

STRUCTURE OF THE INTERVIEW, Continued

NO.	QUESTION	TOPIC
8	• "Is your father living?" (If yes) "How is his health?" • (If no) "Age and cause of death?" • Repeat for mother, siblings, children, and spouse.	family history
9	"Can you tell me something about yourself? Your job, etc.?"	patient profile, open questions at first
10	• "Where were you educated?" • "Tell me about your family." • "Do you recognize any recent stress?"	patient profile, more detailed questions
11	"Can you think of any further information that may help us?"	final reflection
12	"Do you have any questions thus far?"	opportunity for additional discussion
13	"We will now proceed with the physical examination."	end of interview

ORAL PRESENTATION OF A PATIENT

Communicating Effectively	To communicate effectively one must maintain the interest of the audience. When presenting a patient's medical problems on rounds or in seminars, the physician will be addressing groups of intelligent, well-motivated, intrinsically interested listeners. Thus, the challenge is not to get their interest, but to avoid turning them off. A long, drawn-out presentation with misplaced and irrelevant information interferes with communication. It can breed frustration, and it may ultimately destroy one's reputation for competence. It is essential to strive for a clear, concise, and well thought out presentation. Moreover, one needs to use a perspicuous format. Since a significant amount of information must be conveyed briefly, both the presenter and the listener need a logical structure to assist in the retention of detail.
Language	Before consideration of the ingredients of the presentation format, a few general statements should be made about language. In the <u>absence</u> of the patient, one should use specific medical terminology. With the patient <u>in attendance</u>, all statements must be made in a style that maintains the patient's modesty, dignity, and peace of mind.

(Continued)

ORAL PRESENTATION OF A PATIENT, Continued

Format

A presentation format is given below. There are five distinct sections, each fulfilling a specific role.

NOTE:
- The beginning presenter should review this section prior to his or her verbal presentation and organize the presentation accordingly.
- The beginner should practice the presentation before giving it.

---

1. (Mr., Mrs., Miss) ____(last name)________ came to the hospital (when) ago complaining of (chief complaint)________________________.
2. (He/She) is ____ years old, is (marital status), and lives (where)________________. (He/She) (is/is not) employed (as a) ____________________.
3. History of the present illness in a chronological sequence
   - when it occurred
   - what brought it on
   - where it was (anatomical location)
   - mode of onset
   - severity
   - frequency
   - affected by
   - character
4. FH, PMH, PP
   Include only those positive or negative findings that pertain to the problem(s) or that introduce an additional problem(s).
5. Summary
   Summarize by listing the problems numerically.

TEXT OF CASE PRESENTATION

(1) Mrs. Burton came to the hospital on Saturday, June 21, 1983, complaining of pain in the left shoulder. (2) She is 54 years old, is married, and lives in Galveston. She is not employed.

(3) She was relatively well until Friday, June 20, 1983, when--after eating supper at 5:30 p.m. consisting of porkchops and french fries--she noted a pain in the left mid-humerus. The pain began suddenly at about 6:30 p.m., was aching, and persisted for about 1 hour. The pain was relieved by rubbing with alcohol, but it migrated to the left scapula. About the same time that the pain in the arm began, she noted "gas," described as an epigastric fullness. This sensation radiated slightly upward and downward. She drank Alka-Selzer, cokes, and coffee, which resulted in belching. Belching relieved the epigastric discomfort briefly, but it soon returned. Despite the pain in the scapula and the epigastric discomfort, she played dominoes until about 10:00 p.m. She then felt nauseated and vomited several times. Afterward, she felt much worse, but she denies hematemesis or other gastrointestinal symptoms. She denies any other pain. She went to bed but could not sleep on her left side because of discomfort in the left flank and chest. Eventually she went to sleep. Because the pain and gas persisted the next morning, she came to the UTMB emergency room.

(4) Mrs. Burton has 11 children. Three daughters live with her, and two of these have young children. The third daughter is pregnant. This creates a problem because the noise and activity of the children upset Mrs. Burton. In addition, her 21-year-old son has severe juvenile rheumatoid arthritis.

Her father and one brother died of heart disease, and her father had diabetes. In 1978 she had resection of supposedly benign lower abdominal tumors, probably uterine. At that time she had a colostomy. During that hospitalization she was found to have diabetes mellitus. She has taken Diabenese, two tablets per day, since that time. In 1979 the colon was reanastomosed. In the 1960s she fractured several ribs in an auto accident.

(5) In summary, Mrs. Burton's problems are:

- pain in the left humerus and scapula
- nausea, vomiting, and epigastric fullness
- anxiety about her daughters' small children living with her and about her son's arthritis
- abdominal surgery for some type of tumor
- diabetes mellitus

SELF-ASSESSMENT

Mark the single correct answer.

1. This 23-year-old woman was healthy until 3 a.m. on 10/2/76, when she awoke with a sudden stabbing pain in the right upper abdomen that was so severe that she screamed. The pain gradually worsened, and she became nauseated. She vomited once. The pain continued to worsen, and her husband rushed her to the emergency room. Which important historical item has been omitted from the description given above?

   a. mode of onset
   b. time of onset
   c. alleviation or aggravation
   d. location of pain
   e. severity

2. The chief complaint should be:

   a. a paragraph describing the patient
   b. a brief statement of what brought the patient to the physician
   c. a prose-style account of the problem(s), including the symptoms related to the involved organ system
   d. a list of problems that have been identified at the end of the interview.

3. The past medical history should include:

   a. past major illnesses
   b. surgical procedures
   c. hospitalizations
   d. allergies
   e. all of the above

4. Before writing a medical history one must:

   a. interview the patient
   b. organize events chronologically
   c. obtain exact identifying data
   d. all of the above

5. After asking a patient, "What brings you to the clinic?" and obtaining the answer, "Doctor, I have been having pains in the chest," you should next ask:

   a. "When did they begin?"
   b. "What brought them on?"
   c. "Where is the pain?"
   d. "How many times has it happened?"
   e. "Could you tell me more about the pain?"

SELF-ASSESSMENT, Continued

6. The problem list may include:

   a. physical problem, e.g., chest pain
   b. an emotional problem, e.g., depression
   c. a social problem, e.g., illiteracy
   d. an economic problem, e.g., inadequate wage
   e. all of the above

Choose the single correct answer from these possibilities:

   a. Only 1, 2, and 3 are correct.
   b. Only 1 and 3 are correct.
   c. Only 2 and 4 are correct.
   d. Only 4 is correct.
   e. All are correct.

7. Mr. and Mrs. Jones have a 12-month-old child, John, who is mentally at a level of 6 months, and has a heart defect that can be corrected. You are collecting the history about John from his mother. This should include:

   1. age of the mother, father, and siblings and their health
   2. history of similar problems in other family members and siblings
   3. attitude of Mr. and Mrs. Jones toward their son John
   4. history of Mrs. Jones' pregnancy

8. Mr. Green, an 85-year-old widower, is brought in by his son and daughter-in-law, ages 65 and 60. He has had a stroke, cannot speak, has wandered away from home several times, and has been eating very little. The information that is important to obtain includes:

   1. data about his wife
   2. health of his children
   3. history of similar problems in other family members
   4. information concerning his children's health and financial circumstances and their feelings about taking care of him

9. Marian, age 15, is brought into the emergency room at 7:30 p.m. by several friends. She is unconscious, is mildly cyanotic, and has a large laceration over the scalp. She was well until she fell off a motorcycle. Which of the following types of information are important to obtain immediately:

   1. whether there is a history of diabetes, cancer, or heart disease in the family
   2. where and when the accident occurred
   3. how she gets along with brothers, sisters, and parents
   4. who are her next of kin and how they can be contacted

ANSWERS TO THE SELF-ASSESSMENT

1. c
2. b
3. e
4. d
5. e
6. e
7. e
8. e
9. c

CHAPTER FOUR

Types of Interview Responses

Murphy T. Scurry, M.D.

FACILITATION

Introduction

An interviewer can make a number of different responses during a medical interview. These range from the least controlling--facilitation, silence, repetition, and summation--to the most controlling--direct, closed-end questions. An experienced interviewer first uses the least controlling responses necessary to allow patients to tell their own stories. Yet, the interviewer is in charge of the interview and must be alert to instances in which more control is required, based upon the patient's responses and the flow of the interview. In general, the least controlling responses are used at the beginning of the interview, whereas direct questions may be used later in the interview.

Definition

Promoting communication through verbal or nonverbal means is called facilitation. Here, the patient is encouraged to speak, but no direction is provided. The interviewer uses gestures, facial expressions, an attentive manner and a few words to urge the patient to go on.

Nod of the Head

Facilitation often takes the form of a nod of the nead, which indicates, "I'm listening," "you are explaining this well," or "go on; I'm following you." Of course, interviewers can do this too often.

> NOTE: Nervous, inexperienced interviewers may decrease their own tension by nodding their heads constantly. Interviewers should not nod their heads when patients express strong opinions or strong emotions because the patients may think the interviewers are agreeing with them.

Other Cues

Interviewers may also encourage patients by saying "Yes, I see" or "Uh-huh," by leaning toward the patient, or by looking more attentive.

(Continued)

FACILITATION, Continued

"I Don't Understand"	Interviewers may also communicate that they don't understand something through: • perplexed facial expressions • saying, "I can't follow you right now," "sorry, I don't understand that," or a similar expression of confusion
Summary	Facilitation indicates to the patient that the interviewer is interested in his or her story. The patient will feel confident about continuing to talk and about providing more detail about something that has been said.

REPETITION

Introduction	Repetition involves a reintroduction or return to a topic mentioned by a patient.
Reintroduction	When a patient stops discussing a topic but an interviewer needs more information, the interviewer can encourage the patient to supplement the explanation by repeating the patient's last few words or sentence, perhaps in the form of a question. EXAMPLE: "So, it's been hurting for a week?" The patient feels that the interviewer has understood him or her and sees that the interviewer is interested in more information. The patient will then talk more about the topic he or she has just mentioned.
Return	Interviewers can also refer back to words used by the patient earlier in the interview to encourage the patient to provide more information on a certain topic. EXAMPLE: A patient may, in the middle of a description of a pain in his knee that has been bothering him for a month, mention that he had been forced to quit playing college football 3 years ago because of a severe leg injury. When the patient is through with his description, the interviewer can then say, "You injured your leg in college?"

SILENCE

Introduction

The least controlling response is silence; here, the patient talks freely and the interviewer listens. If the patient falls silent, the interviewer may also remain silent briefly. Usually, the patient will soon begin to talk again. If not, the interviewer should use a facilitating response, such as "go on" or repetition. The ability to judge when the silence should be broken increases with experience.

Nonverbal Clues

Not speaking does *not* mean *not communicating*. The interviewer's facial expression, posture, and body movements indicate his or her response to the story and to the patient in general. An attentive facial expression and posture (sitting, rather than standing) tell the patient that the listener is interested. Interviewers should *look at patients but not stare continuously into their eyes*.

Tolerating Silence

Silence can be uncomfortable and can seem to be a waste of time: many interviewers will make a remark just to keep the conversation going. But silence can be so useful that it is worth learning to tolerate.

Of course, patients may also feel uncomfortable with long silences. Silence may stimulate patients to continue, but it may also lead them to feel that the interviewer is cold and nonsupportive. Long silences, therefore, should be used sparingly, especially in the first interview. Silence is less threatening after the patient-physician relationship has been established.

Silence and Emotion

Silence is almost essential when a patient is overwhelmed by emotion or begins to cry. The interviewer may acknowledge the feelings (for instance, by handing a weeping patient a box of tissues), but should maintain a silence that allows the patient to express emotions fully, thus decreasing his or her tension.

Summary

Silence can stimulate patients to expand on their remarks, allow them to discuss new topics, or permit them to give full expression to strong emotions.

CONFRONTATION

Introduction

In confrontation, the interviewer points out something about the patient's behavior. This response exerts more control over the interview because the patient's attention is directed to something of which he or she may be unaware or may be uncomfortable about discussing. Confrontation, therefore, involves a change in direction of the interview.

EXAMPLES:

- "You sound unhappy."
- "You act annoyed."
- "You look confused."
- "I see that you have been scratching those little bumps on your arm."

Effective Use of Confrontation

Confrontation is difficult for beginning interviewers because it is usually not done in ordinary, polite conversation. In fact, confrontation is generally a hostile act; thus, it takes practice to use it to express sympathy or support during an interview. Confrontation is useful when the patient is having trouble providing information. If a pause occurs during which a patient's discomfort is obvious, a confrontation may be in order unless the patient soon begins to describe his or her problems.

Nature

The nature of the confrontation will depend on what has been observed. The interviewer's response may be:

- "You seem to be having trouble talking about this."
- "You appear to be uncomfortable about your actions."
- "I notice you don't say much unless I ask you questions."

These comments do not interpret the patient's motives; they only reflect the interviewer's observations.

If the interviewer has been incorrect about the patient's discomfort, a confrontation will allow the patient to explain why the interviewer's perception is different from his or her own. The explanation usually provides useful information.

(Continued)

CONFRONTATION, Continued

No Questions

A confrontation is never formulated as a question, for the following reasons:

- Questions are based on an assumption that the interviewer's observation is correct.
- Questions put pressure on the patient to agree with the interviewer.
- Questions require that the patient reply. The patient may not yet trust the physician enough to discuss the topic, however, and may give an evasive, incomplete, or false answer.

Crying

Confrontation may be especially useful when patients look as though they are about to cry (moist, wet eyes, trembling lips). A sympathetic comment, such as, "You look as if you are about to cry" may allow patients to release certain feelings by weeping. Although this can be a therapeutic experience, physicians may not encourage a patient to cry because they feel the patient will be embarrassed about it later. Such a view may reflect the physician's own feelings about crying.

Angry or Anxious Patient

Confrontation can also be useful when the tone of voice, posture, body movement, or facial expression of a patient indicate anger or anxiety. The interviewer can say:

- to an angry patient:
  - "I have the feeling that you are angry about this."
  - "You sound angry about your son's reaction."
- to an anxious patient:
  - "You seem quite concerned."
  - "I have the impression that you are tense."
- to a patient with behavior that indicates tension or anxiety:
  - "You raised your voice when you spoke about your husband."
  - "You seem to be smoking a lot."

These kinds of remarks should "give permission" to patients to express their feelings freely. The information needed by the interviewer can be obtained more easily after such an expression of strong feeling. Moreover, if the interviewer handles the situation well, the patient will feel more trust and confidence in him or her.

(Continued)

CONFRONTATION, Continued

Contrasts Between Verbal and Nonverbal Messages	Confrontation is also appropriate when a patient's verbal and nonverbal "messages" seem to contradict each other. EXAMPLE: Patients may speak about: • joyful events with an air of sadness • catastrophic events without expressing anxiety • situations in which they have been wronged without seeming angry An interviewer who remarks on these incongruities may acquire valuable information on the patient's difficulties and conflicts.
Inconsistencies	A confrontation may be attempted when inconsistencies are observed in the patient's story. In this case, a confrontation may help the patient to tell the "whole truth."
Cautions	Confrontations should always be sympathetic. Since, in ordinary conversation, confrontations are often hostile accusations and the term itself connotes anger, interviewers must ensure that the confrontations reflect sympathy with the patient. Sometimes interviewers' irritation with some action of patients may lead them to point out the behavior, but good interviewers should be able to turn that irritation into interest in the patient and the fulfilling of the goals of the interview. Confrontation should not be overused. Even if the confrontation is sympathetic, patients will feel criticized and "nagged" if they are confronted too often. No more than one or two confrontations about the same observations are appropriate in an interview.

SUPPORT AND REASSURANCE

Introduction	Trust and confidence are created when patients are offered support and reassurance. An interviewer's ability to be supportive and reassuring allows a patient to communicate more freely and ensures that a good patient-physician relationship will continue.
Support	Support is an act that communicates the interviewer's interest in, liking for, or understanding of the patient, or that promotes security about the relationship. EXAMPLE: "You must have felt terrible about that." NOTE: Saying, "I understand" may backfire because the patient may feel or say, "How could you possibly understand?" Indicating that what the patient has just said has been comprehended is supportive.
When to Express Support	Support should always be expressed: • after the patient has expressed strong feelings • after a confrontation to which the patient has responded by crying or releasing fear or anger that has been controlled In these cases, expression of support helps the patient to continue the account.
Supportive Attitude	Supportive words must always be accompanied by a supportive attitude. If the interviewer does not have a genuine interest in the patient and a desire to be helpful, the patient will not respond to supportive words.

(Continued)

SUPPORT AND REASSURANCE, Continued

Reassurance

Reassurance involves words or actions that help to restore the patient's sense of well-being, worthiness, or confidence. When patients are frightened, a reassuring remark may be extremely helpful. As with support, reassurance must be genuine to be effective, and it must be based on real evidence.

Caution

Since reassurance assumes acceptance of the physician's expertise, reassurance should <u>not</u> create unreasonable expectations. Thus, the interviewer can be reassuring by sticking close to the facts: citing what has been learned and how it can be interpreted. The interviewer should not say, "There's nothing to worry about" or "Everything is going to be OK" unless the facts clearly support such statements. "You are improving" is reassuring only if the patient understands the basis of such a statement and only if it can be supported by data.

Overuse of Reassurance

Physicians sometimes repeatedly reassure patients who are anxious about their prognosis. Overuse of reassurance can be ineffective because the clinician's statements may lose credibility. In addition, depressed patients may respond poorly to reassurance because they may think, "She doesn't understand how bad I feel."

SUMMATION

Definition

Summation is a review, <u>by</u> an interviewer and <u>for</u> a patient, of information supplied by a patient.

Purposes of Summation

A summation has several purposes:

- It demonstrates the interviewer's interest in the patient's history.
- It lets the patient know exactly how well the inter viewer has understood the patient's account.
- It allows clarification of the patient's history.
- It refocuses some particular aspect of the patient's history.

Techniques of Summation

Summation may consist of restating what the patient has said and reemphasizing certain items.

EXAMPLES:

- "Is this what you mean?"
- "I am interested in your account of the pain; let's explore it further."

A summation may also be used as a transition to a new topic. The following are examples of summation responses.

SUMMATION RESPONSE	EXPLANATION
"Now, as I understand you, the pain is worse after exertion and you never have pain at rest."	indicates the interviewer's understanding and clarifies the history
"You said that you have never had any blood in your urine before the episode last week?"	questions, for clarification, what the patient has said
"Let's see, your first heart attack was in 1973. And the next was in 1981?"	focuses attention on 1973 and provides a transition to 1981

(Continued)

SUMMATION, Continued

Case Study

The 27-year-old wife of a surgical resident and mother of one child says that, after the first 6 months of marriage, she had never attained a sexual climax during intercourse with her husband. During her pregnancy, her husband showed no interest in her but a male friend did; she had a sexual orgasm with him. Her husband was more interested in her after the pregnancy. As far as she is concerned, sexual relations between them now are acts without feeling. She concludes by saying, "He demands to have sex with me. Sometimes I refuse, but other times I let him and then can't wait until it is over. I put on an act so that he thinks I am enjoying it, but I don't enjoy it. If you asked him, he would probably say that I have an orgasm every time."

Possible Responses

SUMMATION RESPONSE	EXPLANATION
"You say that he doesn't know whether or not you have an orgasm."	clarifies the history
"You say that he demands to have sex and you can't wait until it is over."	questions the patient's account
"You say that you put on an act and you don't let him know how you really feel."	focuses attention on another aspect of the history
"Your husband apparently has a strong sexual attraction for you. You get no enjoyment from sexual relations, but you act as if you do."	summarizes and refocuses the husband's behavior in a more favorable light, which may be useful when counseling the couple later. Bias has been inserted for a purpose.

DIRECT QUESTIONING

Introduction

At some point, an interviewer must obtain specific information about a problem that has been mentioned, and asking direct questions may be the only way in which such information can be acquired. As mentioned before, direct questions should not be asked too early in the interview because the patient should be allowed to tell his or her own story.

Appropriate Use

Direct questioning may be used earlier with patients who ramble, repeat themselves, or bring up unrelated topics repeatedly. Questions that clarify topics the patient has just mentioned--about the time sequence of an illness, for example, or the exact amount of a drug taken--will usually not interfere with a patient's spontaneous account if they are introduced during a pause. Such questions may, in fact, increase the patient's responsiveness because the patient will be pleased that the physician is interested in the specific details of his or her problems.

Caution

Questioning too early may cut off communication if the topic is one about which the patient is defensive or if the question interrupts the patient's train of thought. If the interviewer feels that a topic may be one about which a patient is uncomfortable, the specific question should be saved until later in the interview when the patient has developed some feeling of trust in the interviewer.

Avoiding Bias

Direct inquiry should be conducted in a way that does _not_ bias the response. The interviewer's comments, facial expressions, or gestures can introduce bias by conveying:

- moral approval or disapproval
- surprise
- an increase in interest or attention

Introduction of bias may influence what the patient says.

(Continued)

DIRECT QUESTIONING, Continued

Emotionally Loaded Words

One way to avoid bias is to avoid emotionally charged statements.

EXAMPLES:
- "Does your son usually overeat?" will introduce more bias than, "How often does your son have snacks?"
- "Are you a single parent?" is better than, "Are you an unmarried mother?"

Alternatives

In seeking more detailed information, the formulation of open-ended questions becomes more difficult; therefore, alternatives can be given.

EXAMPLE: "Does it hurt after you exercise?" will elicit more "yes" responses than, "Is the pain related to exercise or to other activities?"

An alternative should be given equal weight. Even adding "or not" will decrease the bias somewhat.

Confrontation to Avoid Bias

Questions should be formulated so that they do not suggest a response.

EXAMPLES:
- "Does the pain stay in one place, or does it move about?" is a good question.
- "Does the pain radiate toward your ear?" is more likely to influence the patient's account.

Confrontation may be used to avoid bias.

EXAMPLE: If a patient scratches his arm repeatedly, it is better to say, "I notice that you're scratching your arm" than "Does your arm itch?"

Bias in Summarizing

Bias may also be introduced by incorporating an inference or personal judgment into a summation of what a patient has just said.

Excessive Concentration

A specific line of inquiry should not be pursued longer than necessary or to the exclusion of other areas. Concentration on one area will often convince a patient that something must be wrong. In contrast, rapid shifts in a line of inquiry may suggest to the patient that a certain topic is not significant. Shifting topics or returning to a topic repeatedly can confuse the patient and decrease the accuracy of reporting.

(Continued)

DIRECT QUESTIONING, Continued

General Exploratory Questions

Specific information should be sought by beginning with general exploratory questions about an area of the body.

EXAMPLES: If an interviewer wants to find out whether the patient has pain in the chest that is made worse by respiration, the following sequence of questions might be used:

- "Have you had any trouble with your chest or lungs?"
- (If pain is mentioned) "Could you describe the pain?"
- "Where is the pain?" or "Could you show me where the pain is?"
- "Is the pain always the same or does it change?"
- (If it changes) "What kind of things affect the pain?"
- (If deep breathing is not mentioned) "Does deep breathing affect it?"

At some point in this sequence, the patient might supply all of the necessary information, in his or her own words. If the patient responds to the first question with all the needed information, the skilled interviewer will not ask for any more, which should encourage the patient to respond to other open-ended questions with information that should not be biased by the interviewer's requests for data.

IF	THEN
the patient says "no" to a general exploratory question	the topic can be changed and the interviewer can move on to another area of interest
the specific information sought is of major importance in testing a diagnostic possibility	the interviewer should pursue the line of questioning even if a negative response has been given to the first question EXAMPLE: "Do you have pain in the chest?" "No." "Do you ever have trouble breathing?"
the patient has denied certain symptoms, but such symptoms are essential in establishing the diagnosis	summarize the denial and repeat the question EXAMPLE: "You don't have any chest pains or trouble breathing. Or did I misunderstand you?

(Continued)

DIRECT QUESTIONING, Continued

Pursuing Specific Information	The decision about how far to pursue specific information depends upon knowledge of the importance of the information sought, as well as upon an evaluation of the patient and his or her responses in the interview up to that point.

DIRECT QUESTIONS AFTER THE OPEN-ENDED PART OF THE INTERVIEW

Introduction	Specific information must be obtained about each symptom reported. Thus, after the patient's spontaneous account, necessary information that has not been supplied must be collected by asking direct questions in the following categories.
Location	• Where is symptom located? • If there is pain, does it radiate or move about? Where? Under what circumstances?

Quality	• What does it feel like?
	  • Dull?
	  • Sharp?
	  • Cutting?
	  • Aching?
	  • Throbbing?
	  • Grinding?
	  • Crushing?
	  • Viselike?
	  • Pressuring?

Intensity	How intense is it? NOTE: The patient's response ("mild" to "intolerable") should be evaluated according to what the interviewer knows about the patient. Tolerance of pain or other physical or emotional discomforts varies.
Quantity	• How many? • How much? • How large? • How many times?

(Continued)

DIRECT QUESTIONS AFTER THE OPEN-ENDED PART OF THE INTERVIEW, Continued

Sequence	If several symptoms are reported, what happens first, second, last?
Setting	• Under what circumstances does the symptom occur? • Does it relate to any of the following? • geographical location • physical environment • social environment • food • exertion • body position
Aggravation and Self-Treatment	• Does anything make it worse or better? • Has any medication been used or any other effort been made to relieve the symptoms?
Related Symptoms	Are there related symptoms such as: • limitation of bodily function • sensations of heat or cold • anxiety • depression • dizziness • faintness • weakness

LAUNDRY-LIST QUESTIONS

Introduction

Often patients will reply to a facilitation or an open-ended question by asking interviewers what they mean.

EXAMPLE:
Physician: "Tell me about your pain" (facilitation).
Patient: "It just hurts."
Physician: "It hurts?" (facilitation).
Patient: "Yes!"
Physician: "Tell me about it" (facilitation).
Patient: "How do you mean?"

Technique

When facilitation does not produce a more detailed description, the patient needs guidance. A technique that is frequently used in this situation is a "laundry-list" question that gives the patient alternatives:

EXAMPLES:

- "Does the pain feel like a burn, ache, drawing, pressure, or piercing?"
- "Does it come on every week, hour, month, or every few minutes?"
- "Do you have these pains every day, week or month?"

NOTE: There are two problems with the last question:

- The patient may be reluctant to give an answer that falls outside the suggested range of frequency, i.e., from one per day to one per month.
- If the order of frequency falls into a logical sequence, the patient may be given a hint about the answer that the interviewer expects, perhaps by the inflection in the interviewer's voice.

To avoid bias, a laundry-list question should scramble the logical sequence and give limits beyond those expected of an accurate answer.

EXAMPLE: "Do you have the pain once a week, once an hour, once a month, once every five minutes, or once a year?"

QUESTIONS THAT ANTAGONIZE

Emotionally Charged Words

Some questions antagonize or scare patients, seem to accuse them of wrongdoing, or make them feel defensive. If interviewers ask these kinds of questions, patients will say little, be uncooperative, and even falsify answers. A way to avoid these questions is to use words and questions that are emotionally neutral.

EMOTIONALLY CHARGED WORDS	EMOTIONALLY NEUTRAL WORDS
paralyzed	lost strength
cancer	growth
mad	distressed
pus	abscess
doesn't care	casual
complain	stated
order	ask
blind	loss of vision

EMOTIONALLY CHARGED QUESTIONS	EMOTIONALLY NEUTRAL QUESTIONS
"Why do you continue to eat salt?"	"It's difficult to avoid salt, isn't it?"
"Have you had a stroke?"	"Have you lost any strength?"
"Then you got mad, right?"	"That must have upset you."
"Was the pain _that_ severe?"	"Did the pain force you to stop what you were doing?"
"What drugs have you taken for this?"	"How have you tried to relieve this?"

Key Point

Interviewers must be conscious of how words and language may be perceived and interpreted by patients. An interview must always be characterized by:

- gentleness
- lack of antagonism
- promotion of comfort for the patient

"YES" AND "NO" QUESTIONS

Danger!

Questions that require only "yes" or "no" answers may provide limited, and sometimes biased, data because the patient's answer may depend more on the question than on the facts. When questions are answered "yes" or "no," interviewers cannot be certain what the answer indicates.

- Patients may be giving the answer they think the interviewer wants to hear.
- Patients may be avoiding discussion of a certain topic.
- Patients may be falsifing answers.

  EXAMPLES: The following questions might be answered with "yes" for any of the above reasons:
  - "Have you been able to take the medicine?"
  - "You saw a doctor about that trouble 3 years ago?"
  - "Are you getting along all right with your job now?"
  - "Are you able to stay on the diet?"

"WHY" QUESTIONS

Introduction

"Why" questions require patients to account for their behavior.

EXAMPLES:
- "Why didn't you take the medicine?"
- "Why did you leave work?"
- "Why did you get a divorce?"

Since much of patients' behavior may be unconscious or related to reasons that are not socially acceptable, these questions may:
- antagonize patients because of the implication in the question
- make patients feel that the interviewer is finding fault with them
- cause patients to become irritated or annoyed

The Difficulty of "Why"

Questions that begin with "why" almost automatically contain overtones of accusation. Patients may see "why" questions as resulting from interviewers' feelings of helplessness or angry frustration.

"Because"

The answer to a "why" question is a "because." Since no one is always capable of understanding his or her own behavior, the "because" answer will be the most socially acceptable answer a patient can muster. The answer then becomes an alibi, an excuse, or a rationalization.

Alternative

An alternative to asking "why" is to state, "I am not clear on . . ." or, "I do not understand the situation. Tell me more about how you see it." Such responses:
- do not irritate or antagonize the patient
- show interest and are supportive

NOTE: They may produce a rationalization, but the patient generally does not feel as defensive as he or she would with a direct "why" question.

DOUBLE-BARRELLED QUESTIONS

Introduction

Questions for which two or more answers are required are called double-barrelled questions.

EXAMPLES:

Physician: "Do you take medicine and follow a diet for your blood pressure?"

Physician: "Do your legs swell and hurt in the evening?"

Explanation

The answers to double-barrelled questions are ambiguous. The physician cannot be certain to which part of the question the patient is replying. Two questions have to be asked in order to get accurate answers.

EVALUATIVE OR JUDGMENTAL RESPONSES

Introduction	Patient: "My doctor just leaves or changes the subject when I ask him what's wrong with me." Student: "You'd better just calm down because you'll get better treatment if you just be patient." <u>OR</u> Patient: "I am trying to lose this weight, but it is so difficult." Physician: "It seems to me that someone as overweight as you could at least follow a simple diet."
Explanation	Here, the student or physician has made judgments about the patient's feelings and has suggested what the patient "ought" to feel or to do. The evaluative and judgmental aspects of the responses will probably not allow the patients to express concerns fully or to develop an effective patient-physician relationship.

SUGGESTIVE QUESTIONS

Introduction	Physician: "When you discussed your vaginal discharge, your face became a bit flushed. Were you nervous at the time?" Patient: "Yes."
Explanation	In this exchange, the interviewer suggested the answer to the question. The interviewer should have simply effected the initial confrontation (without a question), i.e., "Your face seemed a little flushed when you discussed the problem," and then allowed the patient to respond. An open-ended question such as, "How did you feel when you discussed your problem?" could also be used.

PATIENTS' QUESTIONS

Reasons for Questions

Patients may ask questions for various reasons. When patients ask questions during or after the interview, they are seldom asking for information. Instead, these questions are usually posed for other reasons, although those reasons are not always clear. If a patient asks, "Are you married? Do you have any children?" for example, he or she may simply want information or may be trying to manipulate the patient-physician relationship.

IF	THEN
a patient asks a question that indicates he or she wishes to know the physician as a person rather than as a physician	a physician should give a simple, direct, honest reply: "yes" or "no" would be appropriate
the physician gives a direct, honest answer to the kind of question mentioned above	the topic will usually change
the physician replies, "Tell me why you ask?"	the patient may become angry because "why" questions can provoke anger
the patient asks more questions designed to make the professional relationship more personal, informal, and social	"yes" might invite more personal questions EXAMPLES: • "Is your wife/husband happy?" • "Does your husband/wife feel lucky to have you?" NOTE: These questions could lead to a nonprofessional relationship. Such a problem could be kept from developing by the following kind of reply: "I believe we're here to discuss *your* problems. Tell me about...

(Continued)

PATIENTS' QUESTIONS, Continued

Referring the Patient to the Physician	Patients frequently ask questions about: • their diagnosis • their prognosis • their treatment If a student (or other health professional) sees a patient only to interview and/or to perform a physical examination and is <u>not</u> involved in the patient's care, the interviewer should refer the patient to the physician in charge for answers to these questions.
Respond Honestly	Patients frequently ask questions for which the answers are unknown. The best response is to admit honestly that the answer is unknown and then to try to find the answer for the patient. Most patients respond favorably to such honesty because they realize that physicians do not know everything.

NONVERBAL COMMUNICATIONS

Introduction

Nonverbal communications usually provide context for verbal communications and reinforce the spoken words. Sometimes, however, nonverbal messages may convey a meaning that is different from that expressed in the words and may thus show what the speaker honestly feels or thinks.

How They Help

Reading a patient's nonverbal messages will help in the interview in several ways:

- The interviewer will have a more accurate understanding of what the patient means.
- Since nonverbal clues give instantaneous information, an interviewer will not have to wait for the end of a statement to learn the speaker's meaning.
- When the interviewer gives the patient the complete attention that is required to read nonverbal clues, the interviewer's care and interest for the patient are apparent. The patient is likely to be flattered and will react positively.
- Information obtained from more than one method of communication is always more reliable than information obtained from only a single method.

IF	THEN
an interviewer's reading of the nonverbal messages tells whether the patient is: • sad • angry • happy • frightened • anxious	the response to the patient can be appropriate to the patient's feelings (affect)
an interviewer does not read nonverbal clues	the interviewer will get an incomplete picture of a patient's affect

(Continued)

NONVERBAL COMMUNICATIONS, Continued

Patient to Physician	Certain information is obtained by observing the appearance of and behavior of patients. EXAMPLES: • posture • mannerisms • dress • voice AND BY • being aware of the interviewer's own reactions to the patient These observations should be recorded in the Patient Profile portion of the medical history.
Physician to Patient	Interviewers should be aware of the nonverbal messages they give to patients. Fidgeting, looking away, reading a chart, and obtrusive note-taking denote a lack of interest. The physician who questions the patient while standing near the door conveys the message, "Hurry up; I'm leaving." Beginning interviewers may not be conscious of their nonverbal communications and must work at recognizing the messages they are conveying.
Posture	When presenting a patient, students are often asked by professors, "Did the patient appear to be sick?" The answer to this question is based on observations of the patient's posture and body movements that signal, "I am sick." EXAMPLES: • gestures (lying still, clinched fist) • gait (slow, deliberate) • facial expressions (frown, wrinkled forehead) • dullness of the eyes • position of the head (bowed) • frequency and speed of movements (few and slow) • overall body position (doubled over and protecting a part of the body) Posture can also serve to corroborate what the interviewer observes are certain emotional states. EXAMPLES: • depression (much the same as "I am sick") • anxiety (fidgeting, wide-eyed, sitting on the edge of chair) • dependency • suspiciousness • elation

(Continued)

NONVERBAL COMMUNICATIONS, Continued

Voice Quality

Voice quality may suggest personality traits:
- a soft, childish tone may suggest dependency
- a loud, combative tone may suggest aggression
- a slow monotone may indicate depression
- a rapid, expressive manner may suggest mania

Interviewers must be aware of:
- the tone
- the inflection
- the pacing
- the emotion behind the voice

Dress

The dress of patients provides clues about their self-image and their manner of conducting interpersonal relationships. The interviewer begins by noting the purpose of the person's dress.

EXAMPLES:
- the appropriateness for the function the dress is intended to serve, e.g., swimsuit for swimming
- the symbol of the dress -- how it is emblematic of a particular group, e.g., conservative suit for an attorney
- the appeal of dress -- the effect the dress has upon others, e.g., the suggestiveness of the Playboy bunny costume

---

Illustration

Assume that a 42 year-old woman judge entered the hospital yesterday after a heart attack and is wearing:

DRESS	INTERPRETATION
a hospital gown and robe	She is wearing this dress for its utility; it is appropriate for her status and circumstance.
plain pajamas and robe	She is wearing clothes that are symbolic of her social group; it also is appropriate.
a "baby-doll" nightie	She is wearing this for its appeal to others. It may be an attempt to be more attractive and pleasing to staff and visitors, or it may be an attempt to deny her illness. In any case, it is hardly appropriate for her status or circumstance.

EXAMPLES OF NONVERBAL MESSAGES

Introduction

Nonverbal clues can be judged in terms of five basic nonverbal messages:

- openness
- closedness
- anxiety
- anger
- grief and sorrow

In general, it is more difficult to read unpleasant states (anxiety, anger) than pleasant states.

Openness

The body postures illustrated below suggest that the person is open to an inquiry.

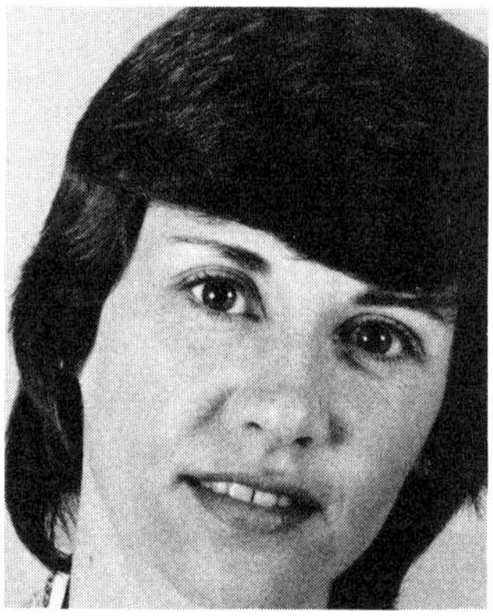

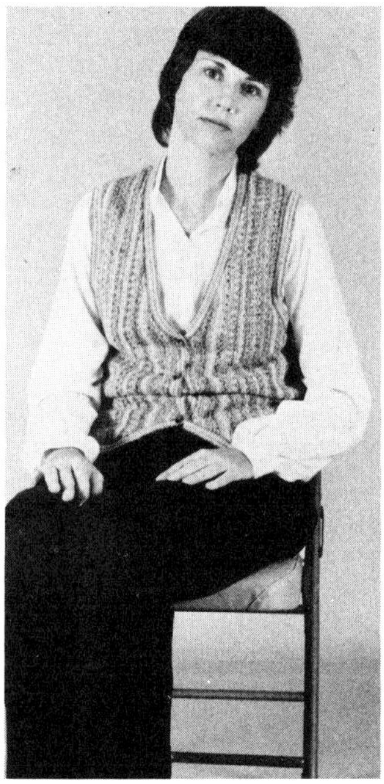

Bodily Expressions

Bodily expressions of openness include:

- inquisitive facial expression
- relaxed posture
- "open" position of arms and legs

(Continued)

EXAMPLES OF NONVERBAL MESSAGES, Continued

Closedness

These postures indicate that the person is closed to an inquiry.

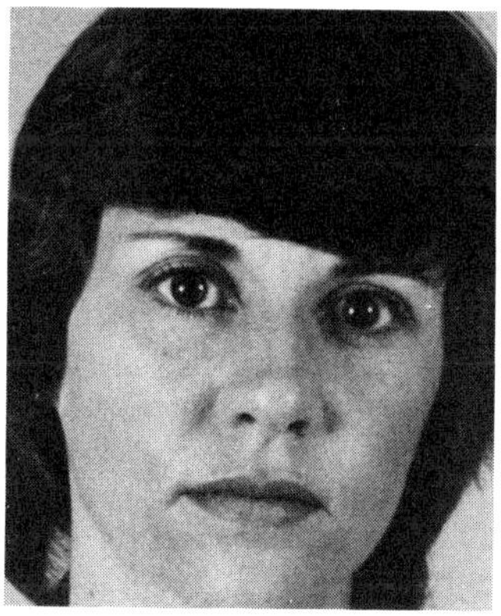

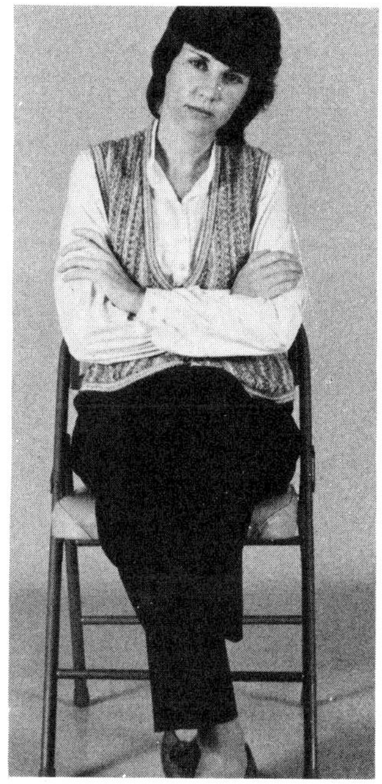

Bodily Expressions

Expressions of closedness include:

- crossed or "closed" legs
- folded or "closed" arms
- tightened muscles and "tightened" posture
- accusatory facial expression

(Continued)

EXAMPLES OF NONVERBAL MESSAGES, Continued

Anxiety

The illustrations below portray anxiety.

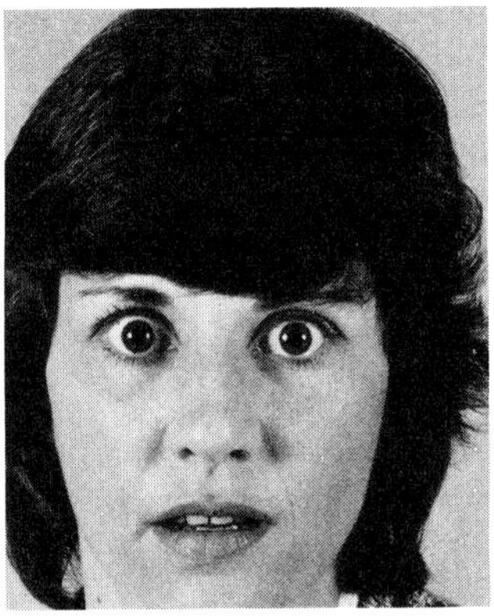

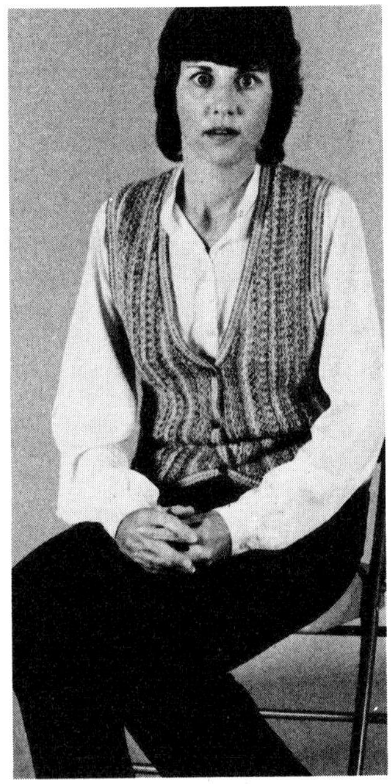

Bodily Expressions

The anxious person's bodily expressions include:

- head in a fixed position
- gestures of self-protection ("guarding")
- trembling
- a position of being about to leave
- trivial, repetitive hand movements
- appearance of being wide-awake and alert

(Continued)

EXAMPLES OF NONVERBAL MESSAGES, Continued

Anger

The following illustrations portray an angry person.

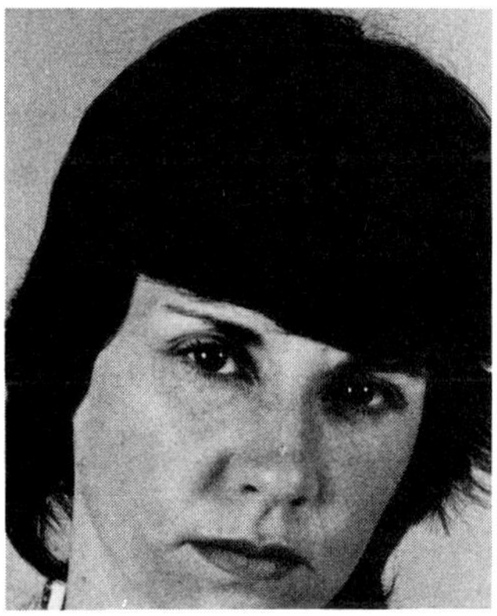

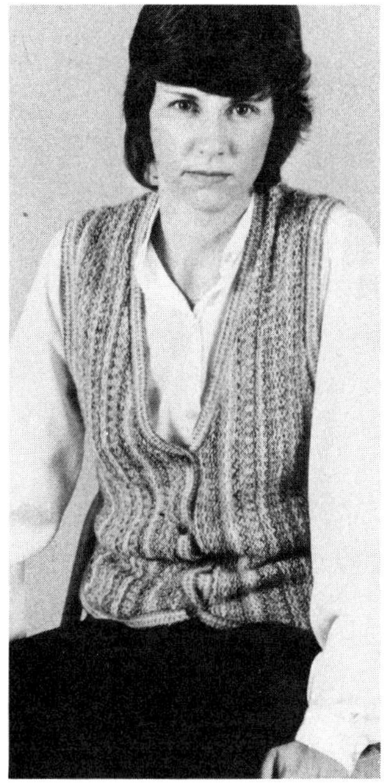

Bodily Expressions

The face of an angry person may have:

- a flushed appearance
- a furrowed forehead
- knitted eyebrows
- narrowed eyelids
- a stare directly at the interviewer
- compressed and retracted lips
- tight masseter muscles
- flared nostrils

(Continued)

EXAMPLES OF NONVERBAL MESSAGES, Continued

Grief and Sorrow

Grief, sorrow, and sadness are the feelings involved in a normal response to loss. The following illustrations portray a person with such feelings.

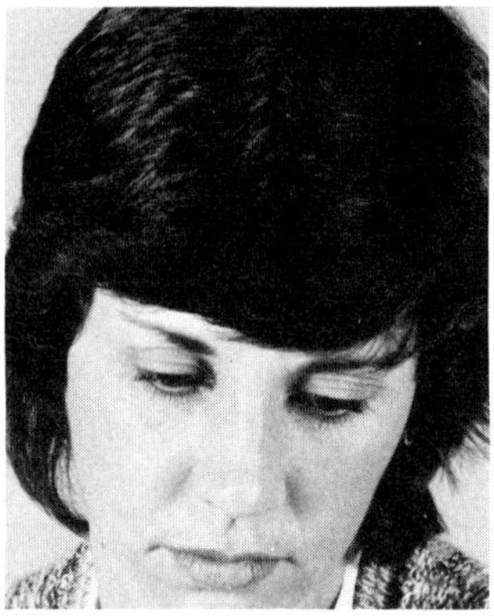

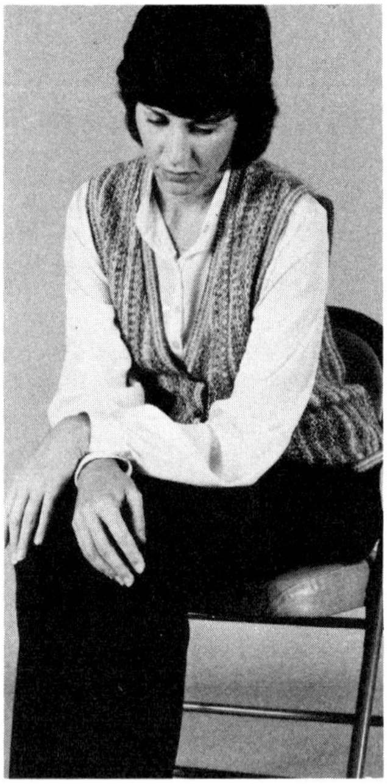

Bodily Expressions

The sad, grieving person may have:

- a flat, nonfurrowed brow
- half-closed and downcast eyes
- red eyes from crying
- a mouth in the form of an inverted crescent
- a pale and lengthened face
- flaccid muscles

INTERVIEWER'S FEELINGS

Introduction

An interviewer can use his or her own reactions to patients to assess them. Patients evoke such feelings as:

- discomfort
- anger
- pleasure
- helplessness
- uneasiness
- tension
- boredom
- embarressment
- sexual arousal

Recognition of Types

By observing the characteristics of patients who generate a specific reaction, interviewers can begin to recognize certain types of patients. This recognition is useful in planning the management of patients.

EXAMPLES:

- A patient who produces sexual arousal may be the type of patient who, purposely or unconsciously, acts seductive.
- The patient who elicits amiable feelings may be the type of patient who overdoes everything and is likely to take more medication than is prescribed.

Awareness

When interviewers are sensitive to the feelings evoked by patients, they can avoid reacting unconsciously toward patients.

EXAMPLE: When anger is engendered by a patient, the interviewer could discharge the feelings by discussing them with a peer or assistant rather then by being abrupt with the patient.

SELF-ASSESSMENT

Answer as directed.

1. Name the three least controlling actions of an interviewer.

2. When is it essential to exercise the technique of silence?

3. Give three reasons why a confrontation should not be initiated with a question.

4. List the four major aspects of observable nonverbal communication and describe how each may be helpful in detecting:

	openness	anxiety	anger	grief
a.				
b.				
c.				
d.				

Mark the single correct answer. Explain why other choices may not be as appropriate.

5. Physician: "Tell me about your headaches."
   Patient: "It is just a pain."
   Physician: "Can you tell me more about it?"
   Patient: "What do you mean?"

   As the physician, your best response would then be:

   a. "I mean, tell me about the headaches."
   b. "Well, for example, would you describe the pain as a burning, throbbing, stabbing, pressing, or sticking pain?"
   c. "Is the pain a severe throbbing ache like a hangover?"
   d. "Where is the pain? What kind of a pain? When did it begin?"
   e. "Well, does aspirin relieve the headache?"

SELF-ASSESSMENT, Continued

6. After the nurse has taken the patient's blood pressure, you comment, "When the nurse took your blood pressure, it was a little high." Which one of the following should be your next statement?

   a. "Were you upset when the nurse took your blood pressure?"
   b. "How did you feel at that time the nurse took your blood pressure?"
   c. "Has your blood pressure been <u>that</u> high before?"
   d. "Have you ever had cardiovascular problems before?"
   e. "You have been taking medication for high blood pressure, haven't you?"

7. A 50-year-old professor states, "Doctor, for the past 2 weeks I have noticed this hard lump on my knee. Even though it doesn't hurt, it bothers me. Do you think it is cancer?" Which one of the following would be the best response?

   a. "Well, I can't be sure at this point, but hard lumps should be investigated."
   b. "Why do you think it may be cancer?"
   c. "Cancer is unlikely; sarcomas seldom occur in your age group."
   d. "How can I answer that at this point? Where does it hurt?"

8. You have been called to the emergency room to see an 18-year-old girl who has cuts over both wrists. After initial treatment, she is sullen but physically well. The surgery resident suspects that the wounds may have resulted from a suicidal gesture. Which one of the questions below would be the most appropriate as the initial inquiry?

   a. "These cuts suggest to me that you may have caused them."
   b. "Were you trying to kill yourself?"
   c. "What's wrong with you? You shouldn't try to kill yourself."
   d. "You should see a psychiatrist because you are apparently suicidal."
   e. "Don't you realize cutting yourself like this will leave scars for life?"

9. If a "laundry-list" type of question must be used to elicit information, which one of the questions below would be the best?

   a. "Do you have the pain every day, week, or month?"
   b. "Do you have the pain once a year, once a week, once a month, or continuously?"

10. Which one of the questions below is best to ask a patient who has just told you that he has abdominal pain?

   a. "Is it a burning pain?"
   b. "What foods aggravate your pain?"
   c. "Can you describe the pain for me?"
   d. "Does the pain go through to your back?"

SELF-ASSESSMENT, Continued

11. Which one of the questions below is best to ask a patient for whom you prescribed Amphojel?

    a. "Have you been able to take the medicine?"
    b. "Could you tell me how the medicine has affected you?"
    c. "Have you improved since taking the medicine?"
    d. "What bad effects have you noticed since taking the medicine?"

12. Which question will likely reveal the <u>least</u> useful information?

    a. "Your pulse was a little rapid; were you calm or nervous at the time?"
    b. "Do you scream at your children?"
    c. "Do you smoke excessively?"
    d. "Do you take sedatives frequently?"
    e. All will probably reveal little useful information.

13. Which one of the questions below is <u>best</u>?

    a. "Is the pain only in your back?"
    b. "You take the pain medicine after every meal, don't you?"
    c. "Has the pain gone into your left arm from your chest?"
    d. "What do you do to relieve the pain?"
    e. "Before taking the medicine, do you always try to relieve the pain by resting?"

14. "Doctor, I have had this cough for 3 weeks, and I can't sleep. It has been so persistent that I can hardly work." Which one of the responses below is now most <u>appropriate</u>?

    a. "You've been unable to sleep?"
    b. "Do you really mean to tell me that you are unable to sleep at all?"
    c. "Have you noticed any other symptoms such as shortness of breath or swelling of your ankles or fever?"
    d. "How do you and your wife get along?"
    e. "Does anything make the cough worse or better?"

15. Which word is most "emotionally neutral"?

    a. cancer
    b. gonorrhea
    c. bleeding
    d. unsatisfactory
    e. mad

16. A 47-year-old man tells you that he has had recurrent severe anterior chest pain associated with dyspnea, diaphoresis, nausea, and weakness for the last 2 weeks. The episodes last 5 minutes, occur while walking up stairs, and are relieved by rest. Choose the best question to ask next.

    a. "Does anyone in your family have heart trouble?"
    b. "Have you ever had similar problems before?"
    c. "Have you ever had heart trouble before?"
    d. "Have you ever had trouble passing your urine?"

SELF-ASSESSMENT, Continued

17. A 39-year-old woman has told you of her headaches, which have been rather severe for 3 months. The last headache occurred while eating dinner at a famous restaurant ("The Four Corners"). She then asks you, "Have you ever eaten at 'Four Corners'?" Your best response is:

    a. "Why yes, have you?"
    b. "No, but I intend to."
    c. "Why do you ask?"
    d. "This has little to do with your problem. Please stick to your medical problems."

Below is a list of questions and statements that a physician might use. Choose the <u>lettered</u> alternative that best describes the question or statement.

a. confrontation
b. summation
c. facilitation

18. ____ "Can you tell me more about that?"

19. ____ "Now as I understand it, you have had three operations on your foot, the first in 1965, the second in 1971, and the most recent in 1982."

20. ____ "You say you have been vomiting after every meal and wake up at night with it also?"

21. ____ "Your voice is shaking, and you are moving around in your chair as if you were really upset."

22. ____ "And then?"

ANSWERS TO THE SELF-ASSESSMENT

1. silence, facilitation, confrontation

2. when the patient stops speaking and is overwhelmed by emotion

3. It assumes that the physician is correct, it requires a reply, and the patient may not be able to answer.

4. (a) posture (b) voice (c) dress (d) interviewer's feelings
5. b
6. b
7. a
8. a
9. b
10. c
11. b
12. e
13. d
14. a
15. d
16. b
17. c
18. c
19. b
20. b
21. a
22. c

CHAPTER FIVE

Physician and Patient Attitudes in the Interview

Murphy T. Scurry, M.D.

THE PHYSICIAN-PATIENT RELATIONSHIP

Introduction

The relationship between physician and patient may be a crucial determinant of the effectiveness of therapy. When the patient knows the physician well, and the physician has the respect, trust, and confidence of the patient, treatment is more likely to be satisfactory than it is in those instances in which the physician does not have the respect, trust, and confidence of the patient.

Degrees of Influence

When the treatment:

- is lengthy
- is unpleasant for the patient
- requires of the patient a high degree of cooperation and self-discipline

the influence of the physician-patient relationship on the outcome is <u>greater</u> than it is in those instances in which the treatment:

- is brief
- is relatively devoid of pain or unpleasantness
- requires little cooperation or self-discipline from the patient

<u>EXAMPLES</u>

- A patient with a high fever due to a "strep throat" can be treated effectively, even if the physician is a perfect stranger to the patient, so long as the patient is willing to cooperate to the degree needed to take an antibiotic four times daily for a period of about 10 days. In this instance a high degree of trust in the physician is not necessary. Nor is a high degree of self-discipline needed on the part of the patient.
- In contrast, consider the patient with third-degree burns over 30% of his skin surface. Such a patient, if he survives, must face weeks or months of hospitalization. Multiple surgical procedures in which skin is cut from the areas of normal skin to graft to burned areas will be necessary. Furthermore, he must undergo daily painful removal of dressings, immersion in a large tank of water containing "Clorox" solution, followed by a re-application of dressings for many weeks. The treatment is painful, and the patient must take, on faith, the physician's reassurances that painful or extended treatment given now can mean relief and improvement sometime in the future.

(Continued)

THE PHYSICIAN-PATIENT RELATIONSHIP, Continued

Categories of Influence

The relationship between the physician and the patient is determined by several categories of influence:

- the behaviors determined by the social role that society assigns to the physician and the social role that society assigns to the sick person
- the rational and realistic personal attitudes and motivations that influence the behavior of the physician and the patient in the physician-patient relationship
- social/economic/educational/ethnic background of the patient and of the physician
- the irrational attitudes and motivations that influence the behavior of the physician and the patient in the physician-patient relationship. These motivations are usually childlike and operate outside of conscious awareness.
- the interpersonal skills of the physician

Models of Interaction

MODEL (PHYSICIAN-PATIENT)	PHYSICIAN ROLE	PATIENT ROLE	APPLICATIONS
active-passive	does something to patient	recipient	• anesthesia • acute trauma
guidance-cooperation	tells patient what to do	obeys or complies	• acute pneumonia • heart attack
mutual participation	helps patient help himself	uses help	most chronic illnesses • diabetes • obesity • glaucoma

THE INFLUENCE OF THE SOCIAL ROLE OF THE PHYSICIAN

Definition

A social role is a configuration of behaviors that are expected of the player of that particular role. These expectations stem from agreements, institutionalized and widely shared within the society, regarding how a person filling a particular social role should behave.

Expectations for a Social Role

Expectations include what a person in a given social role:
- is required to do
- is forbidden to do
- is allowed to do or not to do

according to the individual's personal inclinations.

EXAMPLE: Among the things that a physician is required (generally by law) to do are:
- demonstrate to the state satisfactory completion of a prescribed course of professional training and be licensed by the state to practice medicine
- provide patient care that is generally considered to be acceptable medical practice for comparable practitioners in the geographic area
- maintain in confidence patient information obtained in the course of professional contact with the patient

NOTE: Some states have no privileged communication law, and physicians and their medical records may be subpoenaed into court.

There are, of course, a variety of other behaviors that are required by the role of physician.

Forbidden Activities

There are a number of activities that, by law and custom, a physician is forbidden to carry out in relations with the patient.

EXAMPLE: The physician may not:
- recommend or carry out treatment that is:
  - unnecessary
  - harmful
  - not generally accepted as being good medical practice
- engage with patients in activities that do them harm or have no reasonable probability of being therapeutically beneficial

EXAMPLES:
- providing an addict with addicting drugs
- exploiting a patient's dependency on the physician by becoming sexually involved
- giving a patient a lethal drug to cause the death of the patient

---

(Continued)

THE INFLUENCE OF THE SOCIAL ROLE OF THE PHYSICIAN, Continued

Optional Behaviors

In the mid-range there are a number of behaviors that are optional and that are permitted but not required of the physician.

EXAMPLES:

- belonging to the American Medical Association
- wearing a white coat at work
- being listed in the physicians' section of the yellow pages of the telephone directory

THE HIPPOCRATIC OATH

Introduction

The Hippocratic Oath is a good example of the formalized prescription of behaviors that physicians must exhibit or must not exhibit in relationships with patients. Passed down through the ages and sworn to by countless generations of physicians, it survives because it addresses matters in the lives of physicians and important aspects of the physician-patient relationship so well.

THE HIPPOCRATIC OATH

I swear by Apollo the Physician, by Aesculapius, Hygeia, and Panacea, and I take to witness all the gods, all the goddesses, to keep according to my ability and my judgement the following Oath:

To consider dear to me as my parents him who taught me this art; to live in common with him and if necessary to share my goods with him; to look upon his children as my own brothers, to teach them this art if they so desire without fee or written promise; to impart to my sons and the sons of the master who taught me and the disciples who have enrolled themselves and have agreed to the rules of the profession, but to these alone, the precepts and the instruction. I will prescribe regimen for the good of my patients according to my ability and my judgement and never do harm to anyone. To please no one will I prescribe a deadly drug, nor give advice which may cause his death. Nor will I give a woman a pessary to procure abortion. But I will preserve the purity of my life and my art. I will not cut for stone, even for patients in whom the disease is manifest; I will leave this operation to be performed by practitioners (specialists in this art). In every house where I come I will enter only for the good of my patients, keeping myself far from all intentional ill-doing and all seduction, and especially from the pleasures of love with women or with men, be they free or slaves. All that may come to my knowledge in the exercise of my profession or outside of my profession or in daily commerce with men, which ought not to be spread abroad, I will keep secret and will never reveal. If I keep this oath faithfully, may I enjoy my life and practice my art, respected by all men and in all times; but if I swerve from it or violate it, may the reverse be my lot.

(Continued)

THE HIPPOCRATIC OATH, Continued

Problem of Intense Feelings

Note the emphasis in the Hippocratic Oath that is placed on the necessity for the physician to refrain from sexual or aggressive acts toward patients. There is wisdom in these ancient words. Modern studies clearly indicate that the high degree of intimacy that often evolves between physician and patient stimulates intense feelings in the physician--including sexual attraction and hostile impulses.

Problems of Stress

The problems that such intense feelings pose for the welfare of both the physician and the patient is attested to by numerous articles in the popular press and in current medical literature regarding some of the strains and stresses involved in the practice of medicine, stresses that stem from intense emotions aroused in physicians in the course of their work with patients. Hurtful actions toward patients include mercy killings and sexual involvements with patients, which occur with sufficient frequency to be a cause for concern. Further evidence of the stress of medical practice can be found in the higher rate of drug abuse, alcoholism, and other types of emotional difficulty among physicians than among comparable groups of people in other businesses and professions.

THE SOCIAL ROLE OF THE PATIENT

Introduction

In addition to the institutionalized social role expectations that guide the behavior of the physician, there are reciprocal institutionalized and generally shared expectations that guide the behavior of the person who is in the role of patient.

Components of the Social Role

Among the more important components of the social role of the patient are:

- The patient's status as a sick person must be legitimized either by the presence of an obvious physical disability or of suffering or by the opinion of a physician who states that the person is in fact ill.
- The patient is <u>exempt</u> from expectations to fulfill the usual responsibilities and perform the usual duties during illness.
- Illness, generally speaking, is not considered to be a fault, and the patient is <u>not</u> responsible for its occurrence.
- The patient <u>cannot</u> be expected to get well by personal efforts or will: he or she must be cured either by the physician's intervention or by the illness's running its natural course.
- While ill, the patient should be cared for by others:
  - family
  - physicians
  - nurses
  - hospitals
- The patient is expected to seek competent medical care and to cooperate with the physician in the treatment of the illness.
- The patient is expected to view being ill as undesirable and to want to get well as soon as possible.
- The patient is expected to resume normal duties and responsibilities as soon as recovery permits.

Increased Probability for Success

If both physicians and patient adhere to the behaviors prescribed by their respective social roles, there is an increased probability for a successful therapeutic outcome and the establishment of a mutually helpful relationship between physician and patient.

(Continued)

THE SOCIAL ROLE OF THE PATIENT, Continued

Other Determinants	Other more personal and individualized determinants of behavior in both the patient and the physician also mold the physician-patient relationship. These include: • the logical and realistic attitudes and motivations that both patient and physician bring to the relationship with each other • irrational, unrealistic, and usually childlike and unconscious attitudes and motivations that both physician and patient bring to the relationship with each other

EMOTIONAL RESPONSES OF THE PHYSICIAN

Introduction

Every physician should keep in mind that every new patient evaluates the physician in early contacts, surely as the physician evaluates the patient. If both physician and patient evaluate each other realistically and conclude that the other is reasonably honest, dependable, and considerate, and wishes to work collaboratively toward a mutually shared goal of doing what is necessary to diagnose and treat the patient's illness, then a working alliance is established, and an effective physician-patient relationship begins to develop.

Negative Feelings

A physician is obligated to maintain a professional and nonjudgmental attitude toward all patients and to try to render equally skilled care to all, regardless of whether the physician personally likes them or not. But one can only strive toward the ideal. The fact is, if one really feels dislike, contempt, fear, or another strong negative feeling toward a patient, it is more difficult to be attentive, concerned, effective, and emotionally giving.

Major Safeguard

The major safeguard against such negative feelings toward patients is to be alert to the occurrence of such feelings in oneself.

IF	THEN
these feelings interfere with good care of the patient	the physician is obligated to consult a colleague and attempt to resolve the negative feelings with the help of that consultation
such a resolution is <u>not</u> possible	the physician is obligated to refer the patient to a colleague
a physician finds that such negative reactions toward patients occur with a frequency greater than it does among colleagues	the physician should seek counseling to get help in resolving the emotional conflicts that evoke such untherapeutic attitudes toward patients

(Continued)

EMOTIONAL RESPONSES OF THE PHYSICIAN, Continued

Depends on Type of Patient

In some instances, certain types of patients will regularly evoke negative feelings that interfere with good medical care.

EXAMPLES:

- Some physicians feel anxious, defensive, or hostile toward elderly patients or toward toddlers.
- Some physicians may have negative feelings toward patients who are aggressive and assertive or patients who are passive and dependent.

Almost all physicians do better with certain types of patients than they do with other types of patients, but all physicians should strive to provide good care to the widest possible variety of people.

Being Overly Protective

Being unduly solicitous, concerned, and overly protective toward patients may be as destructive to an optimal physician-patient relationship as being hostile toward patients, albeit in a more subtle and insidious manner. Physicians who behave in an overly protective or solicitous manner toward their patients do so for one or more of the following important and frequently observed irrational attitudes, which are detrimental to the physician-patient relationship.

Inability to Say "No"

Many physicians, often those with large practices, have great difficulty in saying "no" to the demands that patients make on them. Like an overly permissive parent who can set no clear limits on their children's behavior, such physicians unconsciously encourage undue dependence and increasingly impossible demands for:

- time
- attention
- medication

Eventually, such physicians become slaves to their patients and, like any slaves, come to resent the enslaving tyrant. Often the slow build-up of resentment in the physician, because of demands that result from the inability to say "no," results in an explosive outbrust of anger detrimental to all concerned.

(Continued)

EMOTIONAL RESPONSES OF THE PHYSICIAN, Continued

Giving more and more time and energy to patients, such a physician has little time to give to family or to personal recreational needs. The end result is often:

- resentment
- depression
- a turn to drugs or alcohol

As numerous studies have shown, alcoholism and other drug addictions are inordinately frequent among physicians as compared to other occupational groups. The inability to say "no" is probably the greatest occupational hazard that the conscientious physician encounters.

Undue Perfectionism

To be conscientious in the care of patients is an essential characteristic of the good physician. However, carried to an excess, conscientiousness becomes undue perfectionism. Unduly perfectionistic physicians are intolerant of their own shortcomings and failures to an irrational degree. Always falling short of self-imposed perfectionistic goals, such physicians consequently can never feel appropriate pride and sense of accomplishment in a job well done. Always driven to try harder, work longer, do better, such physicians are prey to the endless demands that some dependent patients tend to make.

Difficulty in Dealing With Sexual Stimulation

Difficulty in dealing with sexual stimulation often accompanies the discussion of intimate details of a patient's life. Numerous studies show that most physicians learn to deal effectively with the sexual stimulation involved in the physical intimacy encountered in the physical examination of patients. However, some physicians have difficulty in dealing with the sexual stimulation for both physician and patient that often occurs in the course of discussing the intimate details of sexual problems. Further, some patients will behave in sexually provocative ways toward the physician.

(Continued)

EMOTIONAL RESPONSES OF THE PHYSICIAN, Continued

Dealing with Provocative Patients	It is important to develop a professional reserve in dealing with provocative patients, whether they attempt to provoke a sexual or a hostile response from the physician. To respond in kind to either type of provocation can only disrupt an effective physician-patient relationship. Many patients, especially those with serious disorders, have unrealistic and childishly magical expectations that an omnipotent physician can cure all that ails them. The physician who falls short of this magical expectation will inevitably be the object of anger and resentment. Dealing with anger of this kind can be easier if the physician understands the role that frustrated magical and irrational expectations play in generating anger.
Dealing With an Angry Patient	Patients occasionally become angry because of real or perceived problems with their care. Guidelines for interacting with such a patient include: • allowing the patient to express anger orally without interruption • recognizing that the patient -- not the physician -- is responsible for his or her own anger • acknowledging that the patient is angry, e.g., "I see that you are very upset about that." • refocusing the interaction on the primary problem and possible therapy, e.g., "I can see several possible ways in which we can solve this problem."

SEXUAL ATTITUDES OF THE PHYSICIAN

Introduction	The physician must deal on a personal level with his or her own sexuality. On a professional level the physician can: • discourage patients from discussing sexual problems • apply personal standards to behavior of patients, suggesting that they conform to this standard OR • recognize the variability in expression of sexuality • help patients adjust in terms of their own personal and idiosyncratic life experiences
Statistics	A variable percentage of patients express sexual concerns to their physician under various circumstances: • about 5% if their physicians feel uncomfortable with sexual matters • about 10% if their physicians feel comfortable with sexual matters, but did not ask about their sexuality • about 15% if their physicians inquire about their sexual behavior About: • 80% of physicians believe erotic contact with patients is never beneficial • 5% of physicians engage in sexual intercourse with their patients
Sexual Behavior	Sexual behavior is an interaction among any one or more persons whose goal is pleasurable sexual response, which may or may not be orgasm. The only restraints are: • anatomical • physiological • imaginational • attitudinal

(Continued)

SEXUAL ATTITUDES OF THE PHYSICIAN, Continued

Sexual Norms

Sexual values reflect norms for a given society. They are not absolutes. The sexual attitudes (norms) of a society are determined by historical attitudes toward the:

- culture
- law
- economics
- technology
- religion

  EXAMPLE: Among world religions, Judaism and Christianity have historically been harsh in condemning homosexuality.

Sexual attitudes are not static, nor are all attitudes universal in all segments of a complex society. The persons involved determine their own norms. These norms must conform to:

- anatomical limits (or a person might be physically traumatized)
- rules of the larger group (or a person might be legally or socially traumatized)
- an individual's conscience (or a person might be psychologically traumatized)

Physician as Sexual Counselor

Physicians should consider sexual behavior in a descriptive rather than a prescriptive manner. The physician does not have to approve, but can accept behavior as descriptively normal for that person. The more behavior that a physician rejects (owing to thinking in terms of what people "ought to do"), the fewer patients he or she can potentially help. The physician cannot use personal standards to help patients either restrict or expand their sexual behavior. As a counselor the physician must:

- be comfortable with sexual topics and put the patient at ease
- be aware of the patient's feelings and minimize the patient's embarrassment
- know whether a problem is within one's competence to manage
- know when to refer a patient to a specialist

THE DYING PATIENT

A Special Problem

Dying patients and their families constitute a special problem for health-care workers. Most people try to avoid situations that are unpleasant or difficult for them. One such situation is caring for and developing a relationship with a dying patient. The dying patient represents a failure to physicians and also reminds them of their own mortality. Physicians need to have a sensitive awareness of dying patients and to make a special effort toward them.

Prevalence

A survey showed that:

- most residents find caring for dying patients unpleasant, but say they do not avoid them
- most residents wonder if they could have done anything further when their patient dies
- residents usually seek help from other residents or faculty when having difficulty caring for a dying patient

Remember

The beginning clinician is not unique, and it is appropriate to talk to other students, residents, or faculty about feelings toward caring for a dying patient.

THE REGRESSED PATIENT

Introduction	The phenomenon of regression is an important factor in producing the irrational and often childlike attitudes and behaviors that patients at times direct toward their physicians.
Explanation	Regression refers to the universal tendency of humans who are under stress to revert to modes of thought and behavior characteristic of their childhood years. The patient threatened by the possibility that an illness may be or is in fact serious tends to regress. Childlike hopes for magical cure by an omnipotent, parentlike physician, and childlike rage when those hopes are frustrated, frequently result.
Coping With Regression	If the physician understands the tendency of patients to regress when under great stress, the childlike behavior that results becomes more understandable, and the physician is better prepared to respond rationally rather than with perplexity and frustration.

CHAPTER SIX

The Impact of Social Factors on Medical Care

Murphy T. Scurry, M.D.

OVERVIEW

Introduction

American society continues to set its sights higher in providing health care. This generation of physicians will provide more people with increasingly effective services. In treating the sick they will be called upon to bridge the gaps of misunderstanding, ignorance, and fear that are outgrowths of the varying social, economic, and cultural levels in the U.S.A.

Characteristics of Society

The interview is most effective and professional when the physician has a clear understanding of communication barriers that may exist. This chapter provides an overview of characteristic gaps in society that create differences in personal experience, values, and feelings; the physician's insight into and tolerance of them can make the interview more valuable to both participants.

NOTE:

- Though this chapter attempts to characterize certain societal groups and prototypic behavior, not all individuals within a group fit the description; and, the physician must beware of applying group descriptions to any individual.
- The discussion of these groups is in no way meant to be demeaning. Rather, it is meant to emphasize differences, particularly differences between beginning physicians (who are frequently familiar with upper-level society) and members of the so-called lower societal rank.

Facts

Consider the following facts about health in the United States:

- The United States ranks about 18th in the world in male life expectancy at birth; 11th in female life expectancy at birth.
- The United States ranks 13th in infant mortality.
- The infant mortality rate of nonwhites is double that of whites.
- Health is the third largest industry in the United States.
- About one out of every 20 workers has a job in the health industry.
- Health spending today is five times the spending of 20 years ago.
- Health costs and services are sure to increase during the coming years.

SOCIAL CLASSES

Definition

Social class can be defined as the extent to which individuals and groups in a society have control over the resources in that society. These valued resources include:

- wealth
- power
- prestige

Since life's opportunities and problems are usually defined by one's socioeconomic status, this concept has central importance in any patient's reaction to health and illness.

Common Indicators

In American society the most common indicators of social class are:

- income
- occupation
- education
- residence
- race or ethnic background
- age

NOTES:

- Race refers to a set of biological characteristics.
- Ethnicity refers to cultural heritage or identity. It can be operationally defined by nationality and religious identity.

Social Classes

Indices of social class using occupation and education as criteria depict the following class structure in the United States:

HIGHEST (3%)	HIGH (10%)	MIDDLE (20%)	LOW (47%)	LOWEST (20%)
• physicians • lawyers • professors • executives of large corporations	• nurses • social workers • administrators	• medical assistants • small-business owners • clerical workers • sales • skilled workers	• machine operators • semi-skilled workers	• unskilled workers • unemployed persons

EFFECTS OF SOCIAL CLASS ON PATIENT BEHAVIOR

Introduction	Members of the lower and lowest classes exhibit different behavior in regard to illness and health than that of the higher social classes.
Decision to Seek Medical Care	The poor are <u>less</u> likely to consider a disease serious and are <u>less</u> likely to seek medical attention or take action to prevent disease. The higher a patient's class, the more likely a physician will be consulted for a specific symptom. The lowest socioeconomic class frequently shows indifference to symptoms.
Physician/ Patient Relationship	Lower-class people carry different mind-sets with them to the physician's office. It is not surprising, then, that their ways of adapting to the situation may seem strange to the physician. They tend to personalize all relationships, and therefore they seek highly personalized relationships with physicians when this is possible. This may be satisfying and enjoyable for both the physician and the patient, but that type of relationship may be detrimental to the best interests of both. NOTE: This difference in mind-set can be a source of trouble. Lower-class people may perceive the lack of personalized professional behavior as being: • hostile • indifferent • judgmental • flippant • insincere toward them. They may withdraw quickly into an adaptation of resentful docility or hostility. They then are much less available for any real communication or learning. A natural response to this situation is to retreat or withdraw as soon as possible.
Other Problems	Factors that strongly affect the physician's relationship with patients of low status include: • a marked difference in: • social class • personal compatibility OR • a language barrier between physician and patient Each of these exacerbates what is from the outset a difficult situation.

(Continued)

EFFECTS OF SOCIAL CLASS ON PATIENT BEHAVIOR, Continued

Other Factors

The relationship between a "poverty" or "charity" patient and physician may become more problematic when we consider the career pattern of physicians. The overwhelming majority of medical students belong to families in the two highest social classes. In addition, minorities are underrepresented in medical school relative to their proportions in the population. These facts mean that future physicians are drawn from a homogeneous background and have similar beliefs and modes of interaction that represent only a narrow slice of the population.

Scenario

Often when a physician first goes into practice, a considerable number of his patients are poor. Many of the established physicians in town discourage welfare patients, and so the Welfare Department often sends patients to new physicians who need the money. The new practitioner does not usually like these patients, often feeling that they:

- understand that they were sent to a new physician
- are often inconsiderate and more demanding than private patients, calling more frequently and not being concerned with the hour of the call
- often arrive in the office unkempt and unwashed
- tend to be noisy and rude

It may be difficult to enjoy caring for them. As time goes on, the practice grows considerably, and income rises sharply. The physician buys a lovely home in a desirable neighborhood, and friends and acquaintances begin to include more high-status individuals. The character of the practice also changes, as the prestige part keeps growing. Just as the physician enjoys socializing with higher-status people after office hours, because of more common interests, spending professional hours with them is enjoyable. At first, this insight is upsetting--"it is not right, one should not feel this way. Professional feelings should be separate from social feelings." But then physicians wonder if this feeling might not be natural: as they move up the status scale, they enjoy having a practice that reflects their social life. It seems natural to spend time with a teacher or an executive rather than with a person whose values and life-style are upsetting.

(Continued)

EFFECTS OF SOCIAL CLASS ON PATIENT BEHAVIOR, Continued

Middle- and Upper-Class Patients

Patients of the middle and upper classes can also be difficult to interview. As with lower class patients,

- status incongruity
- personal incompatibility
- language barriers

are obvious things that must be overcome at the outset. In addition, continuous probing from a college-educated patient, or an aggressive business executive accustomed to being in charge of a tight schedule, may create an offensive, threatening situation for the physician. Or a manipulative patient of either sex may challenge professional skills by their skillful avoidance of sensitive topics. Thus, the effect of social class in determining patient behavior is best understood as ranging across a continuum of factors involving:

- age
- occupation
- education
- residence
- economics
- race
- ethnicity

The latter three are stressed because of the special problems of the poor and minorities--problems to which persons from other classes are not often exposed. But that does _not_ mean that an interview between physician and patient of a similar class will be without surprises.

> _EXAMPLE_: A number of people at _all_ income levels express ambivalent opinions about physicians.

RELIGION

Introduction

Religion merits separate discussion because it is an important aspect of the social history. It can be a source of immediate conflict if not handled properly in interviewing patients. Oftentimes, religion plays a major role in how a patient deals with an illness, whether brief or extended. A physician will be called upon to treat patients who hold beliefs different from his or her own. Some patients may believe that illness may be sent by God as punishment for sin. Such illnesses may take any form but are often sudden and severe enough to give the individual time to reflect on his or her transgressions. A stroke, for example, allows the sinner time to think over past behavior and repent. Retardation in children is commonly cited as punishment to the parents, who then spend the rest of their lives contemplating the result of their misdeeds.

Personal Dynamics of Illness

Some religions provide dramatic examples of the personal dynamics that are evident in illness. There appears to be a universal tendency to express feelings about guilt for the occurrence of an illness. "If only I hadn't..." or "I will always blame myself for my child's accident" are familiar comments to physicians and should *not* be ignored in working with the patient's family. Patients' statements about being punished for one's sins should *not* be dismissed as unrelated religious or cultural beliefs but understood as an individual's response to illness.

Nonjudgmental

The physician must be nonjudgmental when dealing with a person's religious views, and must be willing to call in appropriate supportive personnel when needed by the patient. In addition, a word of caution is in order regarding personal religious views and their intrusion into the life of the patient. Many social practices rest on a person's freedom to choose the course of action preferred. The old saying about the difficulty of changing people's mind on questions of religion or politics is appropriate here. *The physician must respect the patient's religious, moral, and ethical views.* The difficult task is to identify these beliefs through a careful and considerate interview, but they become apparent when the data in the patient profile are obtained.

IMPORTANCE OF THE SOCIAL ASPECTS OF THE PATIENT PROFILE

Introduction	Interviewers should gather information on a patient's relations with others and classify those relations as typical or unusual for their social and economic position.
Information Needed	When focusing on the interpersonal aspects of the patient profile in the interview, seek information surrounding: • relations with family and peers • education and occupation • marital history • hobbies and social activities • stress and supportive relationships • the patient's concept of illness • religion

CHAPTER SEVEN

The Complete Medical History

James C. Guckian, M.D.

OVERVIEW

Purposes of the Initial Medical History

Purposes of the initial interview are to:

- establish a relationship and therapeutic contract
- learn of the patient's problems
- evaluate the psychologic makeup of the person
- learn of the individual's or family's reaction to problems
- determine the patient's compliance with suggested care
- begin therapeutic intervention and education of the patient

---

Review

Earlier, the reader learned:

- the technique and the "do's" and "do nots" of interviewing
- the value of initial open-ended questions
- how to proceed from open-ended to more specific questions
- how to write:
  - chief complaint
  - present illness
  - family history
  - past medical history
  - patient profile
  - problem list

(Continued)

OVERVIEW, Continued

Chronologic recording of data in the present illness was emphasized. For each complaint or problem that a patient expresses, the physician must ascertain and record:

DATA	EXAMPLES
date and time of onset	• 3 weeks ago • this morning at 2 a.m.
mode of onset	• sudden • gradual
precipitating or exacerbating factors	• exertion • bending • reaching • lifting
exact anatomical location of complaint	• left upper quadrant of abdomen • anterior chest in midline
severity	• continued until patient reached home • made patient cease inspiration • made patient stop walking
character	• crushing • burning
number of times or frequency	• every day • about every 4 hours
method of relief	• aspirin • baking soda

NOTE: All of these data must be explored and recorded in a chronologic sequence from time of onset until the patient interview.

STRUCTURE OF THE INTERVIEW

Introduction

The developmental, sexual, and psychosocial data integrated into the interview and written history are not fully detailed with each patient. In-depth interviewing or questioning is done in these areas only when the physician senses a problem or when a patient gives a clue that a problem exists. Thus, the interview remains "open," with the physician often following hunches about a problem that is not overt. From each patient, however, a minimal or "screening" set of data is obtained.

Interview Sequence

The open-ended interview and more specific questions related to the present illness are followed by rather direct questions concerning:

- past medical history
- family history
- the patient profile

A sequence of questions is depicted below.

QUESTIONS	TOPIC
"Tell me what brings you to the clinic today."	chief complaint
"Could you tell me more about that?"	present illness, open-ended question
"When did it begin?"	present illness, question directed at obtaining details about each complaint
"You have described the pain in your chest. Does it ever go into your shoulder or arm?"	present illness, specific question to obtain data
"Can you think of anything else that might help us?"	reflection of data obtained in PI

(Continued)

STRUCTURE OF THE INTERVIEW, Continued

QUESTIONS	TOPIC
"Have you ever been hospitalized?" "Have you had any serious illnesses?" "Have you had any serious accidents or injuries?" "Do you take any medication or other treatments?" "Do you have any allergies?" "Are there any medications you cannot take?" (If yes) "For what reason?" "Do you smoke?" (If yes) "How much?" "Do you drink alcohol?" (If yes) "How much?" "Do you have a regular doctor?" "What do you do to stay in good health?" "What immunizations have you had?"	past medical history
"Is your father living?" (If yes) "How is his health?" (If no) "Age and cause of death?" Repeat for: • mother • siblings • children • spouse	family history
"Can you tell me something about yourself? Your job?"	patient profile, open questions at first

(Continued)

STRUCTURE OF THE INTERVIEW, Continued

QUESTIONS	TOPIC
"Where were you educated?" "Where are you employed?" "Tell me about your family." "Tell me about your spouse, (OR, if unmarried) "Do you have a close relationship with someone?" "Do you have any problems regarding sexual matters?"	patient profile (obtain all of these "screening" data for each patient; note general appearance and behavior)
(See next section)	review of systems
"Can you think of any further information that may help us?"	final reflection
"Do you have any questions thus far?"	opportunity for final discussion
"We will now proceed with physical examination."	end of interview

REVIEW OF SYSTEMS

Introduction

The symptoms that frequently occur with disease or dysfunction of each organ system have been discussed. This section details how to inquire about symptoms characteristic of diseases of each organ system and thereby to accomplish a review of symptoms (ROS) by systems. The ROS concerning the system primarily involved should be obtained in the PI when exploring the problem(s) of the PI. These data, whether positive or negative, <u>should be recorded</u> in the PI.

When?

In obtaining the family history, direct questions are asked. The ROS, which is a list of rather direct questions, follows this history and may begin without any further introductory remarks. The physician may, however, wish to say something such as, "I would like to return to <u>your</u> health and ask a few more questions." In any event, the ROS is then begun.

Phrasing of Questions

Since most people have had a symptom of serious disease at one time or another, they might respond positively to such questions as:

- Have you ever had a headache?
- Have you ever had blood in your bowel movement?
- Have you ever had a nosebleed?

The patient may consider these symptoms to represent no problem now, but may feel compelled to answer positively to be completely honest. On the other hand, a history of certain symptoms <u>at any time</u> may be indicative of serious disease, for instance:

- hemoptysis
- hematuria
- nocturnal dyspnea

Thus, how the question is asked will determine the validity and importance of data obtained from the patient.

(Continued)

REVIEW OF SYSTEMS, Continued

Remember!

For each affirmative response in the R.O.S., determine the following:

- date and time of onset
- mode of onset
- contributing factors
- anatomical location
- severity and description
- frequency
- relief

These are particularly important for signal symptoms such as:

- hemoptysis
- hematemesis
- recent severe headaches
- chest pain
- dyspnea
- hematuria
- hematochezia
- personality change

Open-Ended Questions

As in other parts of the interview, open-ended questions are superior to directed ones. Thus, initial open-ended questions are used. If, however, the general or open-ended question is answered negatively, and particularly if the question is answered positively, the physician proceeds to specific questions about each symptom.

(Continued)

REVIEW OF SYSTEMS, Continued

Questions

SYSTEM		QUESTIONS	NOTE
GENERAL		• "Has you weight changed recently?" • "How is your strength or endurance?" • "Do you tire easily?" • "Have you had fever?"	• Emphasize "recently." • One does not say, "Have you ever had . . . ?"
SKIN		• "Do you have any skin problems?" • "Do you have a skin rash?" • "Do you itch?" • "Have you noted any sores on your skin?" • "Have you noted any change in your hair? Nails?"	
HEAD AND EYES	Head	• "Are you bothered by frequent headaches?"	• not, "Are you ever . . . ?"
	Eyes	• "Have you had any trouble with your eyes?" • "How is your vision?" • "Do you see double?" • "Do you have pain in your eyes?" • "Do you wear glasses?" • "Do you see spots or flashes of light?"	• general open-ended question • more specific • direct
EARS, NOSE, AND THROAT (ENT)	Ears	• "Do you have any trouble with your ears?" • "How is your hearing?" • "Do you get dizzy?" • "Do you have pain in your ears?" • "Do you hear ringing or buzzing in your ears?"	

(Continued)

REVIEW OF SYSTEMS, Continued

SYSTEM		QUESTIONS	NOTE
	Nose	• "Do you have any trouble with your nose?" • "Do you have nosebleeds?" • "Do you have a sense of dripping or drainage in the back of your throat?" • "How is your sense of smell?"	
	Throat	• "Do you have frequent sore throats?" • "Do you get hoarse?"	• Note the use of "frequent."
	Mouth	• "Do you have trouble with your mouth?" • "Do you have frequent sores in your mouth?" • "How are your teeth?" • "Do you wear dentures?" • "Do you note bleeding from your gums or mouth?"	
NECK		• "Do you have any trouble with your neck?" • "Have you noted any pain in your neck?" • "Swelling?" • "Knots?"	
CARDIORESPIRATORY		• "Have you <u>ever</u> had any problems with your heart or lungs?" • "Do you have a cough?" • (If yes) "Do you cough anything up?" • (If yes) "What does it look like?" • "Have you <u>ever</u> coughed up blood?" • "Have you had any trouble breathing?" • "Do you <u>ever</u> wheeze?"	• Here the use of "ever" is warranted. • <u>not</u>, "Have you ever had a cough?"

(Continued)

REVIEW OF SYSTEMS, Continued

SYSTEM	QUESTIONS	NOTE
	• "Do you ever get short of breath?"	
	• (If yes) "When do you notice it?"	• after lying down (orthopnea) • exertional • nocturnal
	• "Do you have chest pain?"	
	• "Do you ever note fluttering or pounding of your heart?"	• palpitations
	• "Have you noted any swelling in your legs or ankles?"	
	• "Have you ever fainted?"	
	• "Have you ever had high blood pressure?"	
GASTROINTESTINAL	• "Have you any problems with your digestion or bowels?"	
	• "Tell me about your bowel habits."	
	• "Do you have difficulty swallowing?"	
	• "How is your appetite?"	
	• "Do you have frequent heartburn?"	
	• "Do you have pain in your stomach?"	• or use "abdomen"
	• "Do you ever get sick to your stomach?"	• or use "nauseated"
	• "Do you vomit?"	
	• "Do you have diarrhea?"	
	• "Do you frequently belch?"	
	• "Are there any foods you cannot eat?"	
	• "Have you ever vomited blood?"	
	• "What color are your bowel movements?"	• or use "stools"
	• "Have you ever had tarry-black stools?"	
	• "Have you ever turned yellow?"	• or "been jaundiced"
	• "Are you bothered with hemorrhoids?"	
	• "Do you have pain with your bowel movements?"	

(Continued)

REVIEW OF SYSTEMS, Continued

SYSTEM		QUESTIONS	NOTE
URINARY		• "Have you *ever* had any kidney or bladder trouble?" • "Tell me about your urination habits." • "Do you have pain or burning with urination?" • "Do you have trouble starting your stream?" • "Have you *ever* had blood in your urine?" • "Do you get up at night to urinate?" • "Do you have back pain?" • "Do you *ever* lose your urine?" • "Have you *ever* had a hernia?"	• nocturia
GENITAL	Female	• "How old were you when your periods started?" • "Have you *ever* been pregnant?" "How many times?" "Any miscarriages (abortions)? "How were your children delivered?" • "When did your last period begin?" • "Do you have any difficulties with your periods?" • "How many tampons (or napkins) do you use for each period?" • "How long does your period last?" • "Are your periods regular?" • "Do you *ever* bleed between periods?" • "Do you have a discharge?" • "Do you use birth-control measures? Which?"	• record number • record number and duration of pregnancy • vaginal or cesarean section

(Continued)

REVIEW OF SYSTEMS, Continued

SYSTEM		QUESTIONS	NOTE
		• "How frequently do you have intercourse?" • "Do you have pain or any problem with intercourse?" • "Have you ever had venereal disease?" • "Do you have any trouble with your breasts?"	• sex "screen" • sex "screen"
	Male	• "Have you had any pain or swelling in your scrotum?" • "Do you have a discharge from your penis? • "Have you noted any change in your sex life?" • "Do you have any trouble having an erection?" • "Have you ever had a venereal disease?"	• sex "screen" • sex "screen"
MUSCULOSKELETAL		• "Do you have any trouble with your joints? Muscles?" • "Do you have any back trouble?" • "Do you have any joint pain?" • "Do you have any muscle pain?" • "Do you have pain in your legs?"	
NEUROLOGIC		• "Do you have weakness in any muscles?" • "Have you ever been paralyzed?" • "Have you ever lost feeling anywhere?" • "Do you have numbness or tingling?" • "Have you noted any change in your memory?" • "How is your coordination?" • "Do you have any trouble walking?"	

(Continued)

REVIEW OF SYSTEMS, Continued

SYSTEM	QUESTIONS	NOTE
PSYCHIATRIC	• "Have you ever had any nervous or emotional problems?" • "Do you have any trouble sleeping?" • "Have you noted any change in your personality?" • "Have you ever felt confused?" • "Have you had thoughts that seem strange or troubling to you?" • "How are your spirits or moods?" • "Have you ever had periods when you felt unusually depressed for several days or weeks at a time?" • "Have you ever had periods when you felt unusually optimistic and highspirited for days or weeks at a time?" • "Have you noted any difficulty with your memory such as difficulty remembering people's names, telephone numbers, or the date?"	If any of these questions are answered affirmatively, a detailed "Mental Status Examination" must be done.

Summary

The purpose of the R.O.S. is to:

- remind the patient of any symptoms that may have been forgotten or that may have been repressed
- allow the physician to systematically review symptoms so that none will be missed

The only way to utilize time efficiently in obtaining the R.O.S. is to become intimately familiar with the symptoms by system. Then, a personal design and style can be developed for questions, utilizing the preceding model as a guide. It also is reasonable to have the patient complete a written form before seeing the physician. During the interview, the physician can review any questions answered affirmatively so long as reference to the papers does not disrupt the interview technique.

SUMMARY OF INTERVIEW COMPONENTS

The following table summarizes components of the interview.

Interview Components

Identifying Data	
Chief Complaint	
Present Illness	• time of onset • precipitating event • anatomical location • mode of onset • severity • frequency • method of relief or worsening • character or quality • other symptoms related to involved organ system
Past Medical History	• hospitalizations • serious illnesses • major injuries • operations • allergies • medications and other treatments • regular MD and last visit • health maintenance activities • immunizations • tobacco • alcohol • "recreational" drugs
Family History	• parents • siblings • spouse • children • high blood pressure, heart disease, cancer, diabetes, bleeding disorders in family
Patient Profile	• education • occupation • appearance and behavior • family relationships • social relationships • sexual relationships • stresses
Review of Systems	

THE WRITTEN HISTORY

Introduction	Since history and physical examination forms may be used in the future, one should learn to use them.
Present Illness	The report should be written in complete sentences and should be a prose-style chronologic description of the PI. It should include a complete description of <u>each complaint</u> that is included in the PI.
Patient Profile	The profile should include reference to all of the items listed on the history form.
Past Medical History	The past medical history may be recorded in outline form, but should include reference to all of the items listed on the form.
Family History	The family history may be recorded in outline and phrase form. It should include reference to <u>all</u> of those items listed on the form.
Problem List	Include all of the problems that are elicited during the interview when preparing the problem list.

(Continued)

THE WRITTEN HISTORY, Continued

Summary

Completion of the written history form may be summarized as follows:

IF	THEN
a symptom is elicited in either the PI or ROS	the "Pos" (positive) box is checked in the ROS section
the symptom is described in the PI	merely write "see PI" in the space provided NOTE: Remember, for each positive response you must describe the problem completely: • date of onset • mode of onset • precipitating and exacerbating factors • anatomical location • severity and description • number of times or frequency • method of relief
the complaint was not described in the PI	you should do so in the space provided on the form
a question was not asked about an item NOTE: All items on the inventory of ROS should be covered in a complete interview.	check neither "Pos" nor "Neg"
the response to a question is negative	merely check the "Neg" (negative) box

Example

An example of a written history appears at the end of Chapter 9 as Appendix One.

CHAPTER EIGHT

Psychosomatic Problems

Murphy T. Scurry, M.D.

THE DOCTOR-PATIENT RELATIONSHIP

Introduction

Some patients, because of their behavior, strain the doctor-patient relationship and "get to" the physician. Also, each physician has his or her own way of feeling and behaving. Thus, a kind of "personality clash" can create a difficult situation for both doctor and patient. It is important to recognize that this adds to the stress of the relationship.

Objectives

The purpose of this chapter is to:

- indicate the stress that certain patients place upon the physician-patient relationship
- indicate the problems that such patients present
- introduce concepts of management

Presented in this chapter will be:

- "patient types" that generally stress the physician-patient relationship
- some ways in which physicians can add to the problem
- suggestions and principles for dealing with these types of patients

Definitions

The doctor-patient relationship is basically a contractual agreement between two parties who have distinct roles. Emotions are clearly involved. Three components of the relationship are:

- the contract
- the roles
- the emotions

Emotion

The doctor-patient relationship is subject to most of the emotions that exist between people; to name just some:

- anger
- envy
- joy
- sadness
- lust
- care
- boredom

Some of these emotions must be limited if the relationship is to be a good one.

EXAMPLE: If anger is too intense or lust too strong (and character too weak!), the relationship will become unworkable.

(Continued)

THE DOCTOR-PATIENT RELATIONSHIP, Continued

Emotions that assist the work and the effective completion of the central task are useful and even essential. Emotions that characterize a professional relationship include:

- respect
- concern
- understanding
- trust

Such emotions add to the quality of the relationship, assist in establishing rapport, and even aid in curing the patient.

Role

The roles of the doctor and the patient are often seen simplistically in the following terms:

- The doctor, as a professional, is expected to be:
  - the authority
  - knowledgeable
  - skillful
  - understanding
  - objective
  - competent
- The patient may be:
  - sick and debilitated
  - unable to diagnose or treat himself or herself
  - in need of and the receiver of medical services

Awareness of Roles

This oversimplified characterization of the roles of the physician and the patient is neither accurate nor, in many instances, desirable, for patients have important rights in and responsibilities for their own diagnosis and treatment. Nevertheless, if both parties are aware of the above characterization, certain possibilities for compromising the quality of medical care may be avoided.

EXAMPLE: A physician caring for a member of his own family risks losing objectivity and professionalism. This reduces the possibility of making a calm, accurate assessment of the patient's condition or making the crucial decisions that must sometimes be made.

THE CONTRACT

Definition

The arrangements between a doctor and patient, though unwritten, are operative contracts containing all of the components of a legal business contract between two parties:

- The intention is plain.
- Two distinct acts are performed (making an offer, accepting an offer).
- Each party gains something from the contract.
  NOTE: There is no contract if a person promises to do something for another person for which he is to get nothing in return.
- The parties' minds are in accord.
- The parties accept responsibility for their part of the contract.
- Discharging of the contract is plainly discernible.
- Breach of contract is discernible.

Medical Application

How the above definition of contract translates into medical application is shown below:

CONTRACT DEFINITION	MEDICAL APPLICATION
intention is plain	patient seeks help
involves two distinct acts	doctor offers and patient receives medical services
each party realizes something	patient receives services; doctor receives fee
minds are in accord	doctor and patient agree on the services to be provided
responsibility accepted	the doctor, for the medical services; the patient, for cooperating with the doctor and paying the fee
contract is discharged	treatment is completed and doctor is paid
breach of contract clearly discernible	doctor fails to render agreed-on services OR patient refuses cooperation or payment

(Continued)

THE CONTRACT, Continued

Contractual Strains

It is easy to see in terms of a contractual arrangement how certain situations strain the doctor-patient relationship.

EXAMPLES:

- If the patient does not pay the physician, he violates the contract and creates in the doctor a justifiable feeling of having been cheated.
- If the doctor and patient have not agreed on the medical services to be rendered (their minds are not in accord), one may feel he has fulfilled the contractual obligation, while the other feels he has not been given what he came for.

Limits

The doctor-patient contract has limits: the contract begins when the doctor and patient agree upon the specific kind of medical services to be given and ends when such services have been completed. With human nature as it is, however, such simple and straightforward principles are often quickly forgotten. Irrational features, such as:

- covert goals
- magical expectations
- wishful fantasies

begin to creep in, and an agreed-upon, rational, limited contract can quickly be subverted. Thus, the doctor-patient relationship is stressed. Distortion of the contract is a particular hazard in difficult doctor-patient relationships.

EXAMPLE: The doctor who treats a 20-year-old woman with acute leukemia hopes to get the patient into remission and possibly even to cure her. The patient also has these hopes. When she begins to show signs of incurability, the physician--who may find it hard to face death and his or her own limitations--may make fewer visits. Not wanting to die, the patient becomes depressed or angry or both, and the anger may be directed at the doctor who did not cure her.

REGRESSED AND CHILDISH PATIENTS

Common Reaction

It is common for people to become more childish when they see a physician and particularly when they are hospitalized to undergo treatment for serious illness. It is not only common, but also normal, for regression to occur to some degree. After all, sick, hospitalized people are treated somewhat like babies; they are:

- fed
- bathed
- kept bedfast
- wheeled around

Regression is accentuated when the patient is:

- severely ill
- under personal stress in addition to the physical illness
- placed on sedative drugs

Some patients tolerate stress poorly and regress more quickly and severely than others.

Types of Behavior

Regressed patients present many different kinds of behavior. Some whine and cry, others throw temper tantrums, others get quiet and shy. The type of regression will depend on the patient's personality makeup. Too, the regression may wax and wane, depending on such variables as:

- the amount of sleep the patient gets
- the amount of pain experienced
- the time of day

Irrationality

Irrational concerns become foremost, sometimes taking over all three aspects of the doctor-patient relationship, altering the contract (it is nearly impossible to maintain an adult contract with a child) and sorely threatening the helpful emotions previously discussed.

(Continued)

REGRESSED AND CHILDISH PATIENTS, Continued

Correcting the Problem

The problem can be alleviated by recognizing the phenomenon and taking steps to correct the reaction. Appropriate steps include:

- understanding the reaction and conveying this understanding
- remaining calm and reassuring
- not taking the reaction personally
- discontinuing medication that contributes to the regression
- giving the patient more control over his life, especially informing him about what's coming next and thereby treating him more like an adult
- eventually helping him get physically and mentally well

Regression is almost always self-limiting and corrects itself when the patient feels better and gets back his physical and emotional health. However, some patients may stay in this regressed-dependent role well after their illness has abated enough for them to assume more responsibility for themselves. The physician should recognize this and assist the patient. This is done by gradually making the patient assume more responsibility and independence.

DEPENDENT AND NEEDFUL PATIENTS

Introduction

Patients with continuous strong dependency place demands on the physician. Such patients are to be differentiated from those who become dependent upon the doctor because of severe illness with its associated (and normal) regression, which resolves when the patient recovers.

Chronic Dependency

Dependent patients have more than episodic periods of dependency associated with illness. They seem to be dependent most of the time, even when they are healthy. Their basic problem is that they want to be taken care of rather than take care of themselves, and they often attach themselves to care-giving people like doctors in order to get their needs met. To the extent that the physician has an inner need to take care of others and has difficulty setting limits on himself and others, he will have difficulty with such patients.

Vicious Cycle

With this type of patient, vicious cycles ensue: the patient asks for help, the doctor gives it; the patient asks for "a little more," the doctor gives it too; the patient asks for even more, the doctor gets frustrated but still gives more, and it goes on and on.

Setting Limits

The essential element in dealing successfully with these patients is that the doctor be able to recognize dependency in patients and that the doctor:

- set reasonable but firm limits on them
- not go beyond what he or she feels is his or her part of the contract
- not be seduced into making most of a patient's decisions and providing exceptional support.

Saying "No"

A few patients are not content to live within the boundaries of a healthy doctor-patient relationship. They demand more. If repeated attempts to get the patient to accept the necessary limitations fail, then the physician must be willing to give up the patient. Sensing this willingness, most patients will finally accept the doctor's limits. The stress from these patients relates in large part to this struggle. Some patients continuously "push" at the relationship, asking for more, never content with what exists. It is no wonder that physicians become frustrated with them. Those who learn to turn this frustration into a healthy and firm "no" when appropriate will have success with such patients and will feel less harassed by them.

ANGER AND THE AGGRESSIVE PATIENT

Types of Anger

A frontal attack by a patient whom one wants to help is always distressing. There are many "shades" of angry behavior:

- personal indictment
- harsh criticism
- verbal abuse
- physical abuse
- ridicule of the doctor

Anger can seldom be tolerated by the physician for a long period. It stresses the doctor-patient relationship by negating the positive emotions that are needed for an effective doctor-patient relationship. Anger is best dealt with immediately and rather firmly with open-ended questions, which lead to an understanding of the reason for the reaction. It should not be allowed to go on without resolution.

Objectivity

A crucial aspect of the solution of the problem lies in remaining objective and calm, yet firm, with the goal of reestablishing a workable doctor-patient relationship. This is harder to do if the doctor becomes highly defensive, angry, and irrational. The doctor must realize that this angry reaction is most often an aspect of regressive behavior and a defense against feeling vulnerable in a hospital setting. The patient's words often give this away: "You don't scare me!" "Get out of my room!" "I am leaving this damned hospital!"

The "Why"

The physician must be willing to think about how he or she may have contributed to the problem: has he stepped outside the boundaries of the relationship and, in suddenly deciding to "straighten it out", made the patient angry? Once the reaction is dealt with, a workable and useful doctor-patient relationship will often follow, since both the doctor and the patient have worked through a crisis and resolved it. If the doctor remains bitter and angry toward the patient, even after the problem has been resolved, he should strongly consider referring the patient to another physician, since he can no longer be objective. This latter reaction most frequently occurs when the doctor lets the problem get out of hand and does not deal with it when it first arises.

SELF-DESTRUCTIVE DENIERS

Definition

Self-destructive deniers are patients who continue with self-destructive behavior after they have been well educated to the dangers of their behavior and have usually experienced several life-threatening episodes as a result of their behavior.

EXAMPLES:

- patients with malignant hypertension who repeatedly stop taking their medicine
- alcoholics with cirrhosis, ascites, and bleeding esophageal varicies who continue to drink heavily

The physicians caring for these patients usually become angry and frustrated because their efforts are repeatedly defeated by the patients' behavior.

What to Do

The physician's actions in these situations are severely limited. Consultation with a psychiatrist or a special rehabilitation program may be helpful.

SEDUCTIVE PATIENTS

Their Ulterior Needs

Most seductive patients, although they express overt sexual behavior, are quite needful and demanding. They seek their doctor's affection and attention, hoping thereby to be able to solve various personal problems, such as:

- loneliness
- marital discord
- frigidity

There are numerous kinds of seductive patients, including:

- older patients
- younger patients
- same-gender patients

Depending on age, sex, and physical appearance, they may be very appealing to the needful or naive physician.

Identifying and Dealing With Their Approach

If the physician goes along with one personal question ("Are you married?"), there will be others ("Are you happily married?"). One must decide when to deal with the sequence and how to get to the patient's real difficulty: the loneliness, discord, or whatever lies behind the presenting symptom and the seductive behavior. Two responses to the seductive patient readily come to mind. Depending on how clear the approach is, one can adopt the first or the second, or the first and then the second:

- Avoid the personal questions and continue with the task.
- Pause in the task and wonder aloud if there is not more troubling the patient than the presenting complaint.

One cannot allow oneself to become unprofessionally involved.

Professional Perspective

It is essential to understand that the seductive patient's overtures should not be taken personally. This sometimes flattering response, positive as it may be (compared with the negative response from an angry patient), is a reaction to what the physician represents and is based on wishful fantasies. All physicians must understand that they will be sexually attracted to certain patients and that becoming a professional includes putting one's personal needs aside and attending to the legitimate needs of the patient.

DYING PATIENTS

Definition

The term <u>dying patients</u> is used to describe those patients who have a disease that no longer responds to medical treatment and who, because of the disease, are expected to die within a relatively short time.

Helplessness Versus Support

Physicians often make fewer and shorter visits to the bedside of dying patients in spite of the fact that they know these patients need support during the final days of their lives. They find it too painful and difficult. Who wants to get to know someone and become more attached when one knows the person will soon die? Death is often viewed by physicians as an enemy, as something to be conquered, to be held off. In the face of the impending death of a patient, a physician feels helpless. However, the dying patient needs emotional support. Giving emotional support is synonymous with giving medical services in this circumstance. Providing continued emotional support is a vital part of a physician's work.

Stages of Dying

Dying patients go through several important stages. These stages are similiar to those found in most separation experiences and include:

- protest
- mourning
- acceptance

As shown below, while dying patients proceed through these stages, they demonstrate:

- denial
- anger
- depression
- withdrawal

FIRST STAGE	SECOND STAGE	THIRD STAGE
• denial	• anger • depression	• withdrawal

Positive Results

These stages and their concomitant affects are all part of a natural life-process that unfolds only in this last stage of life. Frequently, patients can deal constructively with this process and gain from it, particularly if they have someone to help them through it.

(Continued)

DYING PATIENTS, Continued

Psychological State	Dying patients are in a different psychological state than healthy patients. They may or may not fear talking about dying, but some want to talk about it, and will talk with the physician who can comfortably do so. Physicians who care for such patients should, therefore, endeavor to understand the psychology of dying and also their own concerns about death so that they can deal effectively with dying patients.

Working With Patients	Practical ideas regarding working with dying patients include:
	• letting them ventilate their feelings and thoughts
	• continuing to visit them for short periods and going through the usual procedures of ward rounds (taking vital signs, etc.)
	• letting them have, as much as possible, their last wishes:
	  • friends to visit
	  • enough (or as little) pain medicine as they need
	  • special foods
	• allowing oneself to be sad over the loss and to get extra encouragement from others if needed
	• getting others to help with the dying patient if one is unable to give adequate assistance

Professional Adjustment	As a student and resident, caring for dying patients and working with their families may be the most difficult tasks that will have to be learned and adjusted to. Most neophytes in this situation may receive help by discussing the problems with another student, resident, or faculty member. Don't be afraid to bring up thoughts and feelings in regard to caring for a dying patient.

BIOPSYCHOSOCIAL SYMPTOMS

Introduction

Biopsychosocial knowledge involves an understanding of illness as the product of interacting dimensions, which are:

- biological
- psychological
- sociological

The utility of this knowledge is most apparent in the care of patients in whom psychosocial factors are the major, if not the sole, features of the illness. Such patients constitute more than half of patients presenting to outpatient medical clinics.

Evaluation of Patients

Physicians must use the three variables (biological, psychological, sociological) to evaluate patients. They must avoid use of the functional-organic dichotomy. The detection of physical illness is of no more help in excluding psychological components of an illness than a "negative workup" is in confirming a psychiatric diagnosis. Physicians must develop a nonjudgmental approach to the patient while understanding their own needs. The latter is of particular importance in the care of a "difficult" patient who is demanding of time or poorly responsive to therapy.

Bizarre Symptoms

When psychological factors contribute to the patient's symptoms, their description becomes more personalized, even bizarre, and thus harder for the physician to understand from a pathophysiologic perspective. A patient may state that the pain is like "flowing hot lava" or like "a million biting fireants." The symptoms and their relation to time or physiological events may be inconsistent. This personalization of symptoms may be a somatic component of a psychological disturbance or may modify the perception of a true somatic disorder.

Persistence Despite Treatment

When a symptom is modified by psychological factors, it may remain unchanged after seemingly specific therapy.

> EXAMPLE: A 30-year-old woman, with right upper abdominal pain continued to have the same symptom after 10 years, despite cholecystectomy, hysterectomy, and lysis of intestinal adhesions.

(Continued)

BIOPSYCHOSOCIAL SYMPTOMS, Continued

Stress

The setting in which an illness began may be associated with a significant stress event. Knowledge of this event can be of particular value when the event is shown to have meaning to the patient.

> EXAMPLE: A 56-year-old woman had recurrent abdominal pain. She was shy and had difficulty expressing appropriate anger. Her mother was an alcoholic who died of liver cancer, and the woman recalled her having severe abdominal pain near the time of death. The woman's pain began on the first anniversary of her mother's death. Although the patient was not aware of it, the onset of the pain also occurred during events that led to anger that she suppressed because she had learned from her mother that this was improper behavior.

Direct questioning about the relation of stress events to the symptoms is seldom helpful; the physician must obtain the data by indirect means.

Patient's Diagnosis

Some patients respond with a "positive review of systems." The patient's diagnosis of:

- sinus headache
- bronchitis

OR

- hiatal hernia

should be viewed as descriptive, and specific symptoms and their physiological relationships determined. Lack of data to explain the symptoms and a review of medical records may reveal that the patient's diagnosis cannot be documented.

Unwillingness to Accept Emotional Factors

When a patient is unwilling to accept the role of emotional factors in an illness, consider this action as a mechanism for keeping these factors from conscious awareness. The patient with organic causes of pain is willing to see a psychiatrist if it will make the patient feel better. Physicians must frequently discuss emotional issues even though this is uncomfortable. If the discussion is avoided overtly or covertly, the patient may not consider such issues further.

(Continued)

BIOPSYCHOSOCIAL SYMPTOMS, Continued

Hypochondriasis	Hypochondriasis is a personality trait in which patients maintain an obsessive preoccupation with their bodily function. They magnify the significance of normal body activity and common everyday discomforts, see themselves as sick, and relate to people through their symptoms. The only significant human relation may be with the doctor who listens to their complaints. This need to relate through their symptoms makes them unresponsive to therapy. Hypochondriacs are intensely concerned about their illness, yet still need to maintain their role as sick persons.
Chronic Pain	Some patients have a lifelong history of pain. Frequently, there is a family history of alcoholism or physical abuse. In this environment, the child is made to feel worthless. The only intimate contact with the alcoholic or abusive parent may be when the child is being punished or abused. Pain becomes a means of atonement for feelings of self-devaluation and guilt. The patient may place himself or herself in troubled or painful circumstances. The patient cannot accept a state of well-being, for to do so would pose the threat of experiencing unbearable feelings of guilt. Thus, the doctor's attempts to make the patient well fail.
Depression	Depression consists of feelings of: • discouragement • loss of interest • worthlessness • sadness • tearfulness • loss of appetite • constipation Yet, the patient may focus concerns on somatic complaints such as headaches or backaches. This misinterpretation may be made by the physician as well, especially when he or she fails to explore the setting and circumstances preceding the onset of illness. These patients respond to antidepressive medication.

(Continued)

BIOPSYCHOSOCIAL SYMPTOMS, Continued

Somatic Delusion	Somatic delusions represent psychotic disorganization and may be the first sign of schizophrenia or a major affective psychosis. Patients have bizarre beliefs about their symptoms. EXAMPLES: • headache is being caused by huge worms migrating through the brain, splitting it into pieces • liver is decaying and beginning to smell The symptoms are not being described metaphorically, but patients truly believe what they say. These patients need psychiatric referral.

BIOPSYCHOSOCIAL TREATMENT

Flexible Approach	Therapy is directed toward modification of psychosocial behavior. The following recommendations may be successful for one patient yet not for another. If one approach fails, another may be tried.
Establish Factors	Establish the significance of psychosocial factors in patients' illnesses. Patients may feel reluctant to discuss certain issues or be unable to acknowledge their significance. Direct questioning is seldom helpful, so the physician must be indirect and flexible in his or her interview, often obtaining the psychosocial data by open-ended questions and questions outlined in the patient profile.
Questioning Technique	Use a symptom-oriented, nondirective interview style, with questions designed to encourage elicitation of spontaneous information through patients' own associations. This allows patients to give the history in their own way. More specific questions can be asked later to fully characterize the symptom. The physician should allow patients to follow their own associations to determine whether the data are significant.
The Somatic-Psychosocial Dichotomy	Do not attempt to separate the somatic from the psychosocial data. Patients will frequently describe their symptoms in the context of interpersonal relations and emotional concerns if allowed to do so. The encouragement of more personal data is best done at the time patients themselves introduce such matters. EXAMPLE: A 38-year-old man volunteers that his abdominal pain begins while driving to work. The physician's questions about his work at this time may disclose conflicts on the job that would not be mentioned later when asked out of context. Attempts later in the interview to elicit psychosocial data should be made by referring to patients' earlier associations. In this way, patients learn to present the history in the most productive manner and to recognize that feelings are as important to the doctor as their symptoms.

(Continued)

BIOPSYCHOSOCIAL TREATMENT, Continued

Physician's Role	Maintain unbiased interest. The physician should communicate nonjudgmental concern. Fear of disapproval prevents patients from sharing intimate feelings. Obtain a complete history and perform an appropriate physical examination. The presence of obvious psychological factors in the problem does not exclude somatic illness.
Avoiding Laboratory Procedures	Avoid unnecessary procedures. After the interview and physical examination, the physician develops an assessment of the problem(s). One must then have the confidence <u>not</u> to order unnecessary diagnostic studies to "rule out organic disease." If the patient presents with complaints that cannot be readily understood, it may be wiser to temporize than commit oneself to a diagnostic plan with uncertain effectiveness and with attendant risks and expense. In time, the issues may become clarified. <u>Do not</u> use symptomatic or psychotropic medications that are not indicated.
Avoiding Reassurance as "Emotional"	Do not attempt to reassure by stating that the problem is "emotional." Patients may be unable to understand the significance of emotional factors in illness. Informing patients that their symptoms are emotional or functional may also anger the patient. To say that the problem has not been clarified and that the problem warrants further visits reaffirms the doctor's interest in the patient. If asked by the patient whether or not the problem is emotional or psychological, it would be appropriate to say that it is important to understand the role of <u>all</u> factors in the illness-- emotional and physical. The patient's awareness of associations between emotional factors and the symptoms is not necessary for improvement and must <u>not</u> be a goal for the physician.
Accepting Symptoms	Accept the symptoms at face value. Patients may be unable to give up symptoms that meet certain needs. Patients should be informed that it would be too ambitious to expect a rapid recovery after months (or years) of illness. Again, the physician should indicate willingness to work with the patient to adapt to and possibly diminish the symptoms. No promises can be made for cure. This approach establishes a contract in which the doctor is not obligated to produce results and the patient is encouraged to actively work on the illness in conjunction with a partner, the physician.

(Continued)

BIOPSYCHOSOCIAL TREATMENT, Continued

Regular Visits	Set up regular visits as the first step in the development of the therapeutic relationship. Scheduling ongoing visits confirms the physician's desire to help the patient. During these sessions, the same symptom-oriented approach is maintained with continued efforts to elicit the patient's own associations. The physician's task is to listen without feeling compelled to remove the symptoms. When the patient recounts continued symptoms, the physician should communicate an understanding of how difficult it must be to go on with such distress. A brief physical examination ("laying-on of hands") also may have therapeutic value.
Building Trust	Build the patient's confidence, so that when a trusting relationship is established, the patient will begin to discuss concerns and feelings that would not previously have been discussed. This is an objective sign of improvement. If the physician continues to provide a nonjudgmental approach to the expression of these concerns, the somatic symptoms will begin to lose their significance. During periods of exacerbation of symptoms the patient may ask the doctor to "do something." Similarly, night calls or "emergency" visits may be demanded by the patient. If the doctor can provide reassurance, the patient's symptoms may be allayed and diagnostic procedures may be avoided.
Physician's Attitudes	Be cognizant of one's own attitudes. The patient's insistence on maintaining a sick role may conflict with the physician's expectations of a symptom-free and compliant patient. Physician's may call these patients "crocks" or "turkeys," terms that attempt to allay the sense of frustration. Physicians must avoid the "dual" concept--organic or functional. Such a concept will cause the physician to view the patient's symptoms with less credibility than those symptoms due to "organic" disease.

(Continued)

BIOPSYCHOSOCIAL TREATMENT, Continued

Evaluating Progress	Progress may be assessed in some patients by their ability to function despite symptoms rather than by the symptoms' presence or severity. Other patients may appear to have improved, though if asked, they will say that the symptoms have not changed or that they are even worse. The physician must remain alert to new developments. Patients with psychosomatic problems may develop organic disease.
Termination	Be aware that treatment may be prolonged. Once a therapeutic contract and relationship is established, ending is difficult. It is best to progressively decrease the frequency of visits when patients are doing well. If a patient suddenly decides to end the relationship, he or she should be seen once more to explore feelings and to be certain that it is not an attempt to test the doctor's interest. Patients should be encouraged to return whenever necessary.

PART TWO

The Physical Examination

CHAPTER NINE

The General Physical Examination

James C. Guckian, M.D.

OVERVIEW

Introduction

In mastering the skill of physical diagnosis, certain techniques must be developed, which are then enhanced by recognition and examination in further detail of a large number of physical abnormalities. Moreover, for maximal effectiveness, the physician must also be able to organize and modify performance according to the demands of the clinical situation. This requires repeated practice of a large number of highly complex manipulative sequences to a point of nearly automatic behavior.

Background

To better understand the performance requirements in this area, a time and motion study of practicing physicians was carried out to determine the:

- content
- sequence
- time

devoted to each aspect of the most commonly practiced routine physical examination. A basic physical examination was designed. This examination contains those steps that are felt by a majority of physicians to offer a high yield of abnormal clues. Moreover, considerable attention was devoted to both timing and sequencing the steps

- to maximize the physician's efficiency
- to reduce to a minimum the chance of overlooking or omitting a data point

The individual maneuvers and sequence of the examination are summarized in this section.

Purpose

While it is obvious that this is only one of many situations within which a physician must function, learning the routine patient examination as a cornerstone provides a framework in which to subsequently organize the many variations and expansions that must be added on demand.

(Continued)

OVERVIEW, Continued

Objectives	The physical examination procedure should be memorized and practiced (on roommate, spouse, etc.) until performance can be demonstrated • quickly • efficiently • completely You must be able to: • describe verbally the maneuvers you are performing and what you expect to find in a normal adult • define the terms used in the physical examination.
Order	The physical examination is NOT recorded in the order in which it is performed: • the record is organized by organ systems • the examination is done by body regions The examination should be done as illustrated on the following pages.
Equipment	The following equipment must be available for the complete general examination: • sphygmomanometer • stethoscope with bell and diaphragm • tongue blades • penlight • otoscope with speculums for ears and nose • ophthalmoscope • percussion hammer • thermometer • watch • gloves • lubricant • vaginal speculum Other equipment may become necessary for more detailed examinations; these items will be described elsewhere in this book.
Important!!	MASTERING THIS EXAMINATION IS THE FIRST PRIORITY.

PREPARATION

Learning Instructions

- Memorize the physical examination sequence.
- Become familiar with the range of normal findings.
- Master the proper use of the examining instruments.
- Review the material until the sequence and procedure of the examination can be recalled.
- Take the self-assessment test at the end of this chapter.

Before the Examination

A few words with the patient in the examining room before beginning the examination sometimes helps relax the patient and allows some observations about his/her general appearance:

- Note the facial expression and apparent age.
- Observe the patient's:
  - ability to arise from a chair
  - gait

    NOTE: Normally one's gait is symmetrical, without a limp and with associated swinging of the arms.

Four Positions

The four-position examination is conducted with the patient:

- seated facing physician
- seated with the back to the physician
- supine with the physician at the patient's right side
- seated on the edge of the examination table

See Figures 9-1 through 9-4.

Remember the Purpose

The purpose of the physical examination, as described in this section, is the detection of conditions that are not producing symptoms. Examinations relevant to a patient's problems and illnesses are adapted from this screening examination.

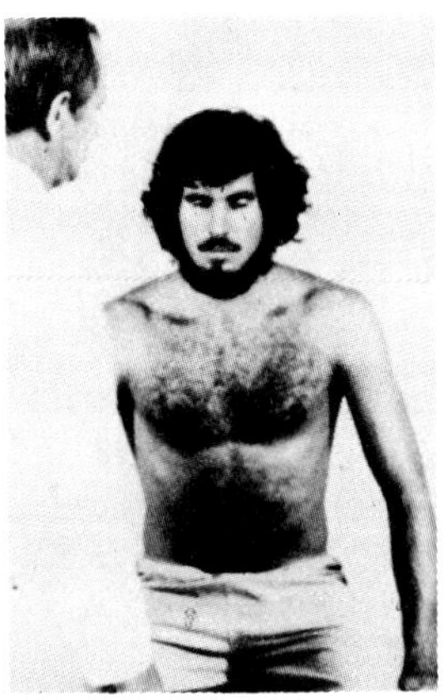

Fig. 9-1

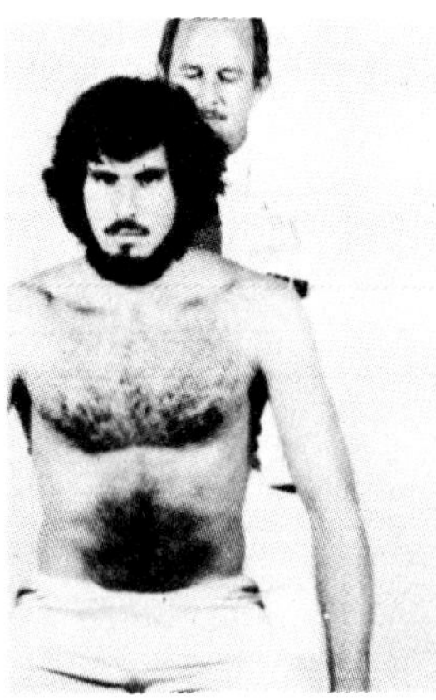

Fig. 9-2

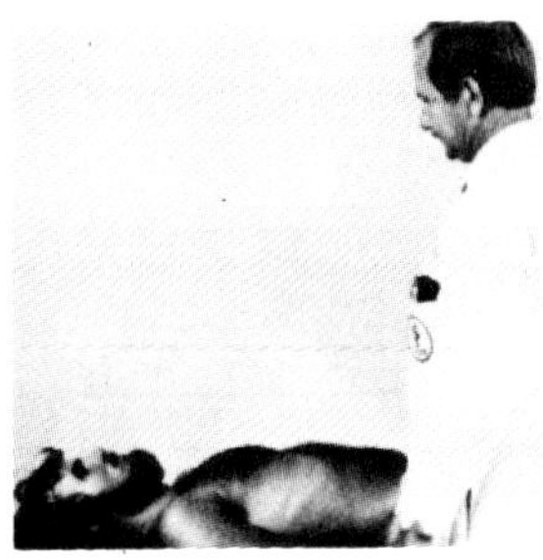

Fig. 9-3

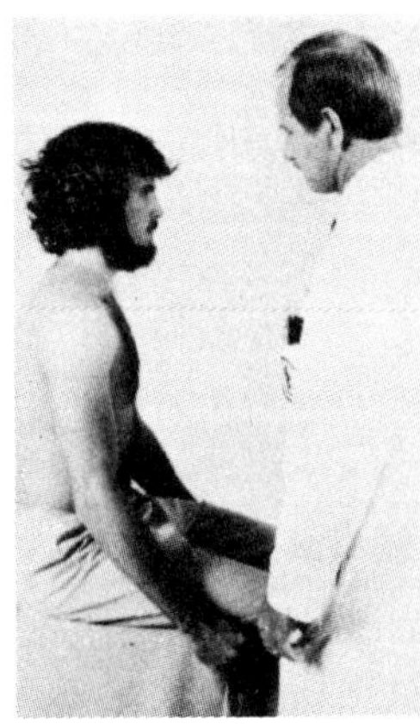

Fig. 9-4.

PATIENT SEATED FACING PHYSICIAN

Introduction

With patient seated facing the physician, the general examination of
- hands and arms
- neck
- head
- eyes
- ears
- nose
- mouth

are performed in sequence.

Procedure

After washing up, start with the patient sitting facing you. Begin with hands and arms.

	STEP	ACTION	NOTE
Hands and Arms	1	Measure the blood pressure with the sphygmomanometer: a. Fit the cuff evenly and firmly around the upper arm. b. Place the stethoscope over the brachial artery. c. Inflate the cuff to 200 mm of mercury. d. Deflate the cuff slowly, auscultating over the brachial artery. e. Note the systolic and diastolic pressure.	See Figure 9-5.
	2	Inspect the nails, observing the sheen and regularity of growth. Check the joints of the hands for mobility.	Fingernails should be: • smooth • translucent • evenly attached to the underlying nail bed Palms should be: • moist • smooth
	3	Palpate the musculature of the arms.	Inspect and palpate the skin in all body regions as you progress through the examination and palpate muscles and joints.

(Continued)

PATIENT SEATED FACING PHYSICIAN, Continued

	STEP	ACTION	NOTE
	4	Take the radial pulse for 15 seconds and multiply by 4.	A sharp, well=defined pulse of 50 to 100 beats per minute is normal.
	5	Palpate for the epitrochlear lymph node.	See Figure 9-6.
	6	Try to palpate the axillary lymph nodes under both arms, noting any tenderness. See Figure 9-7.	Normal lymph nodes may not be palpable; nodes enlarged because of previous inflammation are frequently felt.
Neck	7	Examine the neck.	Palpate the lymph nodes in the anterior triangles, the supraclavicular area, along the carotid arteries, and in the submandibular area. Lymph nodes smaller than 1 cm in diameter may be normal. The carotid pulses should be strong and symmetrical. Note the position of the trachea. It should be in the midline.
Head	8	Examine the head. Inspect the scalp and hair, and note the configuration of the head.	Bones in the adult should be fused into a symmetrically smooth skull.
	9	Observe the texture and color of the hair, and check the skin of the face for symmetry of movement, which is controlled by the facial nerve.	

(Continued)

PATIENT SEATED FACING PHYSICIAN, Continued

	STEP	ACTION	NOTE
Eyes	10	Using the pocket screener: a. determine patient's visual acuity by holding the card 14 inches from the eyes b. with each eye covered in turn, ask patient to read as many lines as legible	If patient wears glasses, check the vision both with and without the glasses. Normal vision is 20/20.
	11	Using a penlight, inspect the conjunctiva. It will be pinkish.	The sclera is normally white. The edge of the eyelids should be at the limbus, the outer most part of the iris.
	12	Determine the extraocular movements in the six cardinal directions of gaze.	Wrinkling of the forehead should occur with the patient's eyes in the upward gaze. This movement is mediated through the facial nerve.
	13	Test the pupillary reaction. Shine the penlight quickly into one eye and observe the reflexes of both eyes.	The illuminated eye shows constriction of the ipsilateral pupil, and the consensually illuminated eye shows an equal constriction of the contralateral pupil.
	14	Shine the light into the other eye.	The reaction should be the same.

(Continued)

PATIENT SEATED FACING PHYSICIAN, Continued

	STEP	ACTION	NOTE
	15	Check the retina: a. Set the ophthalmoscope on +10 and have patient look straight ahead. b. Looking into the right eye, hold the instrument in your right hand and stand on patient's right. c. With the ophthalmoscope 12 inches from patient's eye, move in gradually, decreasing the setting until the retina comes into focus. d. Turn the lens wheel of the ophthalmoscope until the lighter yellow color of the optic disc is seen nasal to the center of the retina. e. Refocus until the margins of the optic disc are sharply defined and the exit of the vessels can be seen clearly.	b. Reverse this procedure for the left eye. c. Look for the arteries, which should be bright red with a reflecting sheen. The veins should be dark red and pulsating with the heartbeat. The size ratio of the artery to the vein should be 2 to 3.
Ears	16	Change the ophthalmoscope attachment to examine the external auditory canal and tympanic membrane.	
	17	Draw the auricle of the ear upward and back, inserting the <u>otoscope</u>. See Figure 9-8.	Observe the major landmarks of the: • tympanic membranes • anterior and posterior folds • pars flaccida • pars tensa • malleus, which is visible behind the eardrum

(Continued)

PATIENT SEATED FACING PHYSICIAN, Continued

	STEP	ACTION	NOTE
	18	Test the hearing using a wristwatch or a whispered number.	
Nose	19	Use a penlight to check the septum of the nose, which should be in the midline. Look at the turbinates.	Turbinates should be pinkish and unclogged. The mucosa of the nose should be smooth.
Mouth	20	Using a tongue blade: a. Inspect the mouth, noting the reddish mucous membranes. b. Note Stensen's duct. c. Observe the tonsils.	In dark-skinned races the mucous membranes may have a black or brown pigmentation.
	21	Inspect the teeth.	Teeth should appear normal, with neither cavities nor discoloration. Gums should be smooth, pink, and not bleeding.
	22	Observe the pharynx.	The pharynx appears red, with small nodules representing lymphatic tissue.
	23	Test the gag reflex by touching the lateral walls, tonsils, or back of the tongue.	This tests the 9th and 10th cranial nerves.
	24	Have the patient phonate, saying "Ah."	The soft palate and vulva should elevate symmetrically.
	25	Have the patient protrude the tongue.	It should do so along the midline.

PHYSICIAN BEHIND PATIENT

Introduction

While patient is seated with back to physician, the
- thyroid
- chest
- spine and flanks

are examined in sequence.

Procedure

	STEP	ACTION	NOTE
Thyroid	1	Try to palpate the thyroid gland: a. lightly place the tips of the first two or three fingers of both hands on either side of the trachea, slightly below the level of the thyroid cartilage b. a light rotary motion, as the patient swallows, should palpate the smooth symmetrical tissue.	The thyroid is frequently not palpable in normal adults and usually not visible. Having the patient swallow may make the gland more prominent.
Chest	2	Examine the chest: a. inspect the skin. b. have the patient inspire deeply, and, as the rib cage expands, feel the movement of the chest for symmetry.	
	3	Percuss the upper, middle, and lower lung fields: a. place the distal two phalanges of the left middle finger firmly against the chest wall b. with the middle finger of the right hand, strike two sharp blows in succession over each lung field and note the resonant sound.	

(Continued)

PHYSICIAN BEHIND PATIENT, Continued

	STEP	ACTION	NOTE
	4	Percuss the lateral aspects of the chest wall.	
	5	Place the stethoscope on the back and have the patient breathe deeply in and out through the mouth. Auscultate the apices, midlung and lower lung.	Breath sounds should increase in intensity as the patient inspires and rapidly decrease in intensity as he or she expires.
Spine and Flanks	6	Percuss the spine and flanks with the hypothenar area of your fist.	There should be little or no tenderness in these areas.

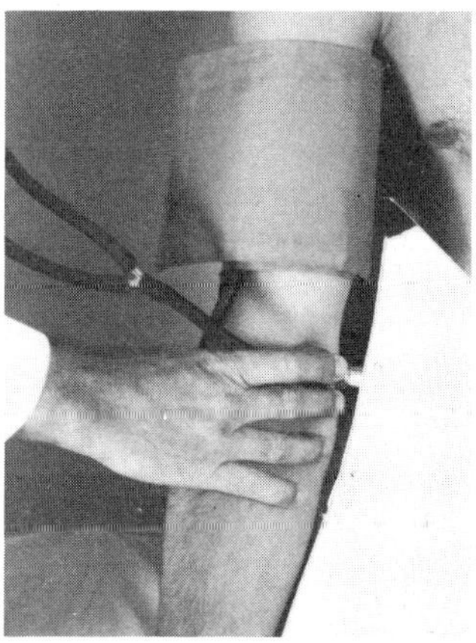

Fig. 9-5.

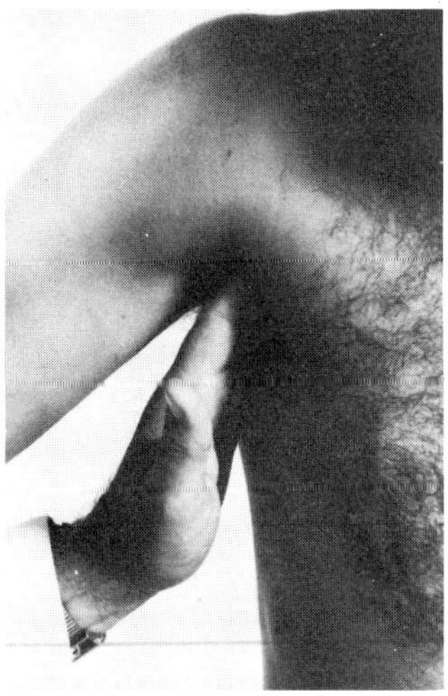

Fig. 9-7.

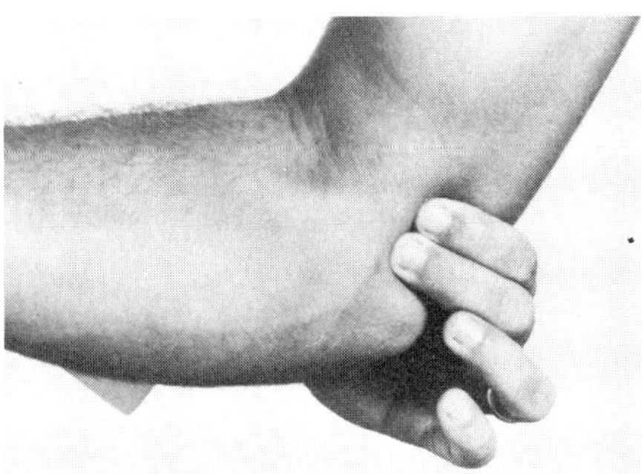

Fig. 9-6.

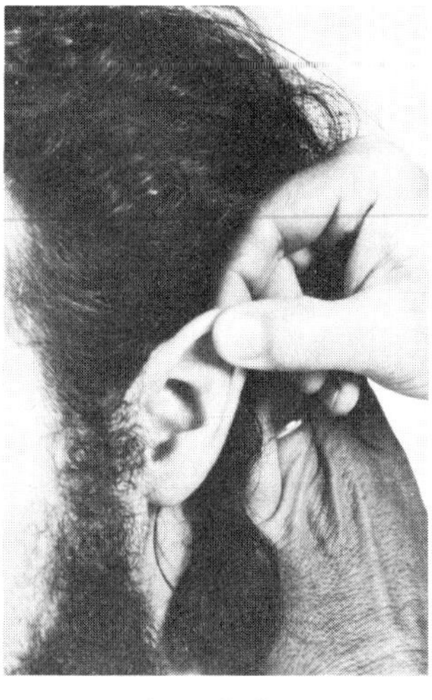

Fig. 9-8.

PATIENT SUPINE

Introduction

From the supine patient's right side, the physician examines:
- chest
- breasts
- heart
- lungs
- abdomen
- legs

in sequence

Procedure

	STEP	ACTION	NOTE
Chest	1	Inspect the skin of the chest.	
Breasts	2	Have the female patient remove the towel for the breast examination: a. starting at the upper-outer quadrant, begin palpating the four quadrants of the breast. b. Palpate the axillary tail of the breast and the nipple. c. Try to express fluid from the nipples.	a.,b. palpate lightly at first, then deeper if any breast substance is encountered. The variation of the consistency of normal breast tissue depends on: • age • obesity • menstrual cycle • pregnancy Normally, there will be a cobblestone feel to the breasts, but no masses larger than 5 mm should be palpable. c. There should be no secretions unless the woman is pregnant or in the immediate postpartum period. Occasionally, breast secretions are noted in pubescent males and females.
Heart	3	Examine the heart: a. Inspect the neck veins.	a. Normally the veins may be visibly full of blood in the supine position. There may also be minimal pulsation with the cardiac cycle.

(Continued)

PATIENT SUPINE, Continued

	STEP	ACTION	NOTE
		b. Place your right hand lightly over the precordium, and, with the middle and ring fingers, palpate for the apical impulse. c. Auscultate in the suprasternal notch. d. Beginning at the apex or mitral area, auscultate the heart in the 5 major positions using the diaphragm. e. Move the stethoscope over the tricuspid area; then to the left sternal border in the 3rd or 4th intercostal space. f. Auscultate the aortic area.	b. Normally, the apical impulse is localized to a 2cm. area in the fifth intercostal space of the midclavicular line. c. You may also hear normal systolic and diastolic heart sounds, but no sounds in between. d. At the apex the first heart sound is definitely louder. e. At the pulmonic area, the second heart sound is definitely louder. f. The second heart sound also tends to be louder in this area also.
	4	Auscultate the apex again, this time with the bell.	You may hear low-frequency sounds not audible with the diaphragm.
Lungs	5	Have the patient breathe deeper and faster than normal through the mouth as you auscultate the lungs laterally and anteriorly	Notice the character of the breath sounds.
	6	Have the female patient drape her breasts.	

(Continued)

PATIENT SUPINE, Continued

	STEP	ACTION	NOTE
Abdomen	7	Examine the abdomen: a. Inspect for: • bulges • masses • skin lesions	
		b. Auscultate for bruits and bowel sounds in the epigastrium.	b. Bruits arising from the aorta or a stenosed branch may be audible. Normal peristalic activity produces gurgling sounds heard every 5 to 10 seconds.
		c. Palpate superficially; then, go back and palpate deeper for organs and other masses. d. As the patient inspires, palpate for the liver in the right upper quadrant. e. When the patient takes another deep breath, palpate for the spleen in the upper left quadrant.	
		f. Percuss over the liver and spleen areas in the upper right and left quadrants.	f. This latter movement will confirm whether the liver and spleen are enlarged; the normal tympanic sound will be obscured by the solid tissue. Percussion in the flanks elicits evidence of ascitic fluid.
		g. Palpate the femoral pulses and the inguinal and femoral areas for lymph nodes. See Figures 9-9 and 9-10.	g. Nodes one centimeter in diameter are often palpable in healthy person.
	8	Allow the patient to cover his or her abdomen.	

(Continued)

PATIENT SUPINE, Continued

	STEP	ACTION	NOTE
Legs	9	Examine the legs.	
		a. Inspect the skin and palpate the muscles and joints.	a. There should be no tenderness, swelling, or fluid present.
		b. Check for edema by trying to indent the skin over the tibia and ankles.	b. Normally the skin cannot be indented.
		c. Palpate the dorsalis pedis pulse.	c. It should have a quick, sharp beat.
		d. Try to elicit the plantar reflex by drawing a blunted point along the lateral border of the foot, from the heel to the little toe. The stimulation should cause plantar flexion of all toes.	d. Coldness of the feet can prevent a response, so repeat the stimulation.

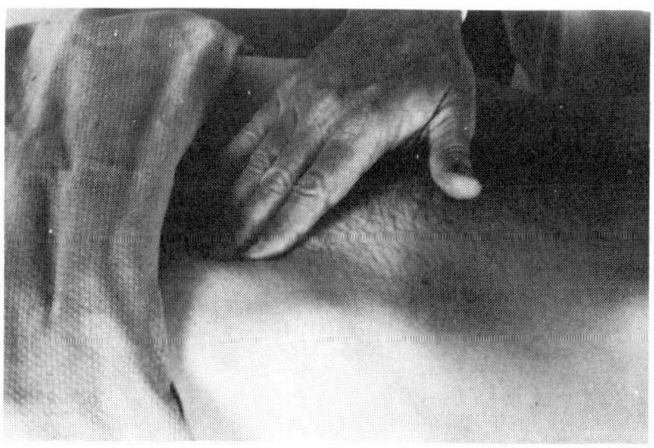

Fig. 9-9.

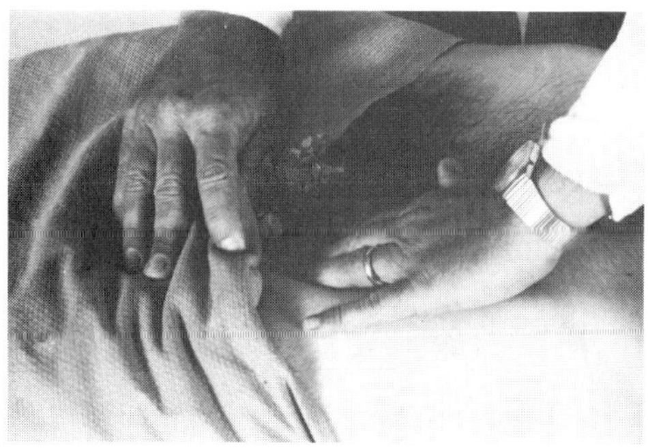

Fig. 9-10.

PATIENT SEATED ON EDGE OF TABLE

Procedure	STEP	ACTION	NOTE
Neuro-logic	1	Test the biceps and triceps reflexes: a. With the patient's arm flexed at a 90° angle, palpate the biceps tendon with your left thumb. b. Strike your thumb with the rubber hammer. See Figure 9-11. c. Strike the triceps aponeurosis with your hammer. See Figure 9-12. d. Check the biceps and triceps jerks in both arms, twice.	c. You should observe a contraction dependent on the reflex arc. The sudden muscle contraction should rapidly return to normal. d. The contractions should be symmetrical.
	2	Test the knee jerk by striking the tendon twice with the hammer. Note the leg's reflex. See Figure 9-13.	
	3	Check the ankle jerk: a. Gently dorsiflex the ankle while the knee is held in slight flexion. b. Observe the reflex of the foot. See Figure 9-14.	b. The ankle jerk should be the same in both feet.

Genitalia and Rectum	Usually, at this point you would examine the genitalia and the rectum, with the male patient standing and the female patient in the lithotomy position. However, these will be discussed later.
After the Examination is Completed	After the physical examination is completed, instruct the patient to dress and join you for further consultation in your office.
Example	The written example of a complete history and physical examination that is Appendix I in this chapter is of a fictitious patient.

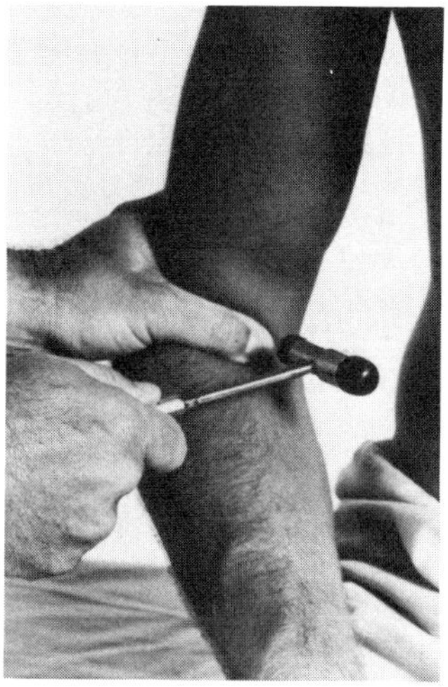

Fig. 9-11.

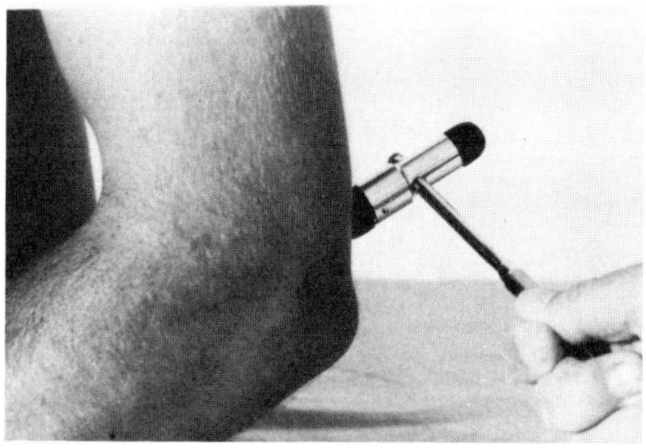

Fig. 9-12.

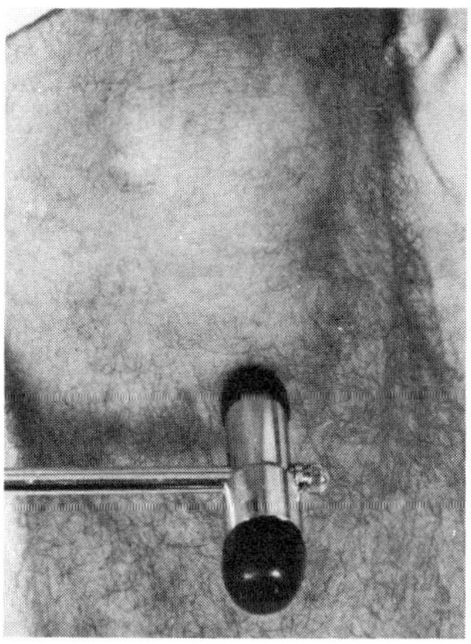

Fig. 9-13.

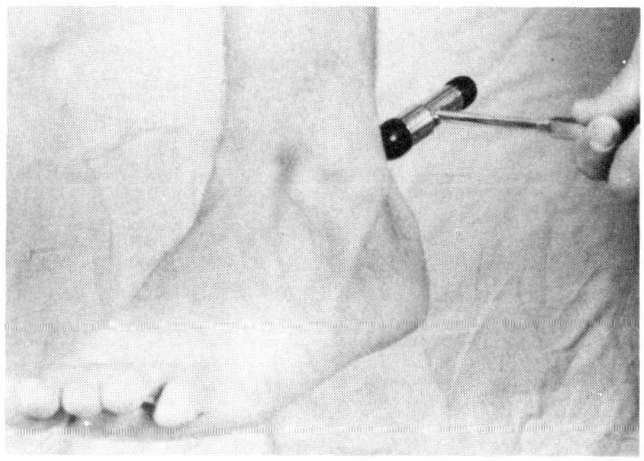

Fig. 9-14.

SELF-ASSESSMENT

Multiple Choice

ITEM	ANSWER	FOR THIS SENTENCE:	SELECT THE CORRECT CONCLUSION
1.	______	When using the oto-scope you should:	a. draw the auricle out and upward b. draw the auricle upward and backward c. draw the auricle upward and forward d. draw the auricle backward and downward
2.	______	In initially auscul-tating the five heart positions you should:	a. tap gently with the reflex hammer b. tap gently with two fingers c. use the stethoscope bell d. use the stethoscope diaphragm
3.	______	Visual acuity is	a. measured with the ophthalmoscope b. measured with the visual screener c. determined by the artery: vein ratio d. normally 20/200
4.	______	In taking the blood pressure the stetho-scope is:	a. over the radial artery b. over the brachial artery c. above the cuff d. under the cuff
5.	______	The gag reflex:	a. is tested by touching the pharyngeal wall with a tongue blade b. is normally absent c. requires intact cranial nerves VII and IX d. is elicited by having the patient say "ah"
6.	______	When using the sphyg-momanometer you should:	a. have the cuff loosely around the upper arm b. loosen the cuff if the diastolic pressure is less than 80 mm Hg c. pump up the pressure to 200 mm Hg d. pump up the pressure gradually to 400 mm Hg
7.	______	The reflex hammer can be used:	a. to check the plantar reflex b. to check the muscle contraction c. to check the knee jerk d. all of the above

(Continued)

SELF-ASSESSMENT, Continued

Matching — For each part of the examination, enter the letter of the normal finding

ITEM	PART OF EXAMINATION	NORMAL FINDING
1	upward field of gaze	______
2	lymph nodes	______
3	palms	______
4	optic disc	______
5	breast	______
6	radial pulse	______
7	aortic area	______
8	tendon reflex	______
9	skull	______
10	movement of arms and legs	______
11	turbinates	______
12	posterior pharyngeal wall	______
13	epigastrum	______

Findings:

a. a sudden variable degree of muscle contraction, rapidly returning to normal
b. All three should be pinkish and unclogged.
c. first heart sound tends to be louder
d. red, with small nodules
e. should be moist and smooth
f. toes flex downward
g. at least 1 cm. in diameter
h. septum should be complete and intact
i. second heart sound tends to be louder
j. cobblestone texture
k. less than 1 cm. in diameter and firm
l. wrinkling of the forehead
m. 50 to 100 beats per minute
n. no defects in bones
o. yellow, with clearly demarcated margins
p. Bruits may be audible.
q. move in association with each other

(Continued)

SELF-ASSESSMENT, Continued

Sequencing	Arrange the following examination steps in the correct sequence on the form.

	STEP
percuss liver and spleen	1
test hearing	2
palpate breast	3
check triceps jerk	4
take radial pulse	5
check for edema	6
auscultate aortic area	7
percuss lung fields	8
inspect scalp	9
palpate carotid pulses	10
inspect mouth	11
inspect conjunctivae	12
auscultate epigastrium	13
inspect turbinates	14
inspect eardrum	15
test ankle jerk	16
palpate precordium	17
percuss spine and flanks	18
take dorsalis pedis pulse	19
inspect nails	20
palpate thyroid	21
auscultate lungs	22

ANSWERS TO THE SELF-ASSESSMENT

Multiple Choice

1. b
2. d
3. b
4. b
5. a
6. c
7. d

Matching

1. l
2. k
3. e
4. o
5. j
6. m
7. i
8. a
9. n
10. q
11. b
12. d
13. p

Sequencing

1. inspect nails
2. take radial pulse
3. palpate carotid pulses
4. inspect scalp
5. inspect conjunctivae
6. inspect eardrum
7. test hearing
8. inspect turbinates
9. inspect mouth
10. palpate thyroid
11. percuss lung fields
12. auscultate lungs
13. percuss spine and flanks
14. palpate breast
15. palpate precordium
16. auscultate aortic area
17. auscultate epigastrium
18. percuss liver and spleen
19. check for edema
20. take dorsalis pedis pulse
21. check triceps jerk
22. test ankle jerk

Sample History and Physical Examination Form

Patient Name: Sarah J. Jones Unit History No. 123456-R

IDENTIFYING DATA:

Age 40 yrs Race W Marital Status M Sex F Occupation Housewife

Residence 1103 Moonbeam, Clute, Texas 77496

Referral Source Dr. J. B. Tone (Clute) Time and Date 10:00 a.m., 1-9-83

CHIEF COMPLAINT: Weakness in right arm - 5 to 6 years.

PRESENT ILLNESS (or PROBLEMS): Five to six years ago Mrs. Jones noted the onset of weakness in right arm and hand. This, in retrospect, is more incoordination than weakness. She could not use right arm and hand as well as left, e.g., coffee cups. She had mild numbness in right arm also. She saw several MDs and had spine x-rays, EEG, etc., but no diagnosis was made. Since then she has had very little problems with arm. She has continued to have these problems but does not believe they are more frequent or more severe.

She was told 8-9 years ago that she had high blood pressure. She was given meds, which she took for only a short while. Six years ago she saw another MD, who said she had hypertension, and she was given meds, which she took for a while. She has a family history of hypertension but denies paroxysms of weakness suggestive of adrenal disease or episodes of headache, flushing, or tachycardia.

For past several months she has noted feeling of faintness and blurred vision on 3-4 occasions lasting several to 30 minutes. These have occurred while walking and do not seem to be positional in nature. She sits for a while, and it passes. They are not associated with tinnitus, vertigo, nausea, sweating, hunger, or palpitations. She has no syncope.

For the last 8 or 9 months she has noted occasional inability to say what she wanted. In addition she has noted inability to follow directions; i.e., she knows what she was asked to do but cannot do it. She has noted that she substitutes inappropriate words.

For the past several months she has had frontal dull aching headache beginning in afternoon and relieved with ASA. She denies nausea, vomiting, or change with Valsalva. However, the onset of headache has been a distinct change.

PATIENT PROFILE: (Personal: education, occupation; appearance and behavior. Interpersonal: family; social; sexual. Stress responses.)

She is married to a full-time Army employee and is a housewife. She has a high school education but no college. She is oriented, speaks softly, and is neatly dressed. Her husband says she is self-conscious about talking because of fear that she may say something wrong. He has noted no inappropriate behavior, staring, or blank spells. She has 3 children (ages 21, 23, and 15) and one grandchild, age 1 year. She is obviously anxious over the impending diagnostic studies, which she has been dreading.

PAST MEDICAL HISTORY: (Indicate date, place and reasons for hospitalizations, significant illnesses, major injuries and operations. Indicate date/reason for last physician visit, health maintenance activities and immunization history. Specify use of tobacco, drugs and alcohol.)

In auto accident 6 years ago and had whiplash injury. This was last physician visit, and she was hospitalized 6 days. X-rays normal. This was 1½ years before problem with arm. Appendectomy at age 15. She does not remember last tetanus-diphtheria booster but has had primary series. She smokes 1½ packs of cigarettes per day and has done so for 23 years. She drinks only beer, usually 3 per night.

MEDICATIONS Past and Present: ASA for headache

Drug Reactions: None

FAMILY HISTORY: (Record age, illness, age/cause of death or current status.)

Father: 66 years, hypertension

Mother: 65 years, living and well

Brothers: one brother, age 45, living and well

Sisters:

Children: Three children living and well, ages 21, 23, and 15

Spouse:

FAMILIAL DISEASES: None

REVIEW OF SYSTEMS

Directions: Check positive or negative only those questions asked. Check nothing if question not asked. Use center area to comment specifically regarding positive symptoms and menstrual history.

	Neg		Pos	Comment
GEN	✓	Weight change		
	✓	Weakness		
	✓	Fatigue		
	✓	Fever or chills		
	✓	Night sweats		
	✓	Heat intolerance		
		Overall status	✓	As noted in neuro.
PSYCH	✓	Anxiety/Depression		
	✓	Mood		
	✓	Sleep disturbance		
	✓	Memory change		
	✓	Suicidal thoughts		
SKIN	✓	Skin change		
	✓	Pruritis		
	✓	Rash		
	✓	Hair change		
HEAD		Headache	✓	See present problems
EYES	✓	Vision change		
	✓	Glasses		
	✓	Diplopia		
		Blurring	✓	
	✓	Scotoma		
	✓	Eye pain		
	✓	Photophobia		
EARS	✓	Hearing loss		Cerumen removed 6 months ago
	✓	Tinnitus		
	✓	Vertigo		
	✓	Ear pain		
	✓	Ear discharge		
NOSE	✓	Epistaxis		
	✓	Nasal discharge		
	✓	Obstruction		
	✓	Sinusitis		
THROAT		Teeth/Dentures	✓	
	✓	Abnormal taste		
	✓	Sore mouth/Tongue		
	✓	Gums		
	✓	Sore throats		
		Speech difficulty	✓	See present problems
	✓	Hoarseness		
NECK	✓	Neck swelling		
	✓	Neck pain		
	✓	Stiff neck		
	✓	Goiter		
	✓	Masses/Nodes		
CR	✓	Cough		
		Dyspnea	✓	For past several years she has noticed dyspnea only on marked exertion, e.g., climbing a hill.
	✓	Wheezing		
	✓	Hemoptysis		
	✓	Chest pain		
	✓	Palpitation		
	✓	Orthopnea		
	✓	P.N.D.		
	✓	Murmur		
	✓	Edema		
	✓	Claudication		
	✓	Syncope		
		Hypertension	✓	8-9 years ago saw Dr. A. B. Simple for hypertension. She took meds for awhile, stopped drugs and again saw him 6 years ago.

	Neg		Pos	Comment
GI	✓	Anorexia		
	✓	Nausea/Vomiting		
	✓	Hematemesis		
	✓	Melena		
	✓	Dysphagia		
	✓	Heartburn		
	✓	Flatulence		
	✓	Abdominal Pain		
		Jaundice	✓	Hepatitis at age six
	✓	Change bowel habits		
	✓	Diarrhea		
	✓	Constipation		
	✓	Hematochezia		
	✓	Rectal pain		
♂♀		Age menarche		Regular menses, 25-30 x 5-6. Gravida 3, para. 3, living children 3.
		Menstrual cycle		
		L.M.P.		
		G./P./A.		
		Age menopause		
	✓	Dysmenorrhea		
	✓	Menorrhagia		
	✓	Metrorrhagia		
	✓	Dyspareunia		
	✓	Contraception		On no contraceptives
	✓	Pelvic pain		
	✓	Sexual dysfunction		
	✓	Discharge		
	✓	Venereal disease		
	✓	Sores		
	✓	Breast mass		
	✓	Breast pain		
	✓	Breast discharge		
URO	✓	Dysuria		
	✓	Frequency		
	✓	Nocturia		
	✓	Hematuria		
	✓	Urgency		
	✓	Incontinence		
	✓	Polyuria		
MS	✓	Backache		
	✓	Joint pain		
	✓	Stiffness		
BLOOD	✓	Lymphadenopathy		
	✓	Bleeding		
	✓	Bruising		
		Anemia	✓	Anemic in past, took iron tabs & anemia was correc.
NEURO	✓	Seizures		
		Paralysis	✓	Present problem
		Muscle weakness	✓	
	✓	Paresthesia		
	✓	Sensation change		
	✓	Tremor		
	✓	Gait		
		Incoordination	✓	
		Headache	✓	

Page 4

PHYSICAL EXAMINATION

Weight 116 pounds	Height 5'4"	Temp. 98.8	
Pulse 88	Rhythm S A		
Resp. 16	Rhythm N		
B.P. 1) Supine: RL 180/?	RA	LA	
2) Standing:	RA 188/112	LA 190/114	
General Appearance: Alert, cooperative, no distress			

MENTAL STATUS		
Affect:	(N)	Ab
Intellectual:	(N)	Ab
Sensorium	Memory	Problems
Abstract	Fund	Intelligence
Thought processes:	(N)	Ab
Judgement, reliability:	(N)	Ab
Insight:	(N)	Ab

Directions: Check normal (N) or abnormal (Ab) only for those areas actually examined. Use the blank area to comment specifically regarding abnormal findings. Draw schematic diagrams and complete charts when feasible. (*) Indicates optional examinations.

N		Ab	
	Appearance	✓	**SKIN** Dry, coarse, scaling skin. Has erythema and scaling in both external auditory canals, left greater than right. Localized area (5x5mm over left anterior superior iliac spine of scaling erythema and lichenification.
✓	Texture		
✓	Temperature		
✓	Moisture		
✓	Color		
✓	Nails		
✓	Hair		
✓	Skull		**HEAD** Seborrhea
	Scalp	✓	
✓	Vision		**EYES** O.D. 20/25 O.S. 20/20
✓	E.O.M.		
✓	Eyelids		
✓	Ocular Tension		O.D. 5 O.S. 6
✓	Conjunctivae		
✓	Cornea		
✓	Sclera		
✓	Lens		
✓	Pupils		
	Fundi	✓	Arteriolar narrowing (grade 2/4 hypertensive retinopathy). No papilledema
✓	Visual Fields		*
✓	Hearing		**EARS**
	Pinna	✓	
	Canals, Drums	✓	See skin
	Rinne, Weber		*
✓	Mucosa		**NOSE**
✓	Septum		
✓	Turbinates		
	Sinuses		*
✓	Lips		**MOUTH-THROAT**
✓	Breath		
✓	Teeth, Gums		
✓	Tongue		
✓	Mucosa		
✓	Tonsils		
✓	Pharynx		
✓	Palate		
	Salivary Glands		*
✓	Motion		**NECK**
✓	Shape		
✓	Trachea		
✓	Thyroid		
✓	Breasts		**BREASTS**
✓	Neck		**NODES**
✓	Supraclavicular		
✓	Axillary		
✓	Epitrochlear		
✓	Inguinal		
	Occipital		*

SCALE: 0 = Absent
↑ = Increased
N = Normal
↓ = Decreased

PULSE	R	L
Carotid	N	N
Radial	N	N
Femoral	N	N
Post.Tibial	N	N
D. Pedis	N	N
* Brachial	N	N
* Popliteal		

PHYSICAL EXAMINATION

N		Ab	
✓	Shape & Symmetry		CHEST
✓	Thoracic wall		
✓	Motion		
✓	Respirations		LUNGS
✓	Resonance		
✓	Breath sounds		
✓	Friction rub		
✓	Rales		
✓	Fremitus		•
	Diaphragm		•
	Voice sounds		•
✓	Pulse character		VASCULAR
✓	Neck veins		
✓	Peripheral veins		
	Inspection	✓	HEART
	Apex impulse	✓	Prominent PMI. No cardiomegaly
✓	Palpation		
✓	Rate, Rhythm		
✓	S_1		
✓	S_2		
✓	Systolic sounds		
✓	Diastolic sounds		
	Percussion		•
	Scars	✓	ABDOMEN
✓	Inspection		
✓	Palpation		
✓	Liver		
✓	Spleen		
✓	Kidney		
✓	Auscultation		
✓	Flanks		
✓	Anus		
✓	Rectum		
	Stool Guaiac		
	Prostate		
	Penis		GENITALIA
	Scrotum		
	Testes		
	Epididymis		
✓	Inguinal canal		
✓	External genitalia		
✓	Vagina		
✓	Cervix		
✓	Uterus		
✓	Adnexa		
✓	Rectovaginal		
✓	Spine		MUSCULO SKELETAL
✓	Back		
✓	Muscles		
✓	Joints		
✓	Extremities		
✓	Cranial nerves		NEUROLOGICAL
	Motor	✓	Receptive aphasia
✓	Gait		
	Coordination	✓	• See special exam
✓	Sensory		•
	Posture		
	Speech		

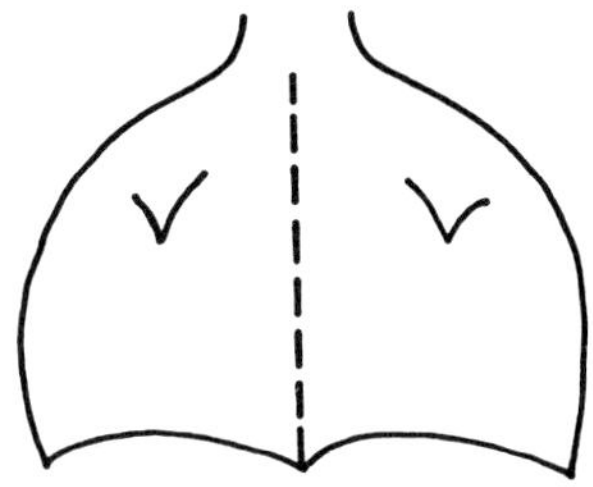

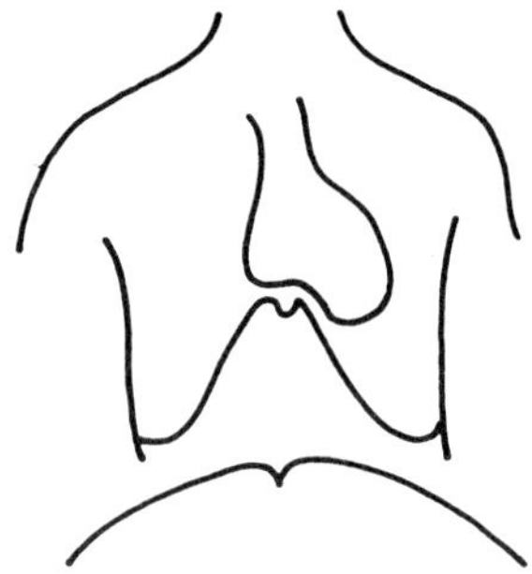

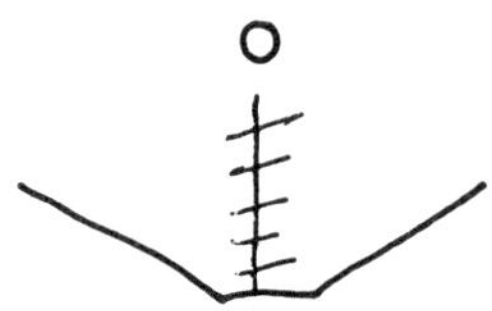

REFLEX	R	L
Biceps	↑	N
Triceps	↑	N
Knee	N	N
Ankle	N	N
Plantar	N	N
• Brachioradialis		
• Abdominal		
• Other path reflex		

SCALE: 0 = Absent
↑ = Increased (or up)
N = Normal
↓ = Decreased (or down)

Page 6

SPECIAL EXAMINATIONS: This space is to be used for special or more detailed examinations. Specify the organ system and/or type of examination. If none is required, check here ______.

Neurological Exam: Poor finger to nose, right arm. Mild adiadokokinesis, right arm.
Motor strength slightly decreased, right arm.
History of expressive aphasia (not definitely demonstrated)
Rerceptive aphasia, mild
Normal stereognosis
Poor 2 point discrimination, right arm
Normal position, vibrating and pain sense
No tremor
Bilateral unsustained clonus in ankles and knees, right greater than left
Hyperreflexia, right arm
Positive Hoffman on right
Normal visual fields by confrontation

LAB DATA BASE:

CBC Hg 13.5 Hct 39 WBC 13.4 N 62 S 1 J 0 My 0 L 21 M 13 E 2 B 1 Other______

Urinalysis normal RPR neg

Chest X-ray pending EKG (over 45 years) normal

SMA 12/60 pending Ca____ P____ Chol____ Gluc____ Bun____ Uric A____ Creat____ Bilirubin____ Alk Phos____ LDH____
SGOT____ SGPT____ PPD Interm (mm induration)

PROBLEM LIST WITH ASSESSMENT AND PLAN

#1. Intracranial lesion. A: The history and physical signs mean left cerebral involvement. This is not due to hypertension, but it could explain the headache. She very likely has a brain tumor or other expanding intracranial mass. I doubt cerebrovascular occlusive disease.

Plan: CT brain scan; No L.P.

#2. Dizziness: A: This may be due to #1 or hypertension

Plan: See #1 and #3

#3 Hypertension. A: She has significant hypertension. Will evaluate kidneys and adrenal cortex and medulla for etiologic factors

Plan: Urinary VMA, serum electrolytes

#4 Headaches. A: Could be #1 or #3

Plan: See #1 or #3

#5 Seborrheic dermatitis

Plan: Steroid ear drops and antiseborrheic shampoo

#6 Skin lesion, left iliac spine. A: This is either atopic dermatitis or tinea corporis.

Plan: Consult dermatologist

#7 Hyperglycemia. A: Must rule out diabetes and pheochromocytoma.

Plan: Await SMA-12

PROBLEM LIST WITH ASSESSMENT AND PLAN
(continued)

#8 Leukocytosis. A: No definable cause.

Plan: Will evaluate other problems that are a greater priority.

Student

Intern

Resident

Faculty

SIGNATURES

APPENDIX TWO

General Physical Examination Checklist

Examiner__________________ Date______ Name of Student____________________

		Completed
I.	**Introduction - in Office**	
1.	Observe patient's ability to rise from chair.	o
2.	Observe patient's gait.	o
II.	**Seated Facing Physician**	
A.	**HANDS, ARMS**	
1.	Determine the blood pressure in arm.	o
2.	Inspect the nails and skin.	o
3.	Inspect and palpate the palms.	o
4.	Determine the range of motion of the joints of the hand.	o
5.	Palpate the musculature of the arm.	o
6.	Determine the radial pulse (15 sec. x 4).	o
7.	Determine respiratory rate.	o
8.	Determine the range of motion of the joints of the arm.	o
9.	Palpate the epitrochlear lymph nodes.	o
10.	Palpate the axillary lymph nodes.	o
B.	**NECK**	
1.	Palpate the lymph nodes in the:	
	a. anterior triangles	o
	b. supraclavicular areas	o
	c. carotid areas	o
	d. submandibular areas	o
	e. posterior cervical area	o
2.	Palpate the carotid pulses.	o
3.	Note the position of the trachea and the size of the thyroid.	o
C.	**HEAD**	
1.	Examine the scalp, the hair, and the bone configuration of the skull.	o
2.	Observe the facial skin and musculature for symmetry of movement (CN VII).	o

	Completed
D. EYES	
1. Test for visual acuity with the pocket visual screener.	o
2. Inspect the eyelids, sclera, and conjunctiva with a penlight.	o
3. Determine extraocular movements in the six cardinal directions of gaze (CN III, IV, VI). Note wrinkling of the forehead with the patient's eyes in upward gaze (CN VII).	o
4. Examine the direct and consensual pupillary reflexes to light in both eyes.	o
5. Examine the retina with the ophthalmoscope.	o
E. EARS	
1. Inspect the pinnae.	o
2. Inspect the external auditory canal and tympanic membrane with the otoscope.	o
3. Check hearing with a wristwatch, whispering, or a tuning fork (CN VIII).	o
F. NOSE	
1. Use a penlight to inspect the septum and turbinates.	o
G. MOUTH	
1. Inspect:	
a. all mucous membranes	o
b. the salivary ducts	o
c. the tonsils	o
d. the teeth	o
e. the gums	o
f. the pharynx	o
2. Test for symmetry of movement of the soft palate and uvula with phonation (CN IX, X).	o
3. Look for deviation on tongue protusion (CN XII)	o

III. Physician Behind Patient

A. NECK	
1. Palpate the thyroid.	o
B. POSTERIOR CHEST	
1. Inspect the skin.	o
2. Examine the symmetry of chest wall movements with breathing.	o
3. Examine for deviations of abnormalities of the spine.	o
4. Finger-percuss the upper, middle, and lower lung fields.	o
5. Auscultate the apices and middle and lower lung fields.	o
6. Percuss the spine and flanks with the fist.	o

IV. Patient Supine, Physician at Right Side

A. BREASTS	
1. Inspect the skin.	o
2. Palpate the four quadrants both superficially and deeply.	o
3. Palpate the axillary tail of the breast.	o
4. Palpate the nipple.	o

	Completed
B. HEART	
1. Inspect the neck veins.	o
2. Inspect and palpate the precordium and the apical impulse.	o
3. Auscultate the suprasternal notch.	o
4. Auscultate the heart:	
a. apex (mitral)	o
b. tricuspid area	o
c. left sternal border	o
d. pulmonic area	o
e. aortic area	o
5. Auscultate the apex with the bell of the stethoscope.	o
C. LUNGS	
1. Auscultate upper, middle, and lower lung fields.	o
D. ABDOMEN	
1. Inspect for bulges, masses, and skin lesions.	o
2. Auscultate over the epigastrium for bowel sounds and bruits.	o
3. Palpate gently.	o
4. Palpate deeply.	o
5. On inspriation, palpate superficially then deeply for the:	
a. liver	o
b. spleen	o
6. Finger-percuss over the liver and spleen.	o
7. Finger-percuss over the flanks.	o
8. Palpate the femoral pulses.	o
9. Palpate the inguinal area for lymph nodes.	o
E. LEGS	
1. Inspect the skin and hair.	o
2. Palpate the musculature of both legs.	o
3. Determine the range of mobility of the joints of the leg.	o
4. Examine the lower legs for edema.	o
5. Palpate the dorsalis pedis pulse.	o
6. Check the plantar flexion reflex.	o
V. Patient Seated on Edge of Table	
A. NEUROLOGIC EXAMINATION	
1. On both sides test the:	
a. biceps reflex. Compare.	o
b. triceps reflex. Compare.	o
c. knee jerk. Compare.	o
d. ankle jerk. Compare.	o
VI. Genitalia and Rectal Examination	
A. GENITALIA, MALE-- STANDING	
1. Penis	
a. Inspect:	
1. skin	o
2. prepuce	o
3. glans	o
4. urethral meatus	o

Completed

- b. Palpate:
  - 1. shaft o
- 2. Scrotum
  - a. Inspect:
    - 1. skin o
    - 2. contour and size o
  - b. Palpate:
    - 1. testes o
    - 2. epididymis o
    - 3. spermatic cord o
- 3. Examine for inguinal hernia.
  - a. Inspect for inguinal area. o
  - b. Palpate the external inguinal ring. o

A. GENITALIA, MALE-- STANDING, BENT AT WAIST, CHEST ON TABLE

- 4. Rectum
  - a. Inspect the anus. o
  - b. Determine sphincter tone. o
  - c. Palpate the rectal vault. o
  - d. Palpate the prostate. o

B. GENITALIA, FEMALE-- DORSAL LITHOTOMY

- 1. Inspect and palpate the external genitalia. o
  - a. perineum, labia majora, and minora o
  - b. clitoris o
  - c. urethral orifice o
  - d. introitus o
  - e. Bartholin's gland o
- 2. Examine the vagina and cervix with a speculum. o
- 3. Examine the vagina and cervix digitally. o
- 4. Examine the uterus and adnexa bimanually. o
- 5. Examine with the two-finger vaginorectal method. o

APPENDIX THREE

Examination of the Bedridden Patient

Introduction

Some patients will be unable to move about as required in the general physical examination.

EXAMPLES:

- patients who are unconscious or deranged (delirious) and are unable to cooperate
- patients who are unable to sit
- patients who are restrained because movement could be harmful owing to:
  - fractures
  - detached retinas
  - spinal injuries
  - recent operations

In these and other instances you must modify the procedures necessary to complete the examination. This appendix will describe the modifications necessary for examination of a bedridden patient (supine position).

Examination Procedure

The examination of patients with an altered state of consciousness should consist in checking:

- blood pressure
- rate and character of pulse
- rate and regularity of respiration
- temperature
- mental status

If patients' conscious states are altered, then describe their:

- response to commands
- response to painful stimuli

Motor Strength

Though gait cannot be tested, an assessment of motor strength can be done. Ask the patient to use various muscle groups against your resistance:

- biceps
- triceps
- wrist flexors and extensors
- quadriceps
- hamstrings
- dorsiflexors
- plantar flexors of the feet

If the patient cannot cooperate, assess the spontaneous movement of the extremities and the movement elicited by response to pain such as pinprick, pressure on the sternum, or firm pressure on the nail beds.

(Continued)

EXAMINATION OF THE BEDRIDDEN PATIENT, Continued

Upper Extremities

Examination of the skin, hands, arms, and axillary nodes is done as described in the general physical examination. The neck is inspected and palpated from the anterior aspect. Note:

- masses
- lymph nodes
- thyroid enlargement
- carotid pulses
- the position of the trachea

If there is no spinal trauma, gently flex the neck and rotate the head to each side, observing for rigidity, pain, or spasm.

Examination of the Head

PART	PROCEDURE
head hair scalp	same as general physical examination Look for signs of trauma.
eyes	same as general physical examination patient cooperation required for: • visual acuity • extraocular movements • wrinkling of the forehead Note the size and symmetry of the pupils and their reaction to light.
cranial nerves III, IV, and VI	Test these nerves with the "doll's eye maneuver": turn the head passively from side to side. Normally the eyes should move as if fixed on an object. See Figure 9-15.
cranial nerve VII	Evaluate by symmetry of the face, forehead, lips, and nasolabial clefts.
ear nose mouth throat	same as general physical examination except that auditory acuity, phonation, and protrusion of the tongue may not be tested if the patient cannot cooperate
cranial nerves IX, X, and XII	Note the presence of the gag reflex (IX and X) and the position of the tongue (XII).

(Continued)

EXAMINATION OF THE BEDRIDDEN PATIENT, Continued

Chest and Back

To examine the chest and back, have an assistant roll the patient to either the right or left. Continue with the examination of the:

- skin
- chest
- lungs
- spine
- flanks

In addition, palpate the sacral area for pitting edema.

Torso

Roll the patient back to the supine position. Continue with examination of the:

- breasts
- skin
- heart
- neck veins
- lungs (anterior)
- abdomen
- legs

Tendon Reflexes

REFLEX TO TEST	PROCEDURE
arms	same as general physical examination
knees	Hold one posterior thigh so that the corresponding knee is flexed to 60°. Strike the patellar tendon. Repeat for the other knee. See Figure 9-16.
ankles	Put one thigh in a "frog leg" position with the knee flexed to 60°. Exert gentle pressure from the plantar surface upward. Strike the Achilles tendon. Repeat for other ankle. See Figure 9-17.

Remainder of Examination

Examination of the genitalia, rectum, and pelvis is done as in the general physical examination except that the examination of the genitalia and rectum is done with the patient in the supine position.

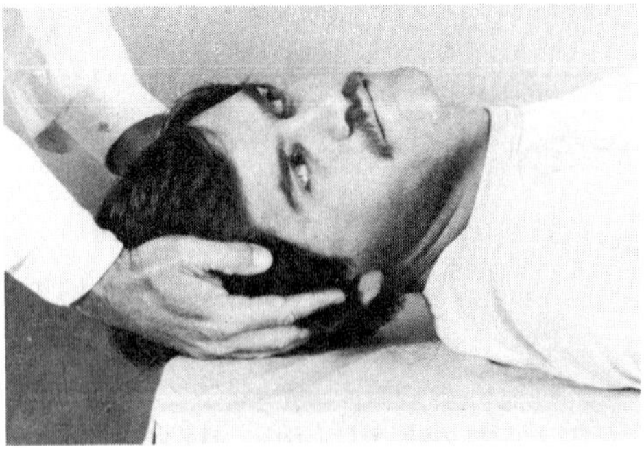

Fig. 9-15.

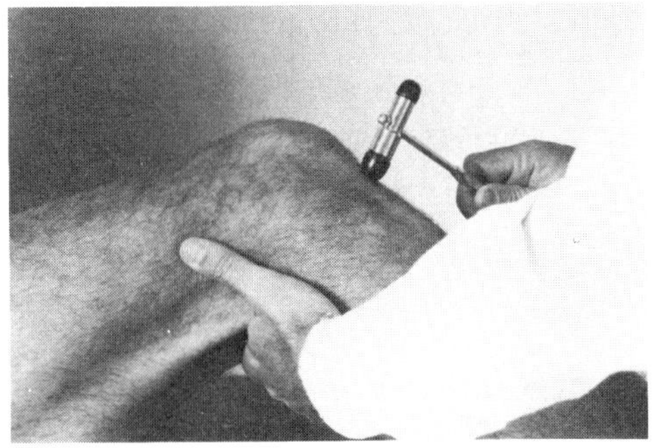

Fig. 9-16.

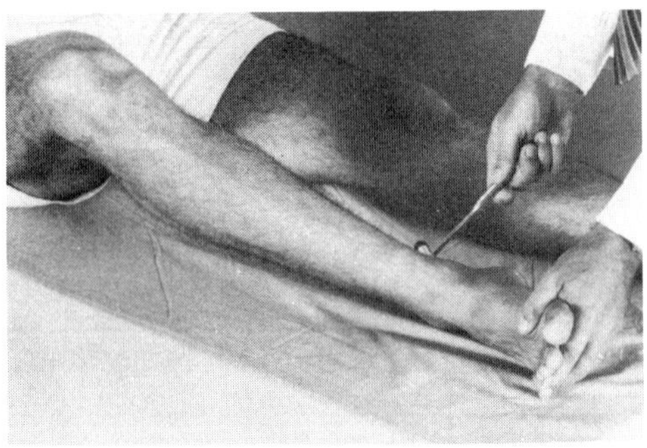

Fig. 9-17.

CHAPTER TEN

Vital Signs and Upper Extremities

James C. Guckian, M.D.

TEMPERATURE

Vital Signs	The vital signs include: • height • weight • temperature • blood pressure • pulse rate • respiratory rate
When Are They Recorded?	These data are recorded together at the top of each record. They are usually taken in advance by an attendant or nurse. Many physicians recheck the blood pressure; this is mandatory if the blood pressure recorded by a paramedical attendant is elevated. The pulse is taken as part of the examination.
How Taken	The temperature may be taken orally or rectally. Axillary temperature is so inaccurate that it will not be considered. The temperature may be recorded on the Fahrenheit (F) or Celsius (C) scale.
Oral Thermometers	The oral glass-mercury thermometer is left in place for several minutes to ensure accuracy, although when fever is present, the mercury column climbs quite rapidly (15 to 30 seconds) to within a few tenths of the final reading. The new digital-readout thermometers with disposable mouthpieces should be left in place until the reading is stable or until the instrument's signal is heard.
Falsely Low Levels	Falsely low levels may result from: • incomplete closure of the mouth • breathing through the mouth • leaving the thermometer in place for too short a time • recent ingestion of cold substances • tachypnea (respiratory rate more than 20/min) NOTE: Rectal temperature, rather than oral temperature, must be taken in these circumstances.
Falsely Elevated Levels	Falsely elevated levels may result from: • inadequate shaking down of the thermometer • previous ingestion of warm substances • recent strenuous activity • a warm bath • a recently smoked cigarette

(Continued)

TEMPERATURE, Continued

Rectal Temperature	Averages 0.5^{o} (C) to 1° (F) higher than oral.
Diurnal Temperature	In most persons there is a diurnal (daily) variation in body temperature of 0.5^{o} to 2°. The lowest ebb is reached during sleep, at which time the temperature may fall as low as 96.5^{o}F (36°C). As the patient becomes active, the temperature rises.
"Normal" is an Arbitrary Value	The normal temperature is 98.6^{o}F (37°C). This arbitrary value, however, applies to patients at bedrest. Normal people may have higher levels when active, or on a hot summer day; readings of 99.4^{o}F (37.5^{o}) are common. Higher values can be recorded in children following hard play.
Fever	If the oral temperature exceeds 99°F (37.5^{o}C) in a patient at bedrest, it is referred to as fever (hyperthermia).
Subnormal Temperature	Subnormal temperatures (hypothermia) are found in patients in coma due to drug intoxication, severe metabolic acidosis, exposure, and immersion in cold water.

PULSE

Introduction

Palpation of the pulse is part of every physical examination.

Absence or Impairment

The pulse is normally equal in the arms, but occasionally the radial artery has an anomalous course. Thus, one must check proximal (brachial and axillary) pulses and the ipsilateral ulnar pulse before concluding that the pulse is absent.

- Thrombosis involving one subclavian, axillary, or brachial artery may result in an absent radial pulse.
- A cervical rib or scalenus anticus syndrome may cause impariment of the pulse.

Palpation

The arterial pulse can be palpated at any point where the arteries lie near the surface and can be palpated against a firmer surface, usually bone. Thus, the pulse can be felt over the following arteries:

- radial
- brachial
- carotid
- femoral
- popliteal
- dorsalis pedis
- posterior tibial

Usually the radial artery is selected because of accessibility over the radial and volar aspects of the wrist.

Taking the Pulse at the Wrist

STAGE	DESCRIPTION
A	Patient's hand is held with the palm upward.
B	Physician places his first three fingers on the patient's radial artery, with the index finger nearest the patient's heart. See Figure 10-1.
C	The radial artery is compressed against the distal radius.
D	The pressure of the fingers flattens the artery during diastole, and the vessel pulsates as it fills with blood during ventricular systole. NOTE: When one is determining the rate, it is desirable to count the pulse for 15 seconds; if any irregularity is felt, it should be counted for 1 minute.

(Continued)

PULSE, Continued

Rate and Rhythm

In addition to noting the presence or absence of the pulse, it is important to note the rate and rhythm. The pulse rate varies with:

- age
- sex
- physical activity
- emotional status

SUBJECT	PULSE RATE
child	varies from 90 to 120 per minute
adult	varies from 60 to 100 per minute, being slightly higher in women than in men
well-conditioned athlete	A pulse rate of 50 per minute is not unusual.

NOTE: If the pulse is rapid during the initial examination, the patient should be rechecked later to ensure a more reliable reading.

Increased Rate

The rate is increased (greater than 100 per minute, tachycardia) in:

- anemias
- fever
- hemorrhage
- various cardiac arrhythmias
- hyperthyroidism

Decreased Rate

The pulse rate may be decreased (less than 60 per minute, bradycardia) by:

- increased intracranial pressure
- obstructive jaundice
- some types of syncope
- heart block
- ingestion of beta-adrenergic blocking drugs

RESPIRATORY RATE

Procedure	The examiner should observe, during quiet breathing at rest, the: • rhythm • rate • depth
Normal Rate	In the adult at rest the normal respiratory rate is about 12 to 18 per minute and is regular in depth and rhythm.
Increase With Fever	The respiratory rate increases with fever, usually about four additional respiratory cycles per minute for each 1°F above the normal temperature. Another way to say this is that the metabolic rate increases by 7% for each 1°F; the resultant increased metabolic demand causes the respiratory rate to increase.
Accessory Respiratory Muscles	Accessory respiratory muscles of the neck may participate in respiration in the patient whose breathing is labored as the result of either strenuous exercise or disease. Under ordinary circumstances there is no evident use of accessory respiratory muscles.

ARTERIAL BLOOD PRESSURE: BACKGROUND

Introduction	Blood pressure, pulse rate, and respiration rate are increased by physical exertion and emotional tension. Therefore, prior to their determination, the patient should be at rest and at ease. The tension produced by visiting a physicain may elevate pulse rate and blood pressure. Thus, if either is elevated at the outset of the physical examination, these determinations should be repeated after the patient has relaxed.
Normal Variation	"Normal" blood pressure varies and depends on: • age • physical conditioning • pulse rate • cardiac output The latter two, as noted earlier, increase with exertion and anxiety.
Instruments	Two types of manometers may be used: • mercury • aneroid

ARTERIAL BLOOD PRESSURE: PREPARATION

Patient Position	The patient may be seated, standing, or reclining during this examination.
Cuff Used on the Arm	• The blood pressure cuff should be deflated prior to its application on the arm. • The cuff is evenly and firmly wrapped about the arm, with the inflating tubes over the brachial artery along the medial arm. NOTE: Failure to apply the cuff properly may result in bulging and slipping, especially in patients with obese extremities. • The lower margin of the cuff should be 2 cm to 3 cm above the antecubital fossa.
Cuff Used on the Leg	The blood pressure can be determined in the leg by cuff: Place the cuff around the lower third of the thigh and the chest piece of the stethoscope over the popliteal artery in the popliteal fossa. NOTE: Generally a cuff larger than standard, ideally 20 cm wide, should be used. See Figure 10-2.
When Is a "Standing" Reading Essential?	If the patient has a history of bleeding, fainting, or hypertension, it is essential that the blood pressure be measured with the patient standing after being in a reclining position. NOTE: Normally there is a fall in cardiac output upon standing, resulting in a fall in systolic pressure of a few millimeters of mercury. With orthostatic hypotension, there may be a fall in systolic pressure of more than 10 mm Hg to 20 mm Hg when the patient stands.
When Is a Leg Reading Essential?	Blood pressure should always be taken in the legs: • when the femoral or popliteal pulses are either weak or absent • in any child or young adult with hypertension, in order to rule out coarctation (congenital narrowing) of the aorta NOTE: Normally there is a higher systolic pressure in the legs than in the arms, primarily because additional pressure in the cuff is needed to compress the larger muscle mass in the legs. In coarctation, systolic pressure in the arms is higher than systolic pressure in the legs because the brachial arteries originate above and the femoral arteries originate below the stenosed segment of the aorta.

ARTERIAL BLOOD PRESSURE: PROCEDURE

STAGE	PRESSURE	DESCRIPTION
A	palpatory systolic	The radial pulse is palpated, and the pressure in the cuff is rapidly increased to a level of about 30 mm Hg above the point at which the radial pulse disappears, or about 200 mm Hg. As the cuff is slowly deflated, a point is reached at which the pulse reappears. The pressure reading at this point is termed _palpatory systolic pressure_.
B	auscultatory	The bell or diaphragm of the stethoscope is placed in the medial aspect of the antecubital fossa over the brachial artery. _NOTE:_ To avoid producing extraneous sounds, it should _not_ touch the cuff or rubber tubing.
C	systolic	The cuff is gradually deflated, several millimeters at a time, until the first sound is heard. This point is referred to as the _systolic blood pressure._
D	diastolic	As the blood pressure cuff is further deflated, the sounds undergo changes in intensity and quality. As the cuff pressure approaches diastolic, the sounds suddenly become dull and muffled and then cease.

IF	THEN
there is complete cessation of sounds	this point is the best index of the _diastolic pressure_
there is _no_ complete cessation of sounds	the point of muffling is the best index of _diastolic pressure_

ARTERIAL BLOOD PRESSURE: PROCEDURE, Continued

IF	THEN
no clear demarcation of the muffling is heard	the diastolic pressure should be left indefinite and so indicated

Auscultatory Gaps

When determining the systolic pressure by the auscultatory method, the examiner may detect heart sounds at a high pressure, hear them disappear, and then hear them reappear at a lower pressure. This is the auscultatory gap.

EXAMPLE: The heart sounds are heard at 182 mm Hg, disappear at 160 mm Hg, and reappear at 124 mm Hg. If the the cuff is inflated only to 150 mm Hg, before deflating, the examiner will assume that 124 rather than 172 mm Hg is the systolic pressure. Thus, the cuff pressure should be inflated to about 200 mm Hg before deflating and auscultating.

ARTERIAL BLOOD PRESSURE: NORMAL FINDINGS

Normal Arm Reading	• Most physicians accept 140 mm Hg systolic and 90 mm diastolic as the upper limits of normal blood pressure. • In persons under 40 years of age the systolic pressure is usually 110 to 140 mm Hg, and the diastolic pressure is 60 to 90 mm Hg. • Obese arms often cause an erroneously high reading because the pressure applied to the cuff must overcome the resistance of the fat before compressing the brachial artery. NOTE: This erroneous reading may be corrected by using a cuff with a width that is half the circumference of the arm.
Normal Reading	The systolic and diastolic pressures in the leg are higher than in the arm, because of the larger muscle masses in the thighs that produce an increased resistance to compression of the artery. Again, wide cuffs should be used to obtain blood pressure in the legs.
Normal Reading in the Upper Extremities	Normally there is little or no significant difference in the blood pressure in the arms.
Normal Pulse Pressure	The pulse pressure is the difference between the systolic and diastolic pressures and normally ranges from 30 to 60 mm Hg. EXAMPLE: If the systolic blood pressure is 130 mm Hg and the diastolic pressure is 76 mm Hg, then the pulse pressure is 54 mm Hg.

ARTERIAL BLOOD PRESSURE: ABNORMAL FINDINGS

Low Blood Pressure

Some patients become alarmed by the presence of low blood pressure. Systolic pressure of 90 to 100 mm Hg, unless accompanied by symptoms and other abnormal signs, is of no clinical importance and requires no specific treatment. Some serious causes of low blood pressure (hypotension) include:

- adrenal insufficiency
- acute myocardial infarction
- hemorrhage
- dehydration

High Blood Pressure

Causes of high blood pressure (hypertension) include:

- chronic glomerulonephritis
- pheochromocytoma
- primary aldosteronism
- renal artery stenosis
- coarctation of the aorta

In most patients with hypertension no cause can be found (essential hypertension).

> NOTE: In some cases, as a result of an increase in cardiac output or of decreased compliance of large arteries, the systolic pressure is high, whereas the diastolic pressure is normal or even low. This is frequently the situation in:
> - anemia
> - hyperthyroidism
> - aortic regurgitation
> - arteriovenous fistula
> - arteriosclerosis

Abnormal Pulse Pressure

PULSE PRESSURE MAY BE INCREASED IN	MAY BE DECREASED IN
• atherosclerosis of the aorta and large arteries • hyperthyroidism • aortic valve regurgitation • arteriovenous fistula • physical exertion • fever • anemia	• aortic stenosis • heart failure • pericardial effusion and tamponade

Abnormal Readings in the Upper Extremities

Occasionally, there may be a significant discrepancy in the blood pressure in the arms.

EXAMPLES:

- aortic aneurysm
- obstruction of one innominate or subclavian artery

UPPER EXTREMITIES: BACKGROUND

Introduction

The arms must be completely exposed. Compare one arm with the other in order to detect:
- asymmetry
- unilateral abnormalities

Inspection

Inspect for:
- symmetry
- size and shape
- muscular development
- prominent vascular structures
- condition of skin, hair, and nails
- joint deformity
- congenital defects
- unusual movements
- condition of regional lymph glands

Palpation

Palpation should assess:
- texture and temperature of the skin
- tenderness
- crepitation (grinding sensation with movement) and mobility of joints.
- abnormalities of the lymph nodes
- pulses

Symmetry

Normally, the arms are nearly symmetric. In right-handed persons the muscles of right arm may be larger than those of the left; the opposite is true for left handed persons. Asymmetry, otherwise, may be due to:
- muscle atrophy
- congenital defects
- traumatic deformities

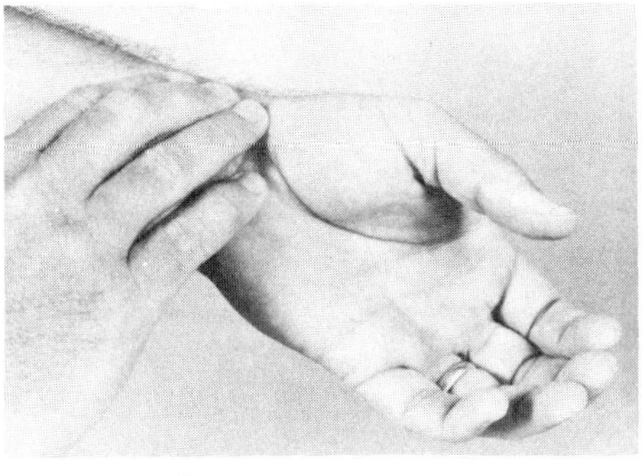

Figure 10-1.

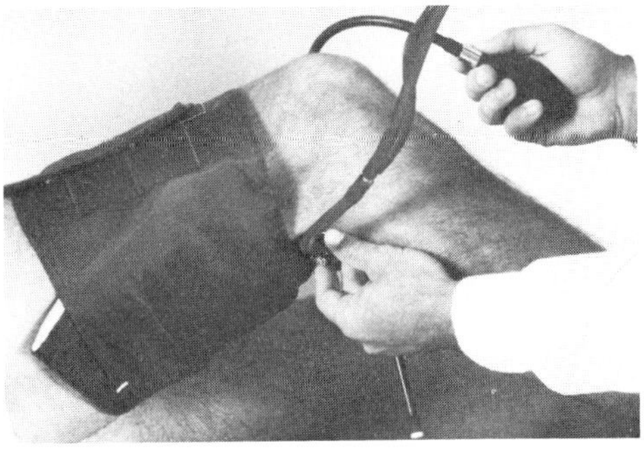

Figure 10-2.

UPPER EXTREMITIES: SIZE, SHAPE, FUNCTION

Abnormalities

A number of diseases alter the appearance of the hands and and arms.

DISEASE	DESCRIPTION
acromegaly	• Hands are large. • Fingers are broad. • Palms are wide. • Skull and mandible are large. See Figure 10-3.
myxedema	• Appearance of the hand is similar to that of acromegaly, as a result of enlargement of the soft tissues.
tetany (due to hypocalcemia or severe alkalosis)	• Wrist and metacarpophalangeal joint are flexed. • Phalangeal joints are extended. • Thumb is adducted into the palm. See Figure 10-4.
digital clubbing	• Tips of fingers are bulbous. • excessive curvature of the nails in all directions • loss of the normal angle at the nail-digit junction NOTE: Although clubbing may be congenital and unrelated to underlying disease, the presence of this finding should prompt a diligent search for pulmonary or heart disease. See Figure 10-5.

(Continued)

UPPER EXTREMITIES: SIZE, SHAPE, FUNCTION, Continued

DISEASE	DESCRIPTION
arthritis	• gnarled appearance of joints See Figure 10-6. • small nodules on the medial and lateral aspects of the distal interphalangeal joints (Heberden's nodes)
Dupuytren's contracture	• One or several fingers of either or both hands are permanently flexed into the palm because of fibrosis and shrinking of the palmar fascia. • The fourth and fifth fingers are most frequently involved. See Figure 10-7.
ganglions	• firm, somewhat cystic swellings that occur on the dorsum of the wrist, arising from the tendon sheaths
wristdrop	• caused by a weakness of the extensor muscles of the wrist and due to radial nerve paralysis • patient unable to extend wrist, hand hangs limp in a flexed position See Figure 10-8.
edema	• Edema, unilateral or bilateral, occurs less frequently in the arms than in the legs, mainly because the legs are usually most dependent.
obstruction of superior vena cava	• bilateral edema of arms and shoulders, face, and neck, and veins are dilated and engorged
unilateral edema	results from lymphatic or venous obstruction caused by: • thrombosis • tumors • lymphangitis or lymphadenitis NOTE: Lymphangitis is detected by the presence of tender, warm, red streaks that are the infected lymphatic channels.

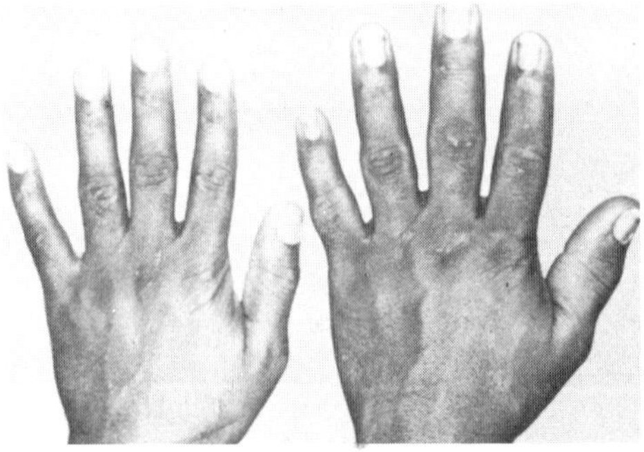

Figure 10-3. Normal hand (left) and a hand affected by acromegaly (right) in identical twins.

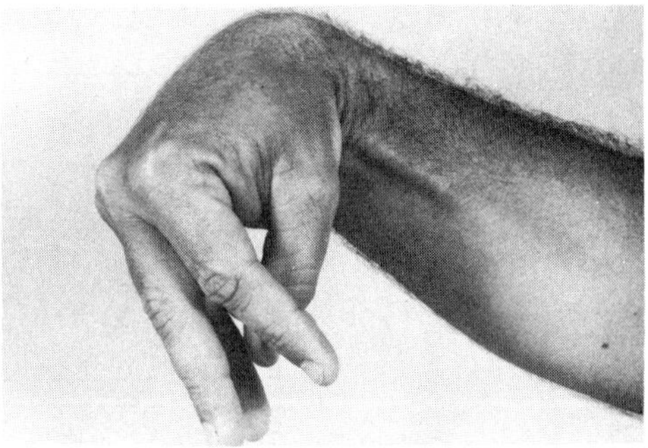

Figure 10-4.

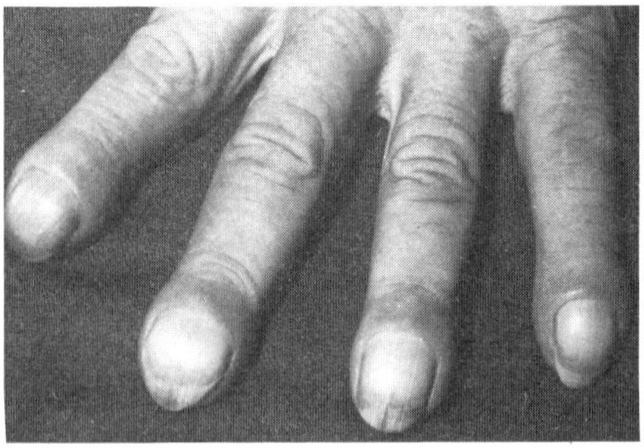

Figure 10-5.

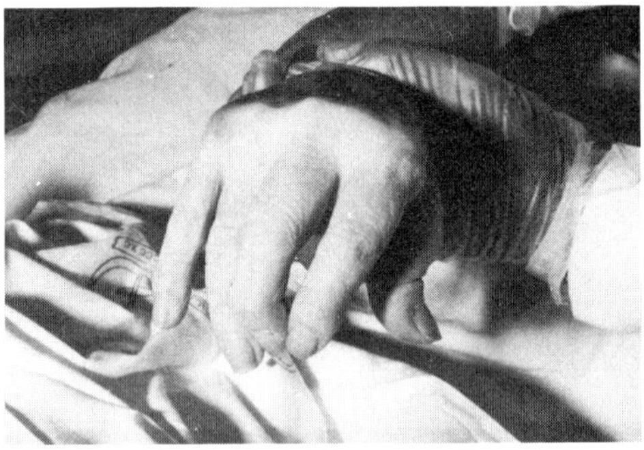

Figure 10-6.

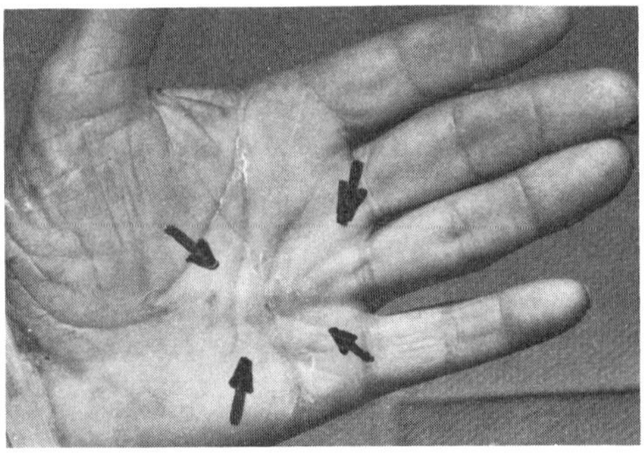

Figure 10-7.

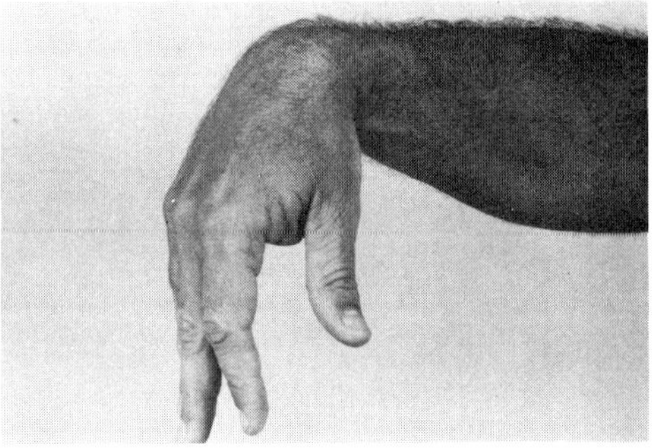

Figure 10-8.

UPPER EXTREMITIES: BLOOD VESSELS

Normal Signs

Veins on the hands and forearms may be distended when the the upper arms are dependent. These veins collapse when the arms are elevated.

Abnormalities

Abnormalities of the blood vessels are summarized below.

DISEASE	DESCRIPTION
thrombosis of deep major veins	• dilated superficial veins that do not collapse • edema • cyanosis
thrombophlebitis (rare in the arm)	• redness • tenderness • edema • increased heat • visible or palpable vein
arteriosclerosis	• visible and palpably tortuous artery
Raynaud's phenomenon	• vasomotor spasm of small arteries in the skin and subcutaneous tissues • fingers cold, pale, and numb • symptoms precipitated by exposure to cold
scleroderma	• frequently associated with Raynaud's phenomenon • Skin over the fingers becomes tight and glistening. • may progress to ulceration and gangrene of the digits

UPPER EXTREMITIES: SKIN AND NAILS

Skin

Skin of the arms should be palpated for temperature and texture. Local and systemic diseases may be manifest on the arms and hands.

CONDITION	DESCRIPTION
hyperthyroidism	• Palms are usually moist and warm. • Skin is smooth and silky.
anxiety	• Palms are moist but cooler than with hyperthyroidism.
myxedema	• Palms are dry. • Skin is coarse, thick, and dry.
chronic liver disease	• redness over the thenar and hypothenar eminences of the palm (palmer erythema or liver palms) See Figure 10-9.
xanthomatosis	• Palms may appear orange. • Nodules (xanthomas) may be present on the elbows and knees. See Figure 10-10.
dermato-phytosis	• scaling on the fingers and palms • red annular areas of scaling in the axillae
petechiae	• small reddish or purplish spots • do not fade or blanch with pressure See Figure 10-11.

(Continued)

UPPER EXTREMITIES: SKIN AND NAILS, Continued

Nails

The nails should be examined for:

- color
- shape
- texture

CONDITION	DESCRIPTION
anemia	• Nails are pale, as are the mucous membranes and conjunctivae.
cyanosis	• bluish tint • due to hypoxia
splinter hemorrhage	• small linear hemorrhages under the nails • occur in subacute bacterial endocarditis or may be due to trauma. See Figure 10-12.
paronychia	• suppurative draining infection involving the soft tissues about the nails. See Figure 10-13.

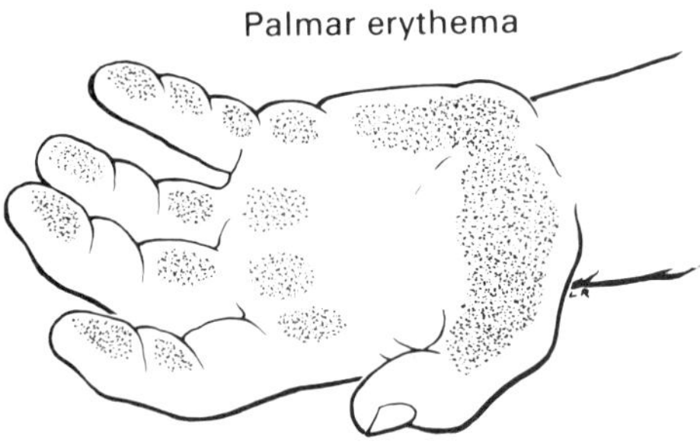

Figure 10-9.

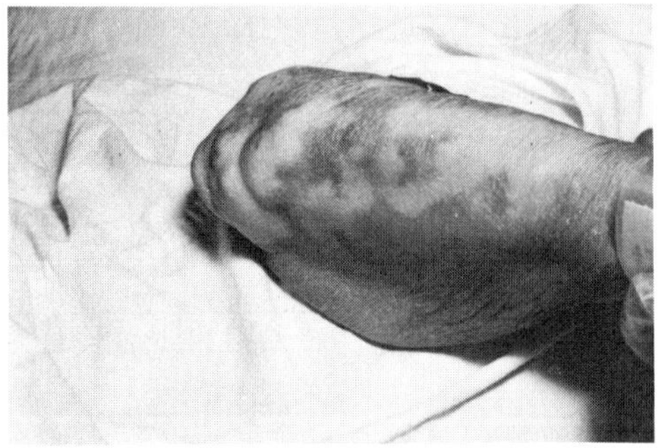

Figure 10-10.

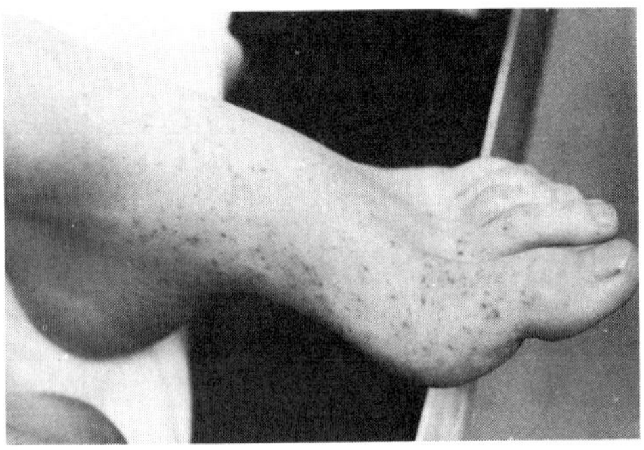

Figure 10-11.

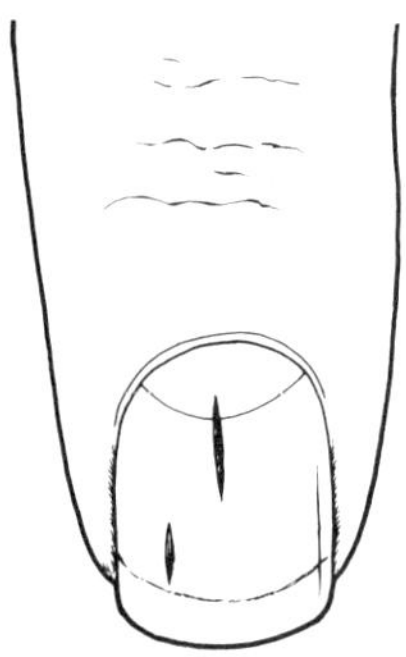

Figure 10-12.

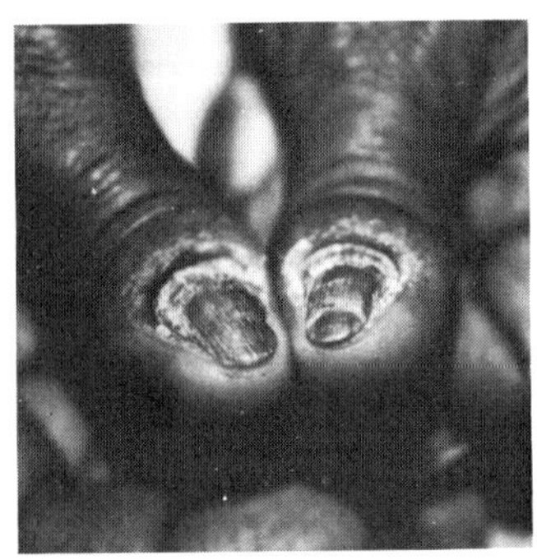

Figure 10-13.

UPPER EXTREMITIES: BONES AND JOINTS

Inspection for Arthritis

Any joint can be involved by arthritis. Joints should be compared for general appearance and symmetry, and should be examined for:

- range of movement
- swelling
- redness
- warmth
- tenderness
- crepitation

Types of Arthritic Involvement

Different types of arthritis tend to involve different joints.

CONDITION	DESCRIPTION
gout	• may involve any joint, but most frequently begins in the big toe • acute gouty arthritis is here termed podagra.
degenerative arthritis	• occurs most frequently in weight-bearing joints (spine, knees, hips) and the distal interphalangeal joints of the fingers NOTE: A common manifestation consists of bony nodules over the terminal interphalangeal joints (Heberden's nodes). See Figure 10-14.
rheumatoid arthritis, acute rheumatic fever and pyogenic arthritis	The involved joints are: • swollen • painful • tender • limited in movement • warm to the touch See Figure 10-15.

Other Signs

Fractures, dislocations, and tumors of the bones and joints may result in obvious deformities.

UPPER EXTREMITIES: UNUSUAL MOVEMENTS

Tremors

Tremors are uncontrollable rhythmic movements. They may be due to the following conditions.

CONDITION	DESCRIPTION
hyperthyroidism	• A fine tremor involving the hands (tongue and legs) NOTE: This can be demonstrated by placing a thin sheet of paper on the dorsal aspects of the extended fingers of the patient's extended hands.
parkinsonism	• A pill-rolling movement in which the thumb rolls over the palmar aspects of the index and second fingers NOTE: This condition is a rest tremor: when hands are relaxed, the tremor is present, but it disappears with voluntary movement.
cerebellar disease	• A shaking, alternating movement NOTE: The tremor may be undetectable with the hand and arm at rest. The tremor is exaggerated when the patient attempts to use the hand and arm in a directed manner.

UPPER EXTREMITIES: REGIONAL LYMPH NODES

Inspection and Palpation

Inspection and palpation of the epitrochlear and axillary lymph nodes is mandatory. If enlarged nodes are present, they should be described:

- location
- size
- consistency
- tenderness
- state of fixation
- whether they are discrete or matted

Description of Axilla

The axilla should be considered a pyramid consisting of an apex and four walls:

- anterior
- posterior
- lateral
- medial

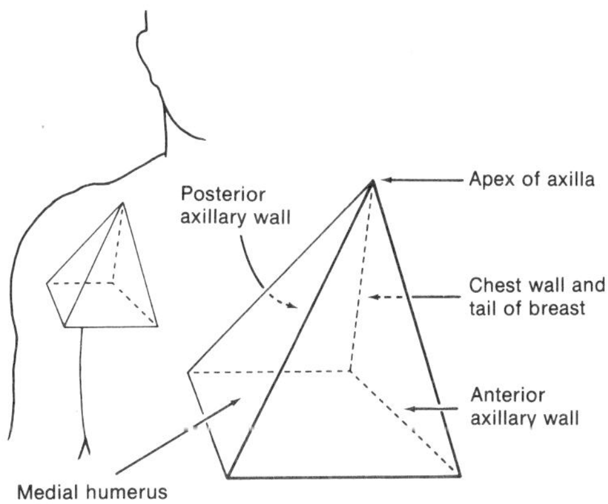

Importance of Axillary Examination

It is essential to inspect and palpate all dimensions of this anatomic pyramid. The axilla should be examined with the arm partially abducted in order to adequately palpate for the presence of enlarged lymph glands. See Figure 10-16.

Epitrochlear Lymph Node

The epitrochlear node is located above and behind the medial condyle of the humerus. This node may be enlarged in inflammation of the hand or forearm and in a number of systemic diseases. See Figure 10-17.

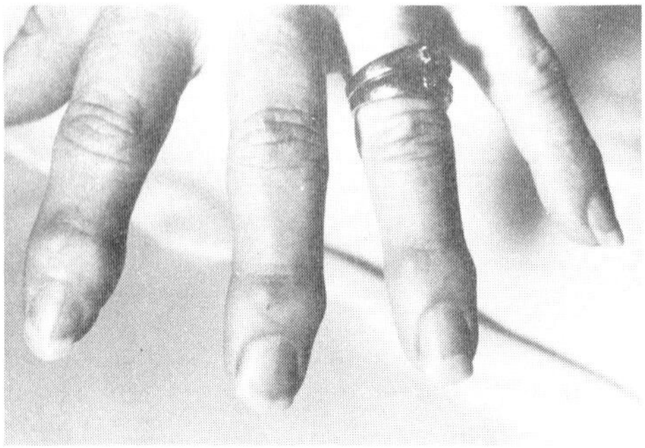

Figure 10-14.

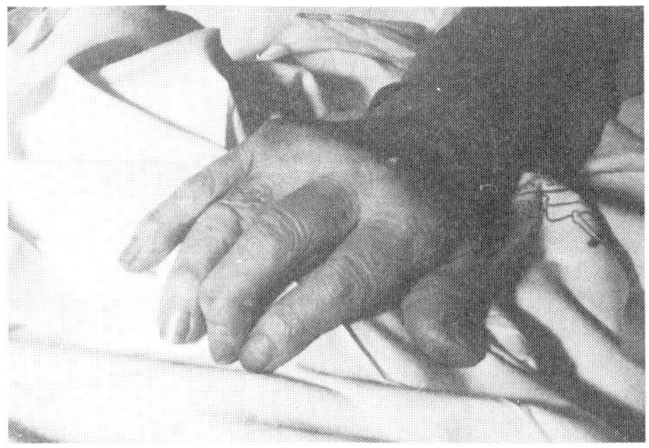

Figure 10-15.

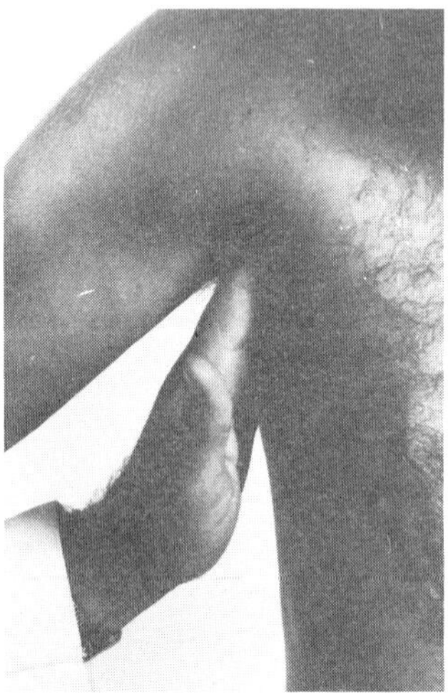

Figure 10-16.

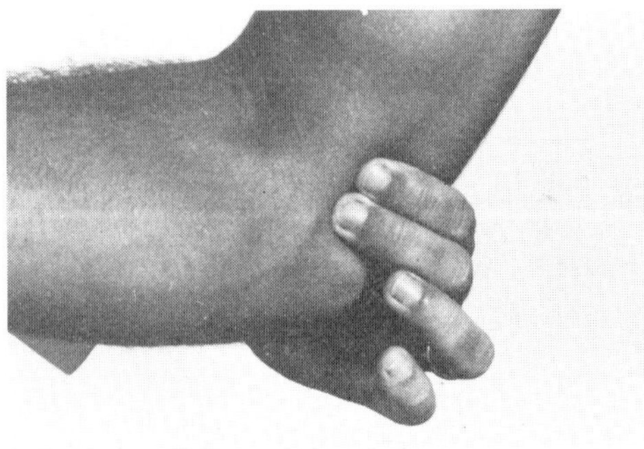

Figure 10-17.

SELF-ASSESSMENT

1. Name the vital signs and the normal range for each.
2. How long does it take for an oral thermometer to register (within a few tenths) the appropriate reading?
3. When does the ebb occur in the diurnal temperature variation?
4. Describe the auscultatory findings when taking the blood pressure. Which point represents the diastolic pressure?
5. What is the normal BP difference between arms? Between the arms and legs?
6. State the average BP change that occurs (in mm Hg) when a normal person assumes an erect position from a sitting or recumbent one.
7. What is the pulse pressure, i.e., how does one derive it?
8. Name five sources of error in taking a blood pressure.
9. Explain how to take a blood pressure.
10. What is coarctation of the aorta?
11. How does one detect orthostatic hypotension?
12. List the points that one must inspect in the upper extremities.
13. List the features that one must describe when a joint deformity is noted.
14. List the features that one must describe if an enlarged lymph node is encountered.

CHAPTER ELEVEN

Head, Eyes, Ears, Nose, Mouth, Throat, and Neck

John C. Barber, M.D., and Roger McNeil, M.D.

MOVEMENTS OF THE HEAD

Determining Range of Motion

Fixation of the head or limited range of motion can be determined by assessing:
- active motion, i.e., voluntary head movement
- passive movement, i.e., movement of the head (in all directions) by the examiner

---

Caution!

No force should be used in moving a patient's head, especially if the neck has been injured: neck injuries make the cervical spinal cord susceptible to permanent injury.

Anterior Motion

If a patient cannot flex the head anteriorly until the chin rests on the sternum, there may be:
- central nervous system disease, with irritation of the meninges (meningitis or encephalitis)
- inflammation of the muscles of the neck
- mechanical limitation of motion as in arthritis of the cervical spine (see Fig. 11-1)

Lateral and Posterior Motion

If the head cannot be rotated 90° to each side, or extend almost to 90°, arthritis of the spine or inflammation of the neck muscles may be present.

Functional Head Tilt

Ocular muscle palsy may cause the head to:
- tilt to one side
- tilt backward or forward
- turn to either side

to obtain a position where double vision is eliminated.

Torticollis

The head may also be tilted to the side if a shortening of the sternomastoid muscle has occurred. This condition, torticollis or wryneck, is usually a congenital defect, but may be caused by muscle inflammation. See Figure 11-2.

(Continued)

MOVEMENTS OF THE HEAD, Continued

Rhythmic Tremor	Many elderly people have a constant, rhythmic tremor of the head, which is caused by ischemic cerebral changes.
Bounding Head	Bounding (a slight up-and-down movement) of the head that follows the rhythm of the arterial pulse may be observed in patients with aortic regurgitation; the bounding is caused by the very wide pulse pressure.

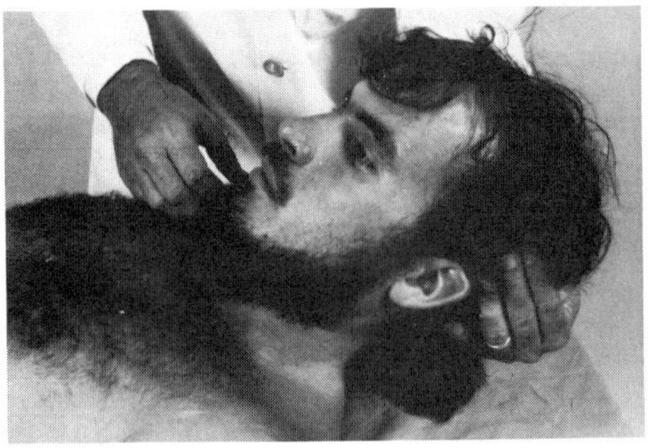

Figure 11-1.

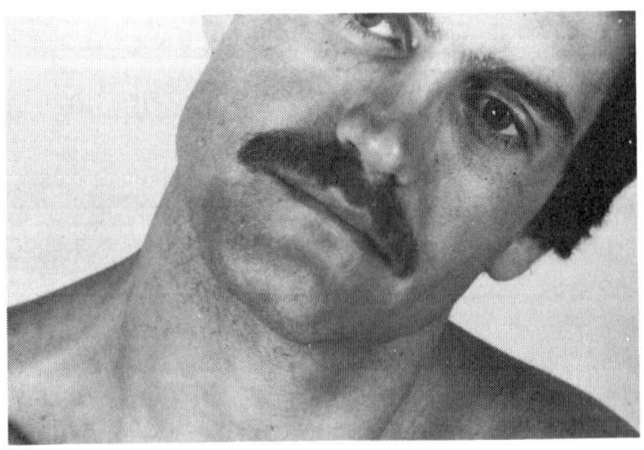

Figure 11-2.

EYES: ANATOMY

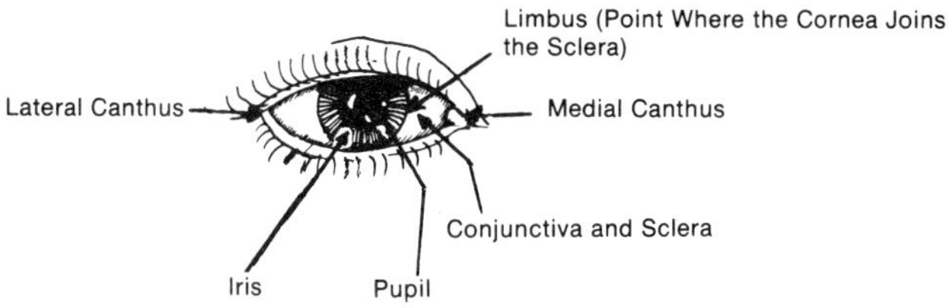

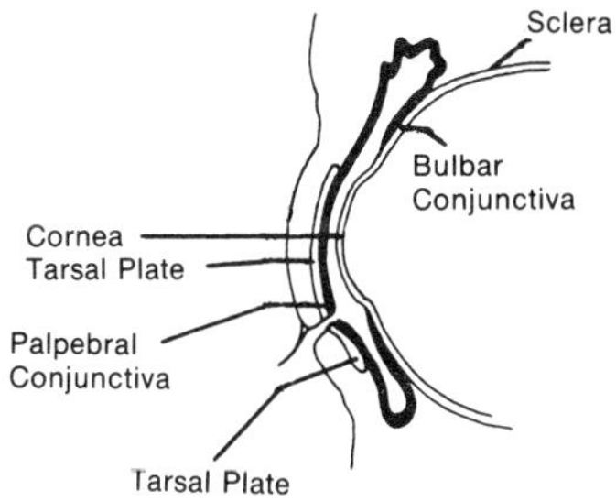

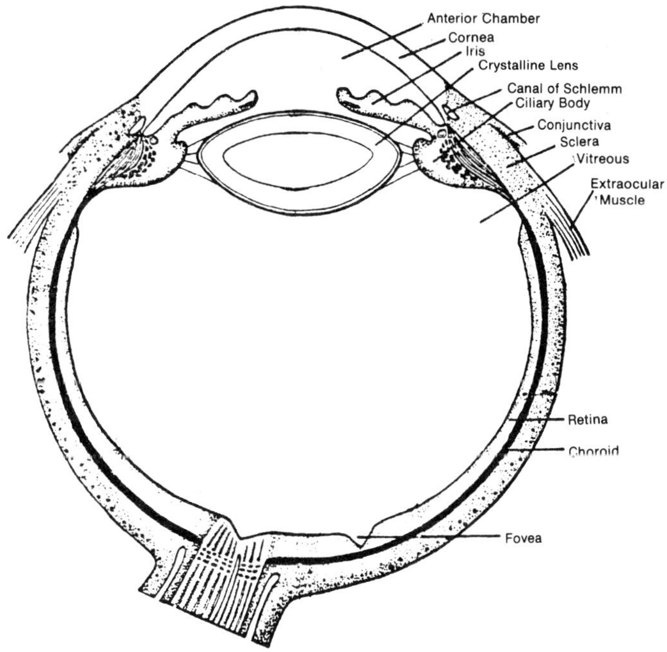

<u>NOTE</u>: The anterior retina and ciliary body can be seen only by special techniques.

(Continued)

EYES: ANATOMY, Continued

PART	DESCRIPTION/FUNCTION
upper eyelid	• covers the upper 1 mm to 2 mm of the iris when open • spreads tears and protects eyes
tarsal plates	• thin strips of firm connective tissue • give eyelids shape and rigidity
conjunctiva	• covers the parts of the eyeball that are visible anteriorly (except the cornea) • joins the corneal epithelium at the edge of the cornea (limbus) • covers the undersurface of the eyelids • mucous membrane
bulbar conjunctiva	• portion of the conjunctiva that lies loosely on the surface of the sclera
palpebral conjunctiva	• portion of the conjunctiva that lines the eyelids
eyeball	• sensory organ for vision containing optical system (cornea and lens) that focuses light and the neurosensory tissue (retina)
iris muscles	• control pupillary size (radial dilator is sympathetic and pupillary sphincter is parasympathetic)
ciliary muscles	• control thickness of the lens, thus enabling the eye to focus upon objects at varying distances
fovea centralis	• a slight avascular depression in the center of the macula • coincides with the center of vision • sharpest visual acuity
macula	• the central retinal area temporal to the optic disc • only portion of the retina with tightly packed, individual neurosensory elements that are responsible for fine visual acuity

(Continued)

EYES: ANATOMY, Continued

PART	DESCRIPTION/FUNCTION
optic nerve	• joins the eye about 5 mm nasal to the fovea, where it appears as an oval white disc (optic disc) • retinal artery and vein enter the eye through the optic nerve
ocular fundus	• portion of the eye posterior to the lens (the ocular fundus in the posterior half of the eye can be seen with the direct hand-held ophthalmoscope)
retina	• lines the ocular fundus • light-sensitive, neurosensory organ

Lubrication

The conjunctiva and cornea are lubricated by tears from the lacrimal gland. Tears drain through the lacrimal puncta (superior and inferior) at the medial ends of the lid margins. The secretions flow through lacrimal ducts to the sac and down the nasolacrimal duct, where they enter the nose. The puncta are papillary structures in the nasal end of the lid margins.

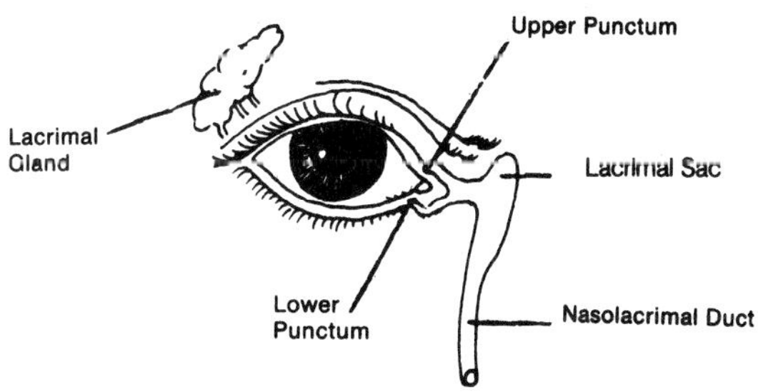

EYES: VISUAL PATHWAYS

DIAGRAM	DESCRIPTION
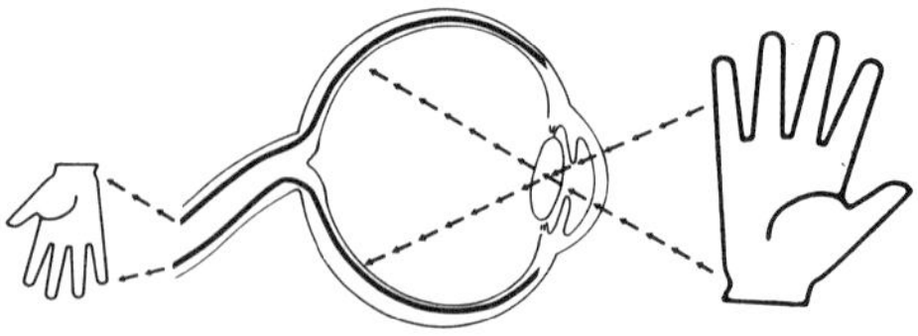	Light that is reflected from an object passes through the cornea and lens to the retina. NOTE: Images are upside-down and reversed, right to left. Thus, light from objects strikes the opposite quadrant of the retina.
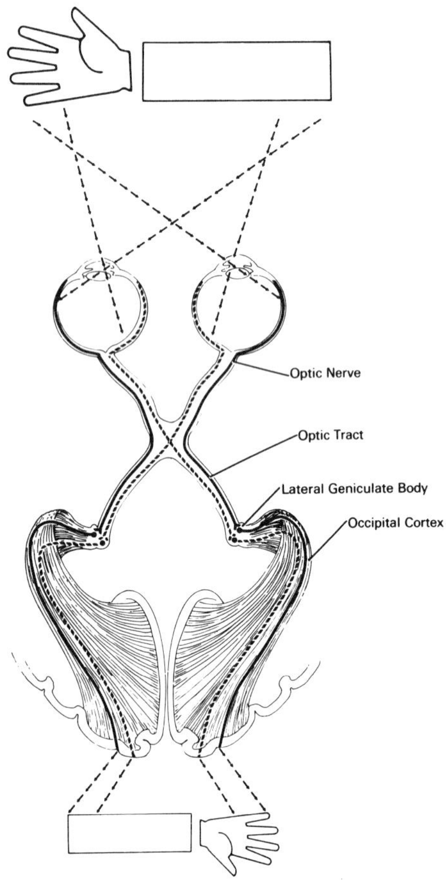	Neural impulses pass through the retina, the optic nerve, and the optic tract to the visual cortex of the occipital lobes. NOTE: The arrangements of nerve fibers in the retina are preserved in the nerves: • temporal fibers run laterally • nasal fibers run medially At the optic chiasm, however, the nasal fibers cross over so that the left optic tract contains only fibers from the left half of each retina, and the right optic tract contains only fibers from the right half. The dividing line passes vertically through the fovea.
	The visual pathway synapses in the lateral geniculate body. The optic radiations then pass through the temporal, parietal, and occipital lobes to terminate in the occipital cortex, along the calcarine fissure.

EYES: REFLEX ACTIONS

Visual Reflexes Aside from producing conscious vision, light rays stimulate two kinds of reflex pupillary actions:
- light
- accommodation

REFLEX	DESCRIPTION	DIAGRAM
light	Light that stimulates the retina causes pupillary constriction (direct light reflex). The sensory pathway is similar to the visual pathway; the pathways diverge, however, at the level of the lateral geniculate body. The light reflex travels through midbrain synapses to the centers of the third nerve on each side, which stimulate both pupils to constrict. Contriction of the contralateral pupil is called the <u>consensual light reflex</u>.	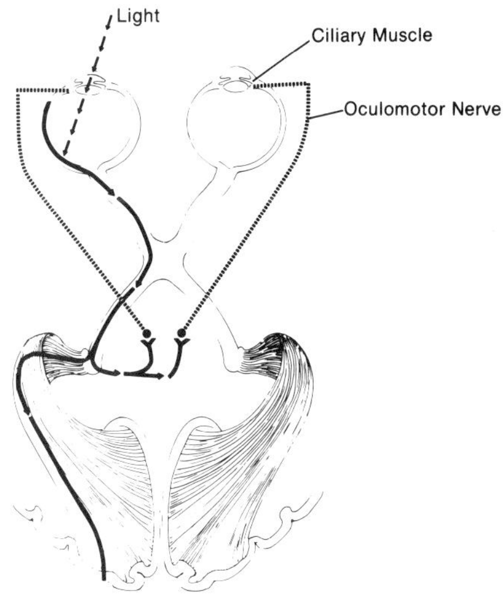
accommodation	Accommodation allows the eye to focus so that a clear visual image is maintained as the gaze is shifted from far to near. Accommodation includes: • convergence of eyes • pupillary constriction • thickening of the lens through contraction of the ciliary muscles Only the convergence and constriction can be seen by an examiner. Sensory pathways for accommodation are similar to the visual pathways. Impulses pass from the occipital cortex to the frontal cortex, then to the midbrain and the oculomotor nerve.	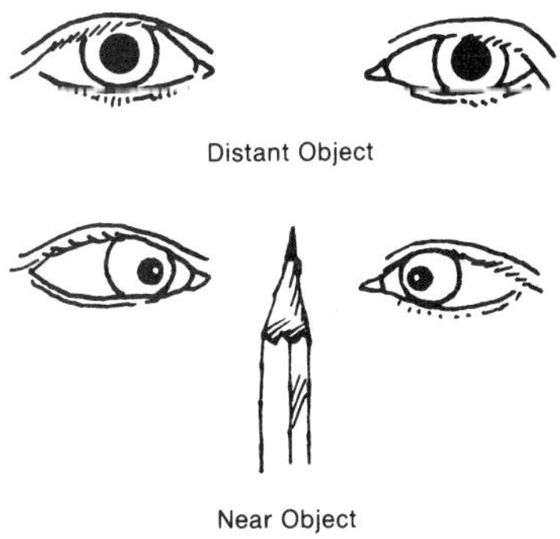

EYES: VISUAL ACUITY

Introduction

Assessment of visual acuity is the most important test of ocular function. Many diseases may decrease acuity, as do problems in refraction. Thus, vision should be evaluated during every screening physical examination.

Important!

Good visual acuity does NOT preclude the existence of ocular disease.

Measurement

- Distance acuity is measured with a letter chart (Snellen chart) placed 20 feet from the patient.
- Near cards can measure distance acuity when placed 14 inches from the eye (see below).
- Special charts are available for testing illiterate patients and children.

  NOTE: Glasses should be worn if the patient usually uses them. Reading glasses will blur distant vision, but are necessary if a near card is used.

Near Card

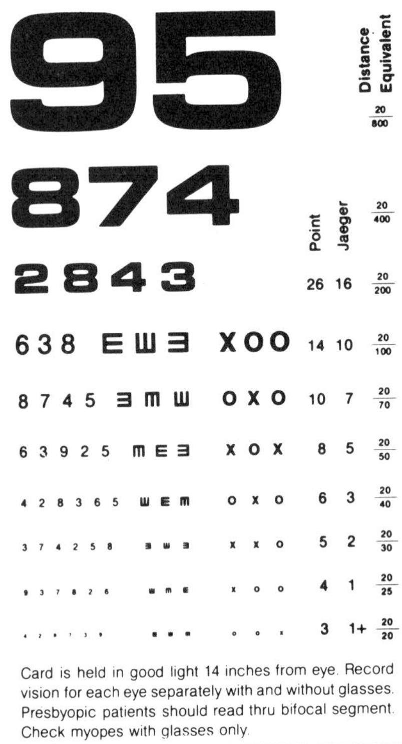
95
Distance Equivalent
20/800
874
Point Jaeger
20/400
2843 26 16 20/200
638 EШƎ XOO 14 10 20/100
8745 ƎmШ OXO 10 7 20/70
63925 mEƎ XOX 8 5 20/50
428365 ШEm OXO 6 3 20/40
5 2 20/30
4 1 20/25
3 1+ 20/20
Card is held in good light 14 inches from eye. Record vision for each eye separately with and without glasses. Presbyopic patients should read thru bifocal segment. Check myopes with glasses only.

(Continued)

EYES: VISUAL ACUITY, Continued

Occlusion	Acuity is measured in one eye at a time. The patient should cover the other eye with the palm by placing the heel of the hand against the nose.
Recording Acuity	Acuity is expressed as a fraction: • The numerator indicates the distance between patient and chart. • The denominator represents the distance at which an eye with normal (20/20) vision can read the line. EXAMPLE: 20/200 means that the patient's eye can read only the 20/200 line at 20 feet, but the normal eye can see these letters at 200 feet. NOTE: When visual acuity is less than can be measured with the chart, it may be expressed as: • the farthest distance at which fingers can be counted or hand movements discerned • the degree of light perception
Presbyopia	Lenses in the eyes of people over 40 years old become inflexible so that accommodation for near vision decreases. This condition, presbyopia, is characterized by difficulty in reading.

EYES: LIDS

Functions

The functions of the eyelids are:
- protection
- cleaning
- wetting
- light control

Purposes of Examination

Lid examination should evaluate:
- the position of the lids in relation to the globe
- the presence and rate of blinking
- completeness of closure
- the presence of inflammation and tumors

Lid closure may be incomplete with abnormally prominent eyes or facial nerve paralysis. Serious damage may occur if eyes become dry because the lids do not close properly.

Systemic Disease

Systemic disease may be present when lid edema is observed. Local inflammation or bulging of the lid skin that results from aging must be differentiated from edema.

Systemic diseases that may cause lid edema include:
- nephrosis
- heart failure
- allergy
- hypothyroidism

Ptosis

Ptosis (drooping of the upper lid) may be due to:
- third nerve disease (see Fig. 11-3)
- loss of sympathetic innervation (Horner's syndrome)

Lid Infections

Common infections of glands of the lid margin include:
- hordeolum (sty): a local infection of the glands around the eyelashes (see Fig. 11-4)
- chalazion: an infection or retention cyst of the meibomian (sebaceous) glands, which lie within the tarsal plates and open on the posterior portion of the lid margins (see Fig. 11-5)
- blepharitis: crusting of the lashes, which indicates that some type of lid infection is present

Abnormal Positions

Examples of abnormal positions of the lids include:
- ectropion: outward rolling of the lids (see Fig. 11-6)
- entropion: inward rolling of the lids (see Fig. 11-7)

Eyelashes normally project away from the eye. If they

EYES: LIDS, Continued

project backward, as in entropion, corneal irritation or abrasion may be produced.

Lid retraction is usually due to thyroid disease.

Palpation

Palpation of the lids is performed by sliding a finger across the surface of the closed lid. Masses (such as chalazion) within the lid may be felt between the finger and the eyeball.

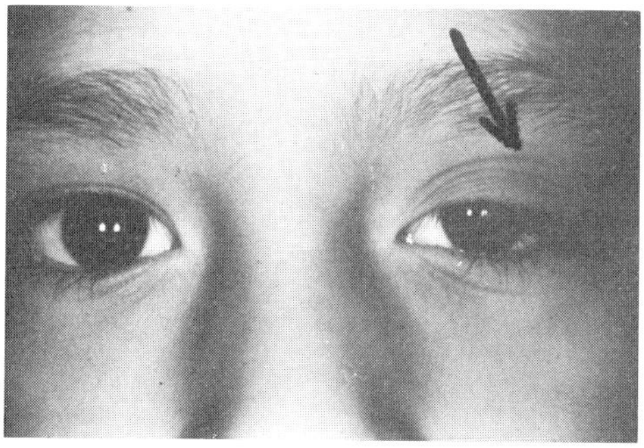

Figure 11-3.

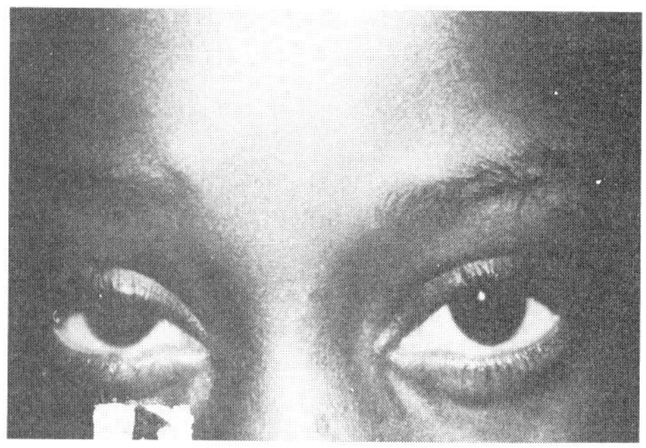

Figure 11-4.

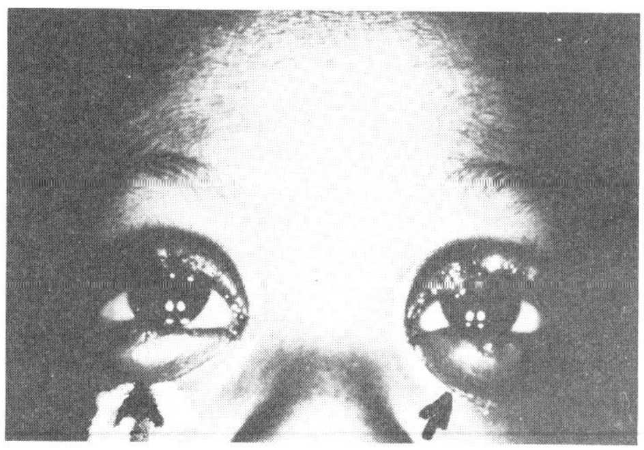

Figure 11-5.

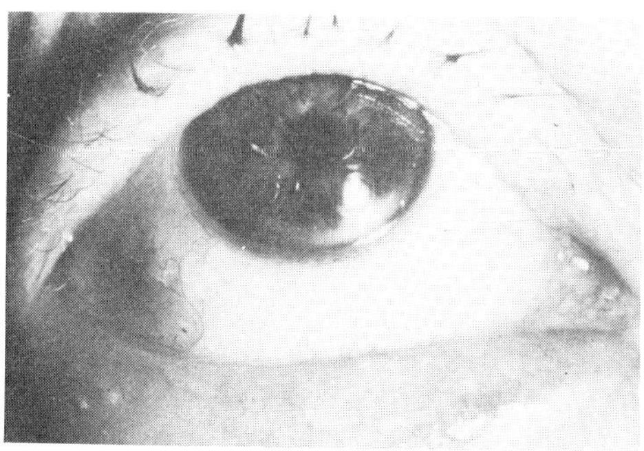

Figure 11-6.

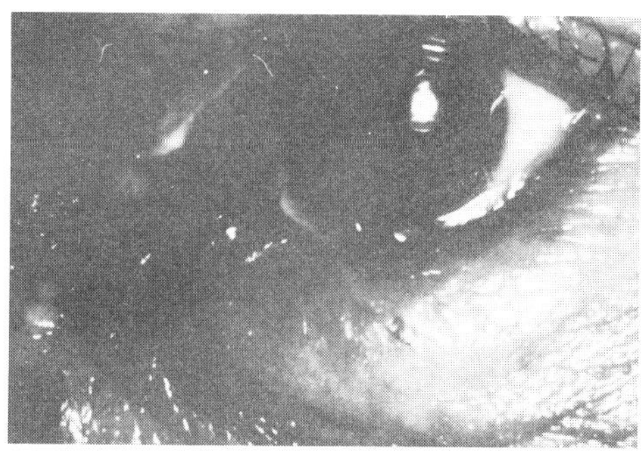

Figure 11-7.

EYES: CONJUNCTIVA

Introduction

Normal conjunctiva is usually transparent (the white color of the eye is caused by the underlying sclera) and has two parts, the bulbar conjunctiva and the palpebral conjunctiva.

Examination of the Bulbar Conjunctiva

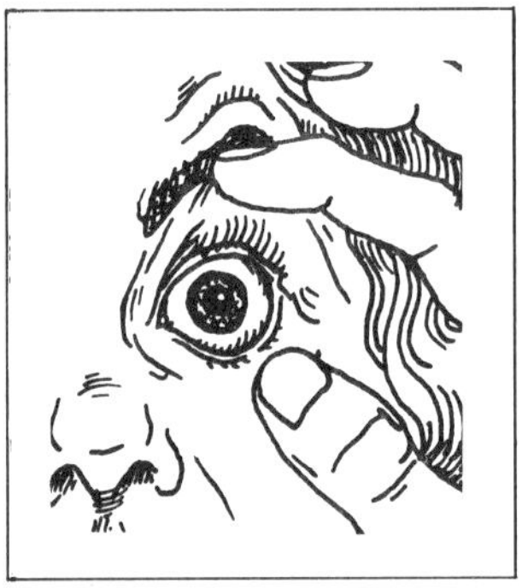

The bulbar conjunctiva is examined by separating the lids widely (without putting any pressure on the eye) and having the patient look up, down, and to each side.

- Small blood vessels are normally visible in the conjunctiva. Dilation of these vessels produces the red seen in many eye diseases.
- Blood vessels and nerves penetrate the sclera at several points about 0.5 cm above the limbus. At these points, particularly in dark-skined persons, uveal pigment often proliferates, and the black dots produced may look like foreign bodies.
- A small, fleshy elevation (the caruncle) is located in the nasal corner of the conjunctiva. Fine hair and tiny yellowish spots (sebaceous glands) are normally present in the caruncle and may be quite prominent in older persons.

(Continued)

EYES: CONJUNCTIVA, Continued

Examination of the Palpebral Conjunctiva

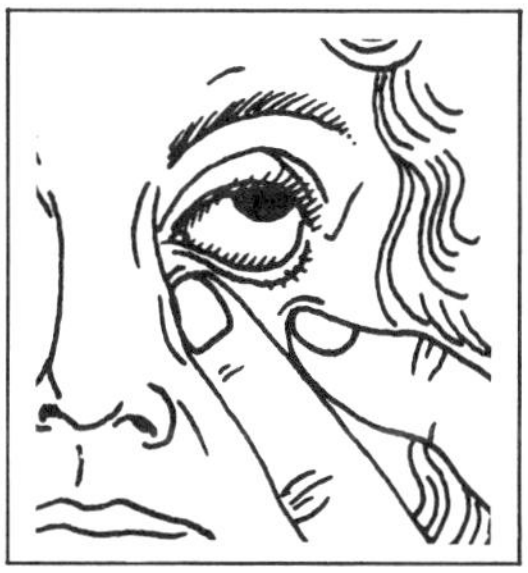

The palpebral conjunctiva cannot be seen unless the lids are everted. The lower lid is everted by sliding the skin that overlies the lower orbital rim downward. The patient should be asked to look upward to increase exposure of the lower conjunctiva.

Because the palpebral conjunctiva rests on fleshy tissue, it is redder than the bulbar conjunctiva. Vertical yellowish striations (meibomian glands) may be seen in the portion of the palpebral conjunctiva that overlies the tarsal plates. If irritation, viral infection, or allergy occurs, the lymph follicles of the palpebral conjunctiva may enlarge and present a nodular appearance that can be seen from the side with a flashlight. See Figure 11-8.

Inspecting the Upper Palpebral Conjunctiva

Inspection of the upper palpebral conjunctiva is necessary to check for foreign bodies. This is done as follows:

- Place a cotton-tipped applicator over the part of the upper eyelid containing the tarsal plate.
- Ask the patient to look down.
- Pull the eyelashes outward and upward, everting the eyelid.
- Inspect the conjunctiva.

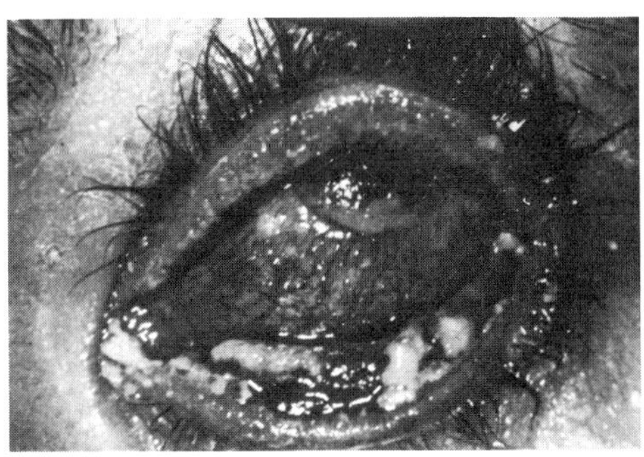

Figure 11-8.

EYES: CORNEA

Introduction

The cornea, which is smooth and transparent, is visible on inspection; bright reflection from its surface can be observed when light is shown into the eye.

Abnormalities

Commmon abnormalities of the cornea are:
- abrasions
- opacities

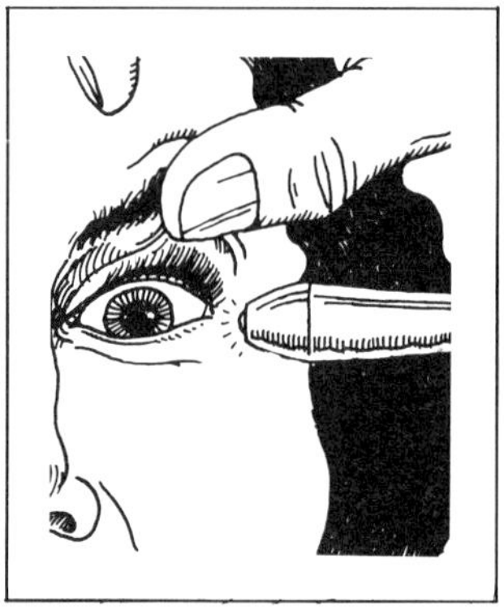

Abnormalities can be detected by illumination with a light. Defects in the light reflections of the normal surface indicate superficial abnormalities. Abnormalities may also cast shadows on the iris, which may be easier to see than the lesions that produce the shadows.
NOTE: Abrasions of the cornea often cannot be seen unless stained with fluorescein.

Sensory Division of Cranial Nerve V

Corneal sensitivity (cranial nerve V) is tested by touching a wisp of cotton to the center of the cornea and observing the lid closure. Brisk lid closure is a normal protective reflex.

> NOTE: The eye should be approached from the side so that the patient cannot see the cotton and blink from fear. Do not touch the lashes, for a touch will also cause blinking.

A great deal of variation exists in corneal sensitivity, so, to assess their normality, the corneal reflexes of the two eyes should be compared with each other (unless the patient has bilateral fifth-nerve loss).

EYES: PUPILS

Introduction

In a normal person, the pupils are round and equal in size, and they constrict when exposed to light and during accommodation.

Pupillary Light Reflex

As noted earlier, pupillary constriction in response to light may be:

- direct, i.e., constriction of the pupil that is exposed to light
- consensual, i.e., constriction of the pupil that does not receive direct illumination

Either optic nerve may transmit the afferent part of the pupillary reflex. Efferent stimuli are distributed evenly to both eyes via ciliary nerves.

> EXAMPLE: If a patient is blind in one eye, the affected eye will exhibit no direct pupil response but will react to the simulation of the normal eye. Stimulation of the blind eye, however, will NOT cause a consensual reaction in the normal eye.

Accommodation

STEP	ACTION
1	Hold one fingertip about 4 inches from the eye being tested.
2	Ask the patient to look alternately at the fingertip and at the wall directly beyond the finger. The eye should not then move.
3	Observe pupillary size as attention is alternated between distance and near.

Accommodation and the Light Reflex

If the pupil reacts to light, reaction to accommodation will most likely be present. Thus, the light reflex should be tested by bringing a light slightly from the side, rather than from the front, while attention is directed at distance.

- Failure to react to light, but preservation of the accommodative response (Argyll Robertson pupil), is characteristic of neurosyphilis.
- The accommodation response must be checked if no light response is observed.
- Accurate determination of the absence of the light reflex requires an examination in a darkened room with a bright light.

(Continued)

EYES: PUPILS, Continued

Size	Although some normal persons (5%) have pupils that are unequal in size (anisocoria), differences in size may be caused by many disorders of the nervous system.
Mydriasis	Mydriasis, enlargement of the pupil, may be caused by: • ocular injury (recent or old) • acute glaucoma • large doses of systemic parasympatholytic drugs • use of parasympatholytic or sympathomimetic drops • paralysis of the third cranial nerve
Miosis	Miosis, constriction of the pupil, occurs: • in iritis • with use of parasympathomimetic drops, e.g., pilocarpine • with use of systemic narcotics, e.g., morphine • in sleep • in interruption of sympathetic nerve fibers
Irregularity of Contour	Irregular pupil contours may indicate: • iritis • neurosyphilis • trauma • congenital defects • a history of ocular surgery
Depth of Anterior Chamber	The distance between the cornea and the iris should be estimated before the pupils are dilated. Eyes with shallow anterior chambers may develop acute glaucoma if the pupil is dilated. A penlight should be shined on the iris from the temporal side. If the eye has a deep anterior chamber, the iris will be is flat, and all of it will be illuminated. If the chamber is shallow, only the temporal half of the iris will be illuminated.

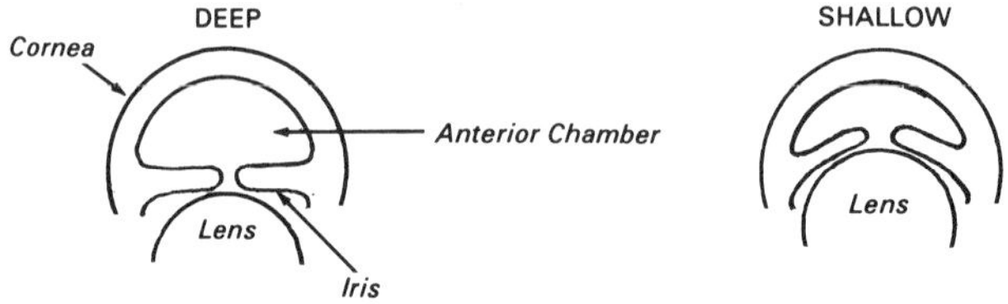

EYES: EXTRAOCULAR MUSCLES

Introduction

To determine straightness of the eyes, a flashlight should be held directly in front of the examiner's eyes, and the patient should look directly at the light. In a normal person, the reflection of light in the two pupils is symmetrical in the center of the pupil. Any displacement of the reflection indicates a deviating eye.

Epicanthus

Many children have skin folds (epicanthus) that curve down from the nasal end of their upper lid and partially conceal their eyes, especially when one eye is turned toward the nose. Epicanthus may be mistaken for crossing of the eyes, but testing for the corneal light reflex allows a quick distinction to be made between epicanthus and crossed eyes. See Figure 11-9.

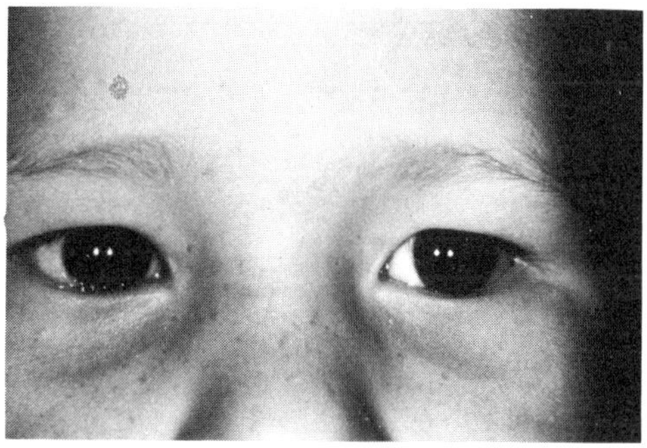

Figure 11-9.

Cardinal Positions of Gaze

Extraocular muscle paralyses are detected by asking patients to move their eyes into the six cardinal positions of gaze. Inability of the eye to turn to a certain position indicates which muscle is paralyzed (see below).

NOTE: Be sure to carry the fixation point out to the extremes of gaze, since this will make a defect more obvious.

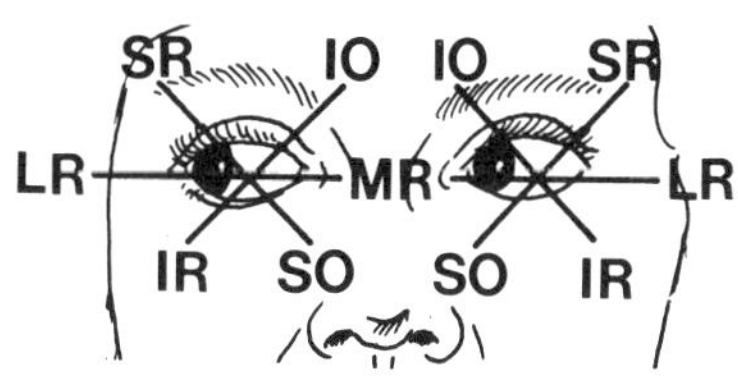

(Continued)

EYES: EXTRAOCULAR MUSCLES, Continued

POSITION TO WHICH EYE WILL NOT TURN	MUSCLE AFFECTED
straight nasal	medial rectus (MR; third nerve)
up and nasal	inferior oblique (IO; third nerve)
down and nasal	superior oblique (SO; fourth nerve)
straight temporal	lateral rectus (LR; sixth nerve)
up and temporal	superior rectus (SR; third nerve)
down and temporal	inferior rectus (IR; third nerve)

NOTE: Straight up and down are not cardinal positions of gaze.

End-Positional Nystagmus

When looking far to the side, some normal eyes develop a rhythmic twitching motion, end-positional nystagmus. Since the the quick portion of this nystagmus is always in the direction of gaze and is followed by a slow drift back, it can be differentiated from pathologic nystagumus, in which the quick component is always in the same direction (regardless of the direction of gaze).

Displacement

The anterior-posterior position of the eye in its bony socket may be changed by:

- exophthalmos-- forward displacement (see Fig. 11-10)
- enophthalmos-- backward displacement (see Fig. 11-11)

Exophthalmos may be caused by:

- retrobulbar infection
- retrobulbar hematoma
- orbital neoplasm
- thyroid disease

Enophthalmos is usually due to sympathetic nerve paralysis or trauma.

Fracture or Notch?

Palpable infraorbital and supraorbital notches can be mistaken for fractures.

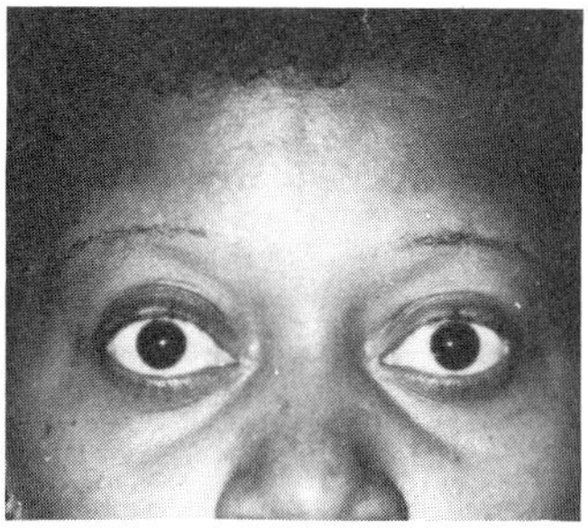

Figure 11-10.

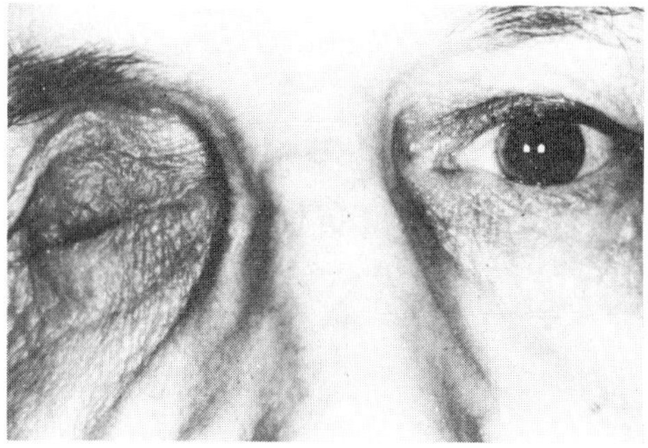

Figure 11-11.

EYES: VISUAL FIELDS

Testing

Confrontation testing is used to test the fields of vision at the bedside.

STEP	ACTION
1	Cover one of the patient's eyes. See Figures 11-12 and 11-13.
2	Ask the patient to look straight ahead, steadily, at a point.
3	Place an object beyond the field of vision and move it forward from the periphery until the patient can see the object. <u>NOTE</u>: The patient must look straight ahead at the fixation point and <u>not</u> at the test object.

Normal Visual Fields

The fields of vision are normally asymmetrical (see below), as measured from the anteroposterior axis of the eye. All four quadrants should be tested for each eye.

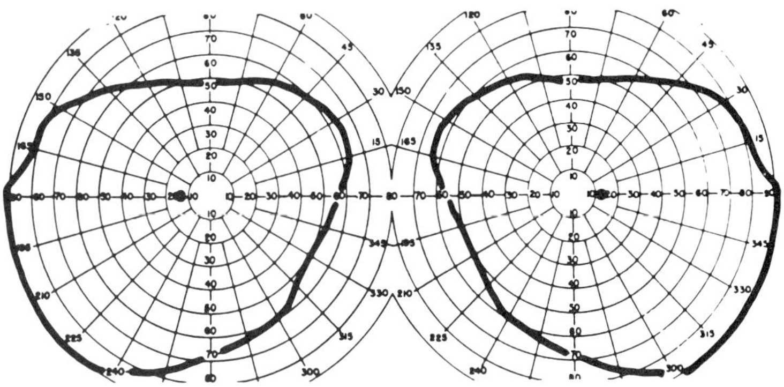

LEFT RIGHT

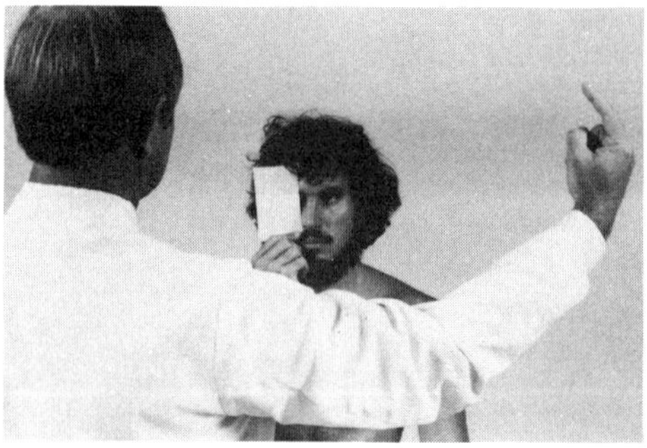

Figure 11-12.

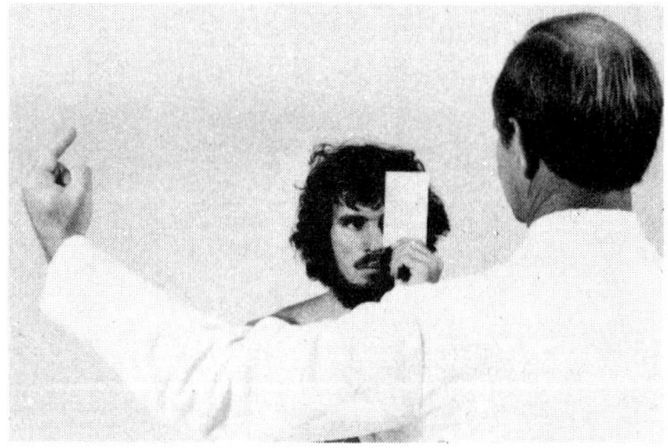

Figure 11-13.

EYES: OPHTHALMOSCOPE

Preparation

Ophthalmoscopic examination requires that the eyes be held still. The patient should be asked to look at a distant object. If the patient is seated and the examiner is standing, the optimal direction of gaze is about 20 degrees upward and straight ahead.

- The examination should be done in a darkened room.
- Dilation of the pupil with 2.5% phenylephrine hydrochloride will make the examination easier and will allow visualization of more peripheral retina.
- Glasses need not be worn by examiner or patient.
- Both examiner and patient should keep both eyes open.

How to Hold the Instrument

An ophthalmoscope is held in front of the examiner's right eye during examination of the patient's right eye and in front of the examiner's left eye during the examination of patient's left eye. The index finger rests on the lens wheel to permit focusing. The head of the ophthalmoscope should be braced firmly against the examiner's brow or nose with the viewing aperture positioned directly in front of the eye. See Figure 11-14.

> NOTE: The relative position of the ophthalmoscope and physician should not change during the examination so that misalignment of the eye and viewing aperture and loss of the fundus from view are avoided.

The free hand may be placed on the patient's forehead and the thumb used to elevate the eyelid.

Light and Focus

The round white light is used most often, at maximum brightness unless the patient cannot tolerate it. In most cases, the ophthalmoscope lens should be set at zero to start.

- Red numbers (minus) will focus farther away.
- Black numbers (plus) will focus nearer.

EYES: OPHTHALMOSCOPE, Continued

Procedure

STEP	ACTION	NOTES
1	Looking through the aperture of the ophthalmoscope, approach to within 1 foot of the patient and direct the light into the pupil.	• A uniform red glow (red reflex) will fill the pupil of a normal eye. Opacities in the clear portions of the eye will appear as black portions within the red reflex. • Absence of the red reflex indicates either abnormal blockage of transmission of light through the eye or that the ophthalmoscope is not on or positioned properly.
2	Always keeping the red reflex in sight, approach the eye until your forehead or the ophthalmoscope touches your hand on the forehead.	Loss of the red reflex during the approach means the light is not directed into the pupil; back away until the red reflex is located again. The light reflex may be lost because of blinking by the patient. To prevent this, the the thumb of the free hand can be used to elevate the upper lid. To prevent bumping the patient's nose with the ophthalmoscope, direct the handle downward and slightly away from the patient by tilting your head slightly.
3	Observe a detail in the fundus such as: • a vessel • a pigment • the optic disc The detail first encountered should be brought into sharp focus by rotating the lens wheel.	Because the patient's eye is only one inch away, your eyes will converge and accommodate. Since this accommodation may be variable, it may interfere with focusing and cause your view to alternately blur and clear. This can be avoided if you pretend to look through the patient's head at a distant landscape. Focusing should be done with the lens wheel, not your accommodation.

(Continued)

EYES: OPHTHALMOSCOPE, Continued

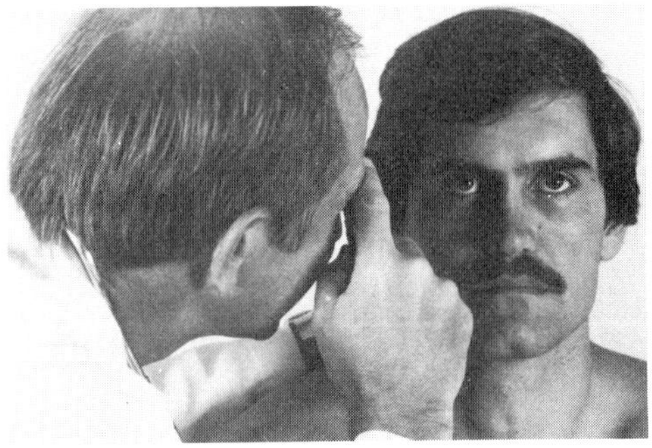

Figure 11-14.

Observing Different Areas of the Retina

When the ophthalmoscope light is moved from one part of the retina to another, the fundus view may be lost if the light no longer enters the pupil. To change the area of retina that is illuminated, the ophthalmoscope must be moved in the opposite direction so that rotation of the light beam is centered at the pupil.

Light Reflections

Dazzling light reflections from the corneal surface may be avoided by moving the ophthalmoscope slightly to one side, up, or down, or by tilting the ophthalmoscope.

EYES: EXAMINATION OF THE OCULAR FUNDUS

Optic Disc

An examination of the ocular fundus begins by locating the optic disc. It is important to remember that all portions of the fundus appear magnified 15 times because of the focusing by cornea and lens.

IF	THEN
the ophthalmoscope light is directed into the eye from about 15° temporal to the straight-ahead gaze of the patient	the optic disc will be the first detail seen
the disc is <u>not</u> located immediately	it may be found by following down the bifurcations of the visible vessels

Features of the Disc

The optic disc is the most conspicuous feature of the fundus, and an examiner should observe its characteristics:
- size
- shape
- color
- physiologic depression in the center (the "cup")
- margins

Size of the Optic Disc

Normal discs are uniform in size, and about 1.5 mm in diameter. High myopic refractive errors in the patient magnify the disc; hyperopic errors make it appear smaller.

> <u>EXAMPLE</u>: After cataract extraction, the disc looks very small because of the loss of the manifying ocular lens.

Fundus Distances

Fundus distances are estimated in terms of disc diameters.

> <u>EXAMPLE:</u> A lesion larger than the disc and located in the lower fundus may be described as being 2 disc diameters in size and one disc diameter from the disc at 6 o'clock.

Shape Optic Disc

Normally, discs are round or oval. Irregularities in shape and size are not defects of the disc itself, but are the effects of disease in surrounding structures.

(Continued)

EYES: EXAMINATION OF THE OCULAR FUNDUS, Continued

Color	• Normal discs are pink-white to pale yellow. • The center of the disc may be more pale than the periphery because a "physiologic cup" exposes the lamina cribrosa.
"Physiologic Cup"	Discs have a depression just temporal of the center. Normal depressions: • vary in size, but they never extend all the way to the margin of the disc • may be deep enough to permit a clear view of the fine fenestrations of the lamina cribrosa • are usually symmetrical in both eyes NOTE: Important indicators of glaucoma are: • asymmetry of cups • cup larger than half of disc diameter
Margins	The disc margin is normally quite regular, although dense pigment is often scattered over the margins. If it is possible to focus clearly on irregularities of the edges, edema or inflammation is probably not present. A crescent of sclera or choroid (dark color) is often visible right next to the disc.
Vessels	The central retinal artery and vein emerge from the center of the disc. Bifurcations may occur in the disc or after the vessels reach the retina. Each major vessel should be observed along its visible length (disc to periphery).
Arteries	Arteries are usually about 35% narrower than veins. Their size varies with the number of branches. A narrow band of light (arteriolar light reflex) is reflected from the longitudinal axis of an artery. Arteries and veins frequently cross, but normal arteries do not indent or displace veins. Arteriovenous crossings should be observed; indentations or displacement of the vein where the artery crosses are due to arteriolosclerosis or hypertension.

(Continued)

EYES: EXAMINATION OF THE OCULAR FUNDUS, Continued

Veins	Veins are darker than arteries and have no prominent light reflex. Veins overlying the disc pulsate slightly (spontaneous venous pulsation), synchronous with the arterial pulse. The pulsation is caused by forcing of venous blood out of the globe with systole. Gentle external pressure on the globe during ophthalmoscopic examination will collapse veins (at the disc end of the vein only) in normal eyes when intracranial pressure is normal.
Macula	The macula (located about 2 disc diameters temporal to the disc) has the greatest acuity of any part of the retina. The "spot" in the center of the macula, a pinpoint depression, is the avascular fovea centralis. Tiny vessels run toward the fovea from all directions but do not enter it. Fine-pigment granularity is normally seen in the macula, as well as in the periphery of the retina. NOTE: If the macula is difficult to locate, the patient should be instructed to look directly at the light, so that the macula is placed in the center of the examiner's field of vision.
Periphery	To see the periphery of the retina, the examiner should instruct the patient to look upward as the ophthalmoscope beam is directed upward, to the left as the beam is directed to the left, to the right as the beam is directed to the right, and downward as the beam is directed downward. The periphery is usually lighter in color than the center of the retina. NOTE: The periphery of the retina can be visualized best by dilating the pupil.
Normal Variations	• Normal fundi can be darkly pigmented except for prominent, crisscrossing, light orange streaks, which represent choroidal vessels. • Fundi of dark-skinned people may be uniformly dark.

(Continued)

EYES: EXAMINATION OF THE OCULAR FUNDUS, Continued

Normal Fundus

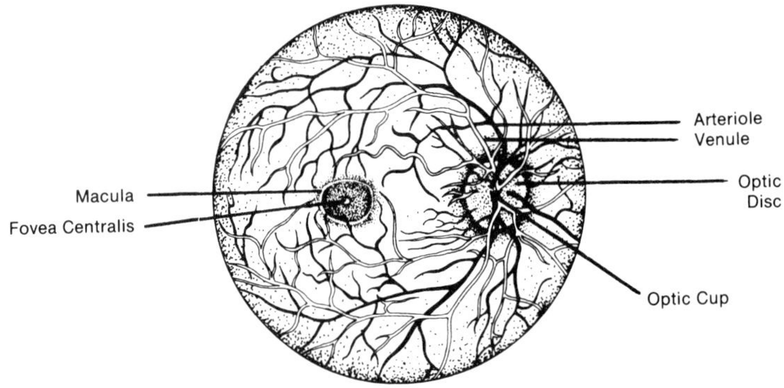

Light Reflexes

Light reflexes are glistening, movable reflections from waves in the smooth surface of the retina. They usually parallel the vessels and encircle the macula, and they are more prominent in young persons than in older persons.

Media

The more anterior portion of the eye (media) may be examined by turning to the higher-plus (black) lenses of the ophthalmoscope.

- This will focus on the posterior vitreous, the anterior vitreous, and the lens, which are transparent and invisible in the normal eye.
- Usually a +15 or +20 lens will be needed to see the iris and cornea.

EARS: INSPECTION OF THE PINNAE

Congenital Deformities	Congenital deformities of the pinnae occur alone or associated with anomalies of the facial bones or temporal bone.
Cauliflower Deformity	Cauliflower deformity indicates previous trauma to the pinna.
Tophi	Uric acid deposits, tophi (which are secondary to gout) are sometimes seen along the margins of the pinna as small, hard, white nodules.

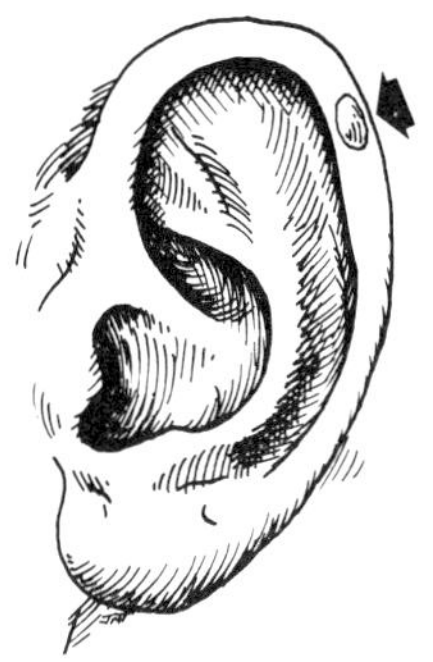

Tenderness	Tenderness when the pinna is moved usually indicates inflammation of the ear canal (external otitis).
Skin Cancer	Ulcers or elevated scaly patches may indicate skin cancer, which often occurs at this site.

EARS: INSPECTION OF THE EXTERNAL EAR CANAL

Procedure

STEP	ACTION
1	Tilt the patient's head slightly to the opposite side and pull the pinna gently backward and upward to straighten the cartilaginous ear canal.
2	Insert the speculum into the meatus. Rotate the instrument slightly to allow the speculum to slide gently into the canal. NOTE: To maximize the view, the largest speculum that will fit the canal should be used.

Deep Inspection

The deep half of the external ear canal in the adult is bony and has a pink lining.

NOTE: Pressure of the speculum in this area is painful and should be avoided.

IF	THEN
the tympanic membrane is to be visualized	the otoscope must be directed slightly forward (rather than at right angles to the sagittal plane) because of the oblique direction of the ear canal
the instrument is pointed in the direction of the opposite ear	the examiner will usually see skin of the posterior bony canal instead of the tympanic membrane

Wax

Visualization of the ear drum may be blocked by wax (cerumen) or pus in the ear canal.

(Continued)

EARS: INSPECTION OF THE EXTERNAL EAR CANAL, Continued

Cleaning of the Ear Canal

The ear canal may be cleaned by several methods.

- A cerumen spoon may be used under direct vision through the ear speculum. See Figure 11-15.

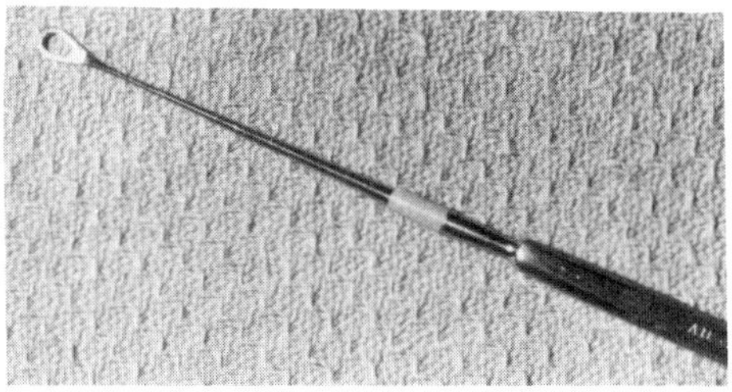

Figure 11-15.

- The ear canal may be irrigated with water at body temperature.

  NOTES:
  - Irrigation is a safe and simple procedure but should not be performed if the ear drum has a perforation.
  - Water is used at body temperature to avoid causing vertigo and nausea due to labyrinthine stimulation.
  - Hard, impacted wax may be softened before irrigation by having the patient put mineral oil or dilute hydrogen peroxide solution into the ear nightly for 3 or 4 nights.

Pus and Inflammation

Pus in the ear canal indicates either otitis media, with perforation of the drum, or external otitis. Inflammation of the external canal may be accompanied by redness and swelling of the lining, which makes insertion of the speculum difficult and painful.

Anatomy

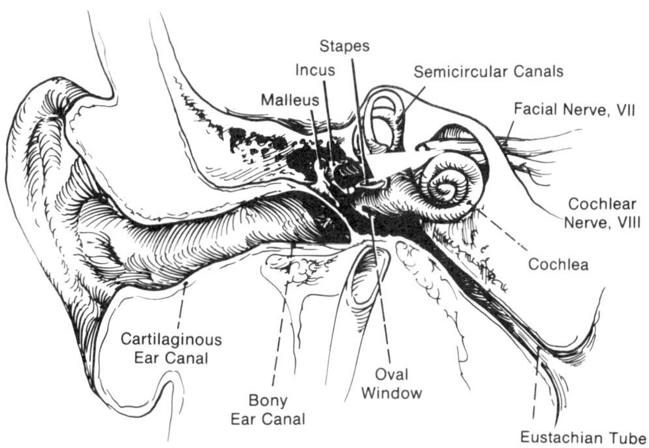

EARS: THE TYMPANIC MEMBRANE

Normal Right Tympanic Membrane

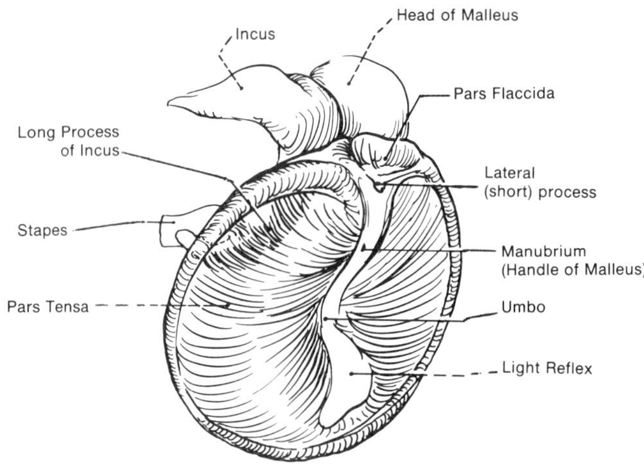

Pars Tensa

The pars tensa constitutes the major portion of the tympanic membrane and consists of three layers:

- outer squamous epithelium
- inner cuboidal epithelium
- middle fibrous layer

Malleus

The handle of the malleus (manubrium) is attached to the pars tensa and has a bony, white appearance. At the upper end of the manubrium, the short or lateral process projects outward. The short process and manubrium should be identified to ensure that the drum is being inspected. The pars tensa is usually pearl gray; it should be examined completely by rotating the otoscope and speculum.

Light Reflex

The light reflex is in the anteroinferior quadrant, issuing from the lower end (umbo) of the manubrium. The importance of this landmark is overemphasized, and attempts should be made to identify more consistent landmarks such as the manubrium and short process.

Long Process of the Incus

If the pars tensa is transparent, the long process of the incus may be seen behind the posterosuperior quandrant of the membrane.

(Continued)

EARS: THE TYMPANIC MEMBRANE, Continued

Head of the Malleus and Body of the Incus	The head of the malleus and the body of the incus lie in the upper part of the middle-ear cleft (attic). The pars flaccida and adjacent bone of the ear canal prevent visualization of these structures.
Inspection of the Tympanic Membrane	Four important characteristics of the ear drum should be ascertained: • color • position • integrity • mobility
Color	The normal tympanic membrane is pearl gray. Dense white plaques (tympanosclerosis) indicate past inflammatory disease. A healed perforation may appear as a transparent area of the pars tensa because the middle fibrous layer does not heal during the repair process. • Red indicates the presence of otitis externa or otitis media. The membrane appears partially or diffusely red due to hyperemia. See Figure 11-16.

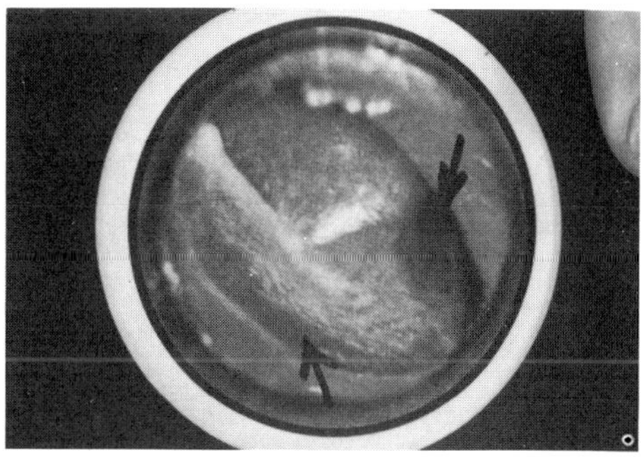

Figure 11-16.

• Yellow or amber indicates serum in the middle ear (serous otitis media); sometimes a level of fluid or bubbles of air may be observed behind the drum.
• Blue indicates blood in the middle ear (hemotympanum).
NOTE: The recognition of minor variations in color of the membrane may be difficult for the inexperienced observer.

Position	The upper posterior part of the membrane should be closer to the speculum than the lower anterior part. This obliqueness is more pronounced in children.

(Continued)

EARS: THE TYMPANIC MEMBRANE, Continued

Outward Bulging

Bulging usually indicates the presence of pus under positive pressure in the middle ear (acute otitis media). The tympanic membrane is usually diffusely red, and landmarks are difficult to identify. See Figure 11-17.

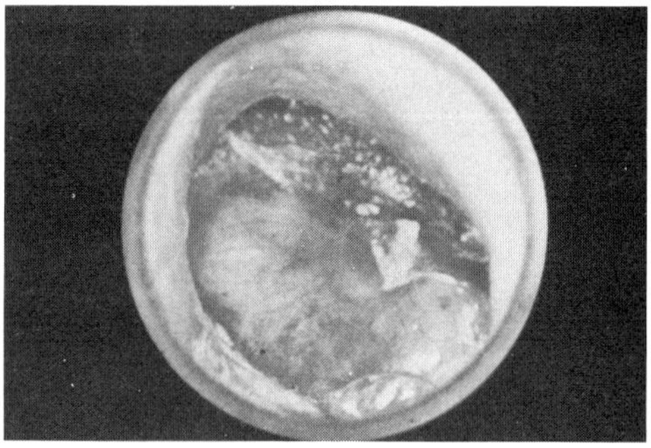

Figure 11-17.

Retracted Ear Drum

A retracted ear drum (Fig. 11-18) occurs when middle-ear pressure is decreased (negative). Negative middle-ear pressure results from eustachian tube blockage, which may be caused by:

- adenoid hypertrophy in children
- upper respiratory infection
- rapid descent during air travel

Stages in Retraction

STAGE	DESCRIPTION
1	Oxygen is absorbed, and a negative pressure behind the drum is produced.
2	The tympanic membrane is pressed inward by atmospheric pressure, which makes the malleus more prominent.
3	The handle of the malleus, because it is attached to the drum head, may come to lie in an almost horizontal, rather than vertical, position.

Perforation

Perforation of the drum may result from trauma or middle-ear infection. Small perforations can be missed easily during an examination; therefore, the pars flaccida, as well as all four quadrants of the pars tensa, should be inspected carefully.

(Continued)

EARS: THE TYMPANIC MEMBRANE, Continued

Pus	Pus in the external canal always suggests that a perforation may exist. The ear should be swabbed clean to permit examination of the tympanic membrane. If white, skinlike debris (cholesteatomas) are seen in the middle ear, an otologic consultation is advisable. See Figure 11-19.
Mobility	Mobility may be assessed by using the pneumatic head attachment of the otoscope. A speculum that is large enough to permit a tight seal of the ear canal must be used, and the bulb should be squeezed lightly in order to apply gentle pressures.
Fluid in the Middle Ear	If fluid is present in the middle ear, movements of the drum become sluggish, and greater than normal pressure is required to produce movements of the tympanic membrane.
Important!	Testing drum head mobility is especially important in children because serous otitis media (fluid behind the ear drum) is the most common cause of hearing loss in children. The change in the drum color may be minimal in serous otitis media, and retraction of the membrane may be difficult to observe. NOTE: Inability to move the drum with pressure may also be the result of an improper seal caused by: • too small a speculum OR • perforation of the drum head

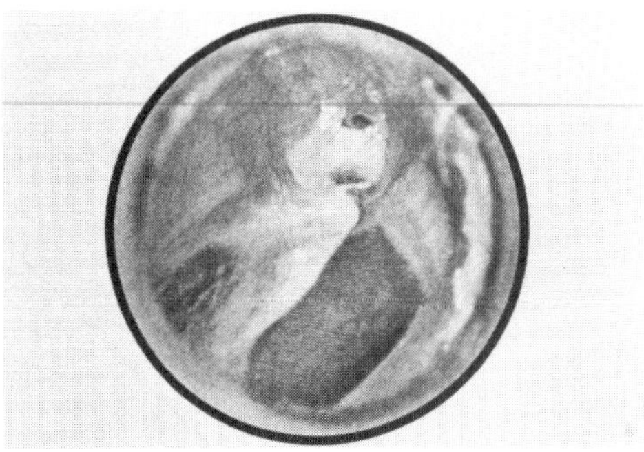

Figure 11-18.

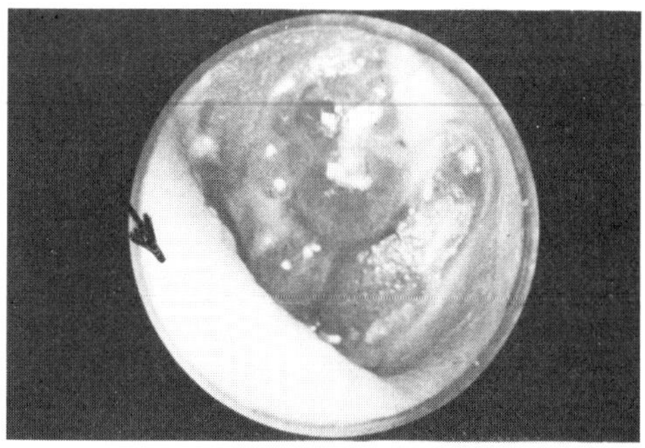

Figure 11-19.

NOSE

External Nose	The skin of the nose is a common site for skin cancer. Cosmetic deformities produced by trauma may also be present.
Nasal Vestibule	The vestibule is the skin-lined, hair-bearing area inside the nares.
Nasal Chamber	Examination of the nasal chamber is performed by inserting a nasal speculum into the vestibule.
Nasal Septum	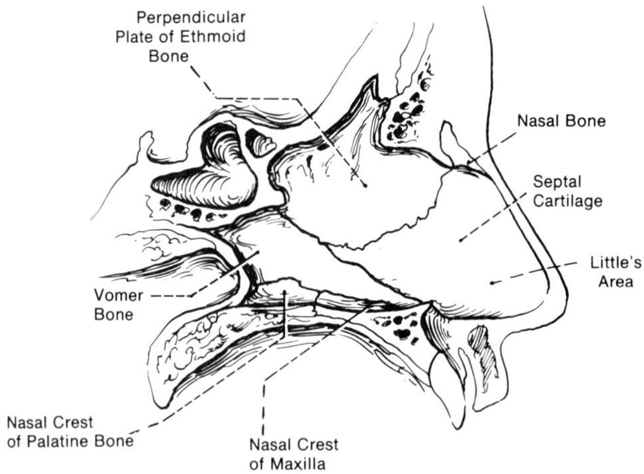
Septal Deviation	Deviations of the septum are common and not important unless nasal obstruction is produced. Prominent blood vessels can usually be seen on the lowermost anterior aspect of the cartilaginous septum, a common site for nosebleeds. This area is easily accessible if cauterization or pressure is necessary.

(Continued)

NOSE, Continued

Lateral Nasal Wall

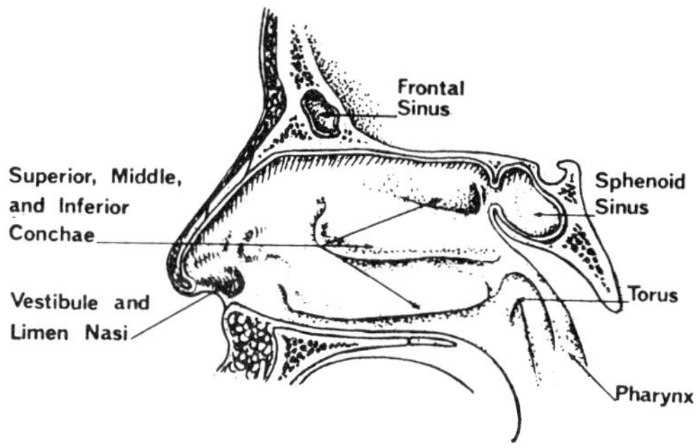

Lateral Nasal Wall

Turbinates — The turbinates (conchae) project into the nasal cavity from the lateral wall of the nose. The inferior turbinate, the largest of the three, is the easiest to see.

Secretions in Nasal Chamber — An excessive amount of watery or white secretions inside the nasal chamber, associated with swelling of the turbinates, usually indicates infectious or allergic rhinitis. Yellow or green pus usually indicates a sinus infection.

Inspection Instruments — Inspection of the posterior nasal chamber usually requires a headlight and mirror, or other special instruments.

MOUTH AND OROPHARYNX

PART	DESCRIPTION	NOTES
mouth	extends from the lips to the anterior tonsillar pillars	
gingivo-buccal sulcus	area bounded by the gums and the inner aspects of the lips and cheeks	The ducts of the parotid glands open into the gingivo-buccal sulci opposite the upper second molars on either side. When the parotid glands are pressed, clear secretions may be seen issuing from duct opening in a small papilla.
oral cavity	extends from the anterior teeth to the anterior tonsillar pillars; roof is formed by the hard palate	
torus palatinus	a bony submucosal protuberance found in the midline of the hard palate	

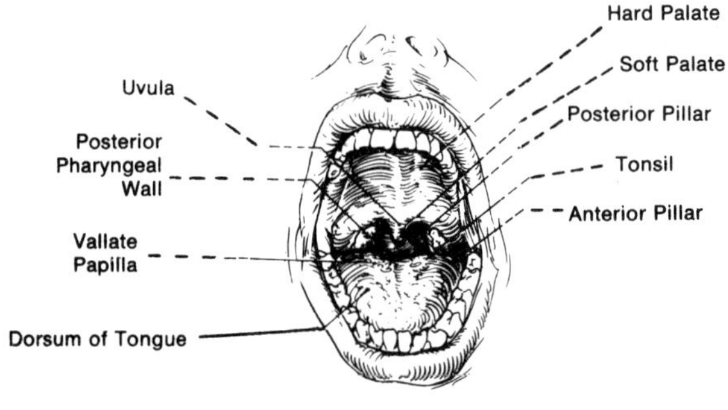

(Continued)

MOUTH AND OROPHARYNX, Continued

Tongue

- The anterior two thirds of the tongue lie in the oral cavity.
- The dorsum of the tongue is covered by papillae, which give it a roughened appearance. Occasionally, a white coating may be observed.

  NOTE: Because of chronic irritation, the papillae may be hypertrophied or nicotine-stained, which gives the tongue a hairy or shaggy appearance (hairy tongue, coated tongue).

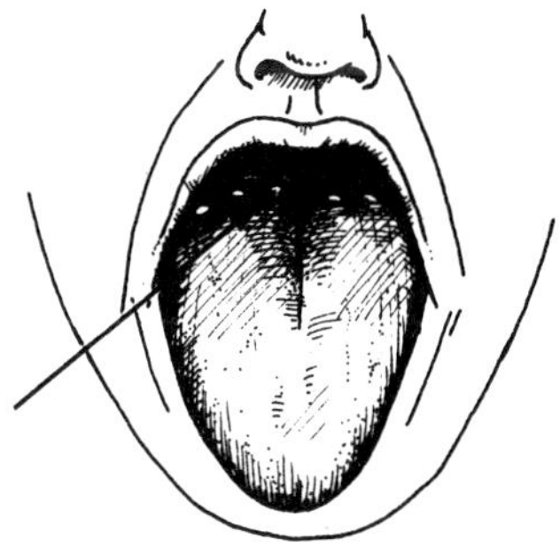

The junction between the anterior two thirds and the posterior one third of the tongue can be identified as the site of the large, round vallate papillae.

Undersurface of the Tongue

The undersurface of the tongue is smooth and overlies the floor of the mouth.

NOTE: This region, which is often ignored during routine examinations, may be the site of cancer.

(Continued)

MOUTH AND OROPHARYNX, Continued

Floor of the Mouth

- The floor of the mouth is bounded by the inner aspects of the mandible and the root of the tongue.
- Anteriorly, near the midline, the submandibular (or submaxillary) ducts open on either side of the frenulum of the tongue. The orifice of the duct may be located by observing the flow of saliva when pressure is applied the submandibular gland.

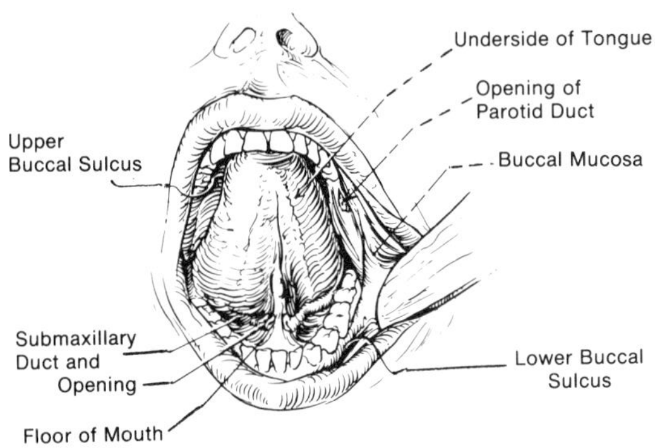

Oropharynx

The oropharynx extends from the anterior tonsillar pillars anteriorly to the posterior pharyngeal wall. The soft palate and the tip of the epiglottis form the upper and lower limits, respectively.

Tonsils

The tonsils can be seen in the fossae between the anterior and posterior tonsillar pillars. Numerous crypts exist in the tonsils, and they may exude a white keratin debris. The tonsils vary in size and may be asymmetric. After tonsillectomy, small remnants of lymphoid tissue (tonsillar tags) may be seen in the fossae, and scarring of the pillars may occur.

(Continued)

MOUTH AND OROPHARYNX, Continued

Parts of the Oropharynx

PART	DESCRIPTION
posterior pharyngeal wall	• part of the pharynx visible to an examiner using the tongue blade • lining appears nodular because of deposits or aggregations of lymphoid tissue underneath the mucosa
posterior third of the tongue	• lies in the oropharynx • The large lymphoid masses (lingual tonsils) on the dorsum have a nodular appearance.
uvula	• extends from the free edge of the soft palate • varies greatly in length and thickness
mucosa	• of the oral cavity and oropharynx is pink, except over the hard palate, where it is whitish (with transverse-running rugae) • Yellowish glandlike structures that may be seen shining through the oral mucosa in some areas are the normal sebaceous or minor salivary glands that lie under the epithelium.

Inspection

The oral cavity and oropharynx are inspected with a tongue blade and flashlight. All areas should be examined carefully, and particular attention should be paid to the teeth and gums. The anterior part of the tongue should be raised so that the floor of the mouth can be inspected.

Placement of the Tongue Blade

When inspecting the oropharynx, the examiner should avoid placing the tongue blade too far back because the patient will gag. The tip of the blade should be at about the level of the vallate papillae, and should depress the anterior part of the tongue downward and forward gently. This can be done more easily if the patient does not stick out his or her tongue. See Figure 11-20.

(Continued)

MOUTH AND OROPHARYNX, Continued

Children	Children will often not permit the tongue blade to be used, but usually an adequate view of the oropharynx can be obtained if they simply open their mouth and protrude their tongue, which they think is fun.
Presence of Inflammation	The oropharyngeal mucosa is normally pink. A fiery red color indicates acute inflammation.
Palpation	Bimanual palpation of the floor of the mouth can detect abnormalities not detectable by external palpation. The finger of a gloved hand is used to explore internally while the ungloved hand explores the submandibular area. See Figure 11-21. • Induration around an ulcer usually indicates malignant neoplasm.

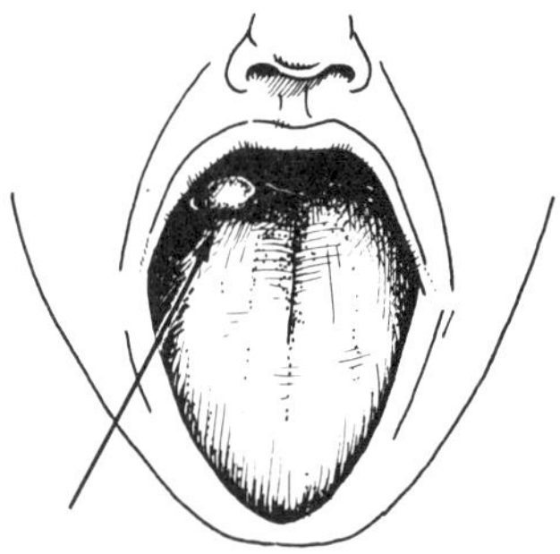

- Tumors in the posterior third of the tongue are often more easily felt than seen.
- Calculi in the submandibular ducts are best felt by bimanual palpation.

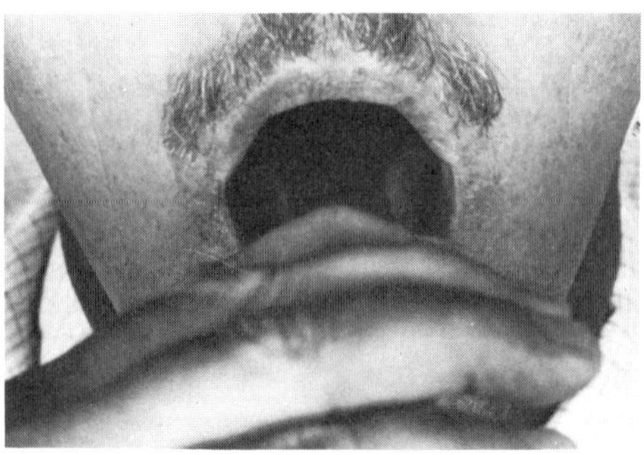

Figure 11-20.

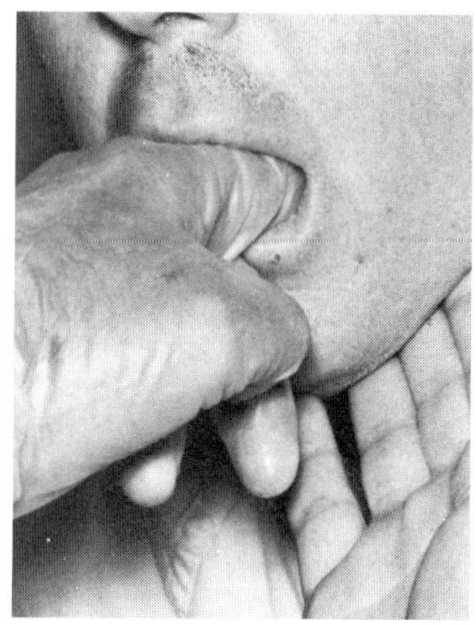

Figure 11-21.

PARANASAL SINUSES

Introduction	Bedside assessment of the condition of the paranasal sinuses is done by: • palpation for tenderness • inspection of the nasal chamber for secretions that may drain into the nose
Tenderness	If pressure over the sinus produces pain, an infection is usually present.
Frontal Sinuses	The frontal sinuses are palpated by pressure above or under the medial aspect of the eyebrow. See A, below.
Anterior Ethmoidal Sinus	Tenderness may be elicited by inserting the index finger along the medial orbital wall and pressing in the direction of the nasal chamber. See B, below.
Maxillary Sinus	Tenderness over the maxillary sinus may be elicited by exerting pressure over the anterior wall (just above the canine tooth). See C, below.

Palpation of Sinuses

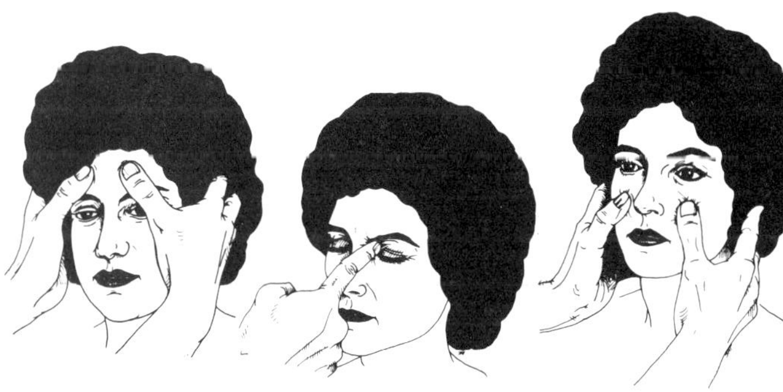

A B C

NECK: BACKGROUND

Introduction

The neck extends from the lower border of the mandible to the upper border of the manubrium and clavicles. It is divided arbitrarily by the sternomastoid muscle into two triangles:

- anterior
- posterior

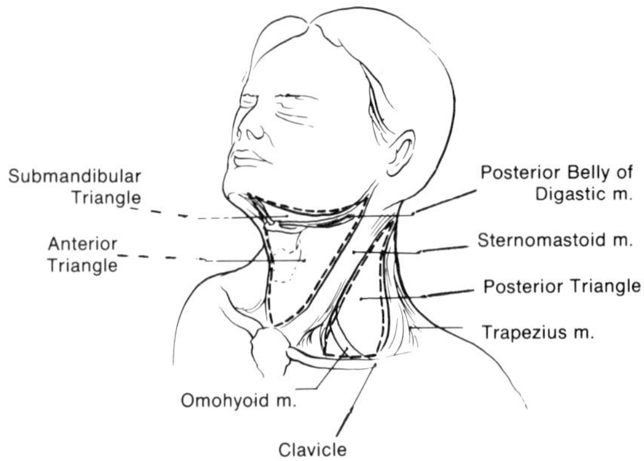

Palpable Structures

The following structures may be palpated easily in the midline:

- the hyoid bone, best felt with the neck extended, just below the mandible
- the thyroid cartilage, with its prominent notch
- the cricoid cartilage, just below the thyroid cartilage
- the tracheal rings.

  NOTE: With the neck extended, the cricothyroid membrane may be felt under the skin between the lower border of the thyroid cartilage and the upper border of the cricoid ring in the midline.
- The internal and common carotid arteries can be palpated deep beneath the bulky sternomastoid muscles.
- Numerous groups of lymph nodes are present in the neck. Small nodes (up to 1 cm in diameter) are often palpable in normal subjects and are usually the result of previous inflammatory disease (tonsillitis, viral infection).

(Continued)

NECK: BACKGROUND, Continued

Anterior Neck Anatomy

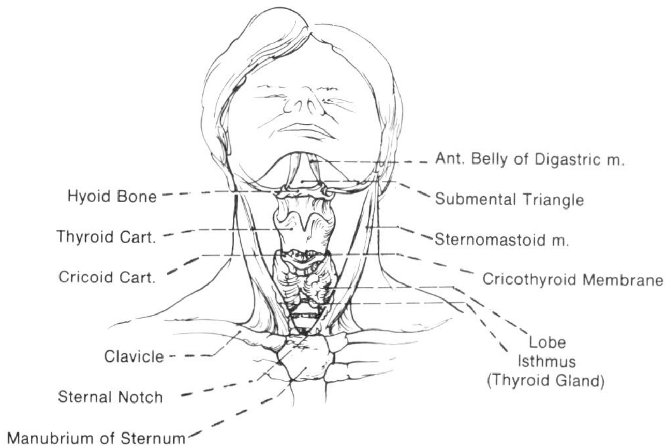

Lymph Nodes

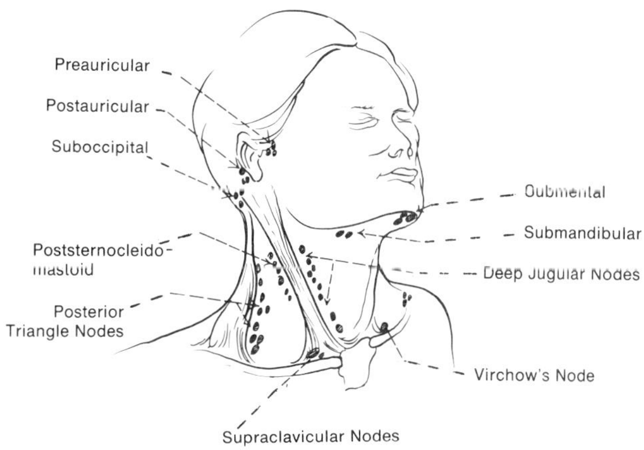

Thyroid Lobes

The thyroid lobes lie on either side of the trachea and may not be palpable in normal subjects.

NECK: EXAMINATION

Position

Examination of the neck begins by inspection from the front, with the patient either sitting or supine.

Asymmetry

Asymmetry may indicate an underlying mass.

Swellings

Swellings in the neck are most commonly:
- enlarged lymph nodes
- thyroid masses (usually identified by their upward movement during swallowing) (see Fig. 11-22)
- cysts (see Fig. 11-23)
- abscesses
- aneurysms

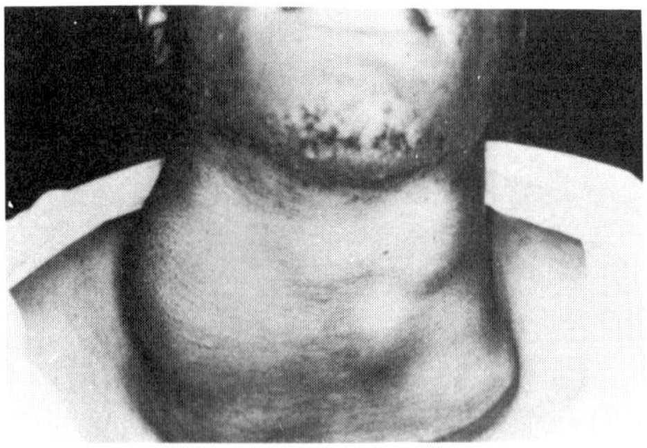

Figure 11-22.

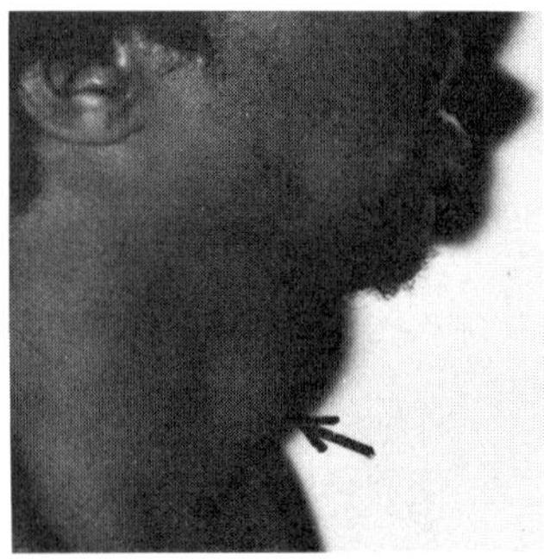

Figure 11-23.

Distended Veins

Distended veins that are observable when the patient is seated indicate obstruction of the venous return that may be caused by:
- heart failure
- constrictive pericarditis
- pericardial tamponade
- mediastinal tumors (superior vena cava obstruction)
- tricuspid valve incompetence

Arterial Pulsations

Arterial pulsations in the neck may be seen in thin patients. A pulsating mass may be an:
- aneurysm
- a tumor of the carotid body

Prominent arterial pulsations are often seen in:
- aortic valve insufficiency
- anemia
- thyrotoxicosis

NECK: PALPATION

Introduction

Palpation is usually performed with the patient sitting. The examiner may stand in front of or behind the patient. One side of the neck should be palpated at a time while the examiner rests the opposite hand on the occiput to control the head.

Trachea

The trachea is palpated for evidence of deviation, preferably just above the suprasternal notch. The trachea may be displaced laterally by:

- an aortic aneurysm
- a mediastinal tumor
- a unilateral thyroid enlargement

A large amount of fluid or air in the pleural space will push the trachea and other mediastinal structures toward the opposite side. Conversely, in the following conditions, the trachea may be displaced toward the affected side:

- unilateral pleural fibrosis
- unilateral fibrosis within the lung
- atelectasis

Lymph Nodes

Palpation of the neck is performed chiefly to check for enlarged lymph nodes or abnormal masses. The examiner should develop a routine whereby the regions of the neck are sequentially palpated on either side.

Palpation

STEP	ACTION	NOTE
1	Palpate the submental and submandibular nodes.	These nodes are felt most easily by curling the fingers under the lower border of the mandible while keeping the thumb of the same hand against the lateral surface of the bone. The lymph nodes in these areas may be felt by squeezing them against the inner surface of the body of the mandible. See Figure 11-24.

(Continued)

NECK - PALPATION, Continued

STEP	ACTION	NOTE
2	Palpate the preauricular nodes by pressing the palmar surfaces of the fingertips over the parotid gland, and moving them gently to and fro.	See Figure 11-25. In these locations, enlarged lymph nodes can be felt easily because they can be pressed against the firm underlying tissues.
3	Postauricular and posterior triangle nodes are palpated in a similar manner.	See Figure 11-26.
4	Palpate enlarged nodes in the deep jugular chain as follows: a. To relax the sternomastoid muscles on the side that is being examined, turn the patient's chin slightly to the *opposite* side and tilt the head so that the ear on the side to be examined lies closer to the ipsilateral shoulder. b. Pick up the sternomastoid muscle between the thumb and fingers. c. By gently placing the thumb and fingertips deep to the muscle, pick up enlarged nodes or masses along the deep jugular chain.	Deep (internal) jugular node enlargement may be missed because of the overlying sternomastoid muscle. a. These nodes *cannot* be felt easily as described above because they will be pushed medially in the direction of the pharynx. The absence of a firm underlying surface against which they may be palpated makes their detection difficult. b. See Figure 11-27. c. Masses in the lateral lobe of the thyroid gland can be palpated in a similar manner.

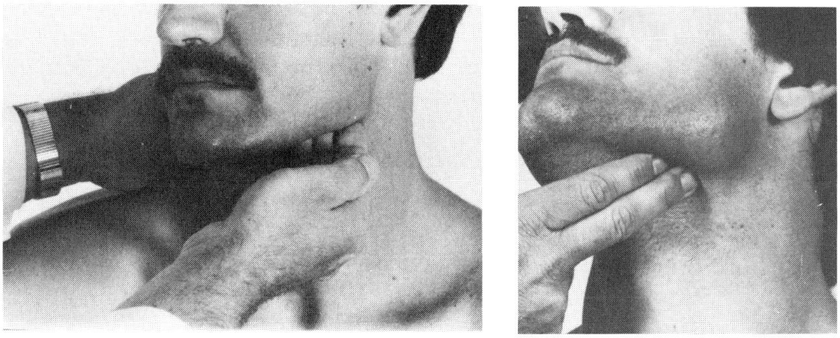

Figure 11-24.

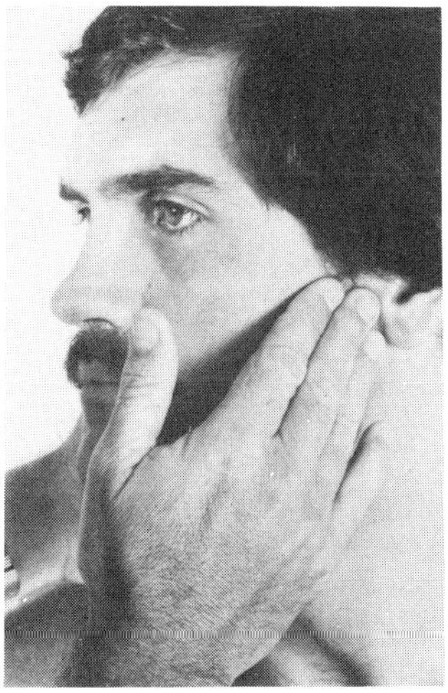

Figure 11-25.

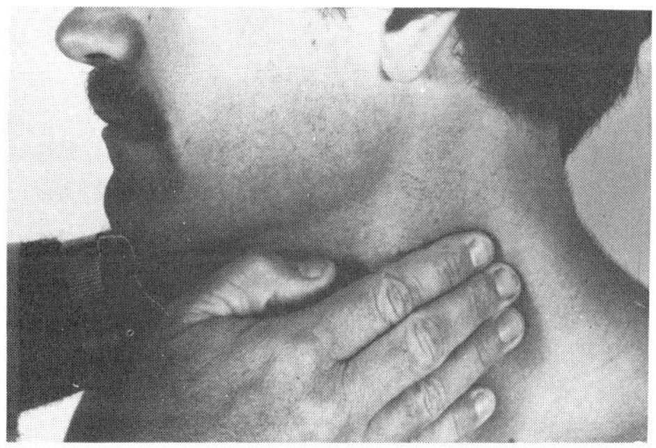

Figure 11-26.

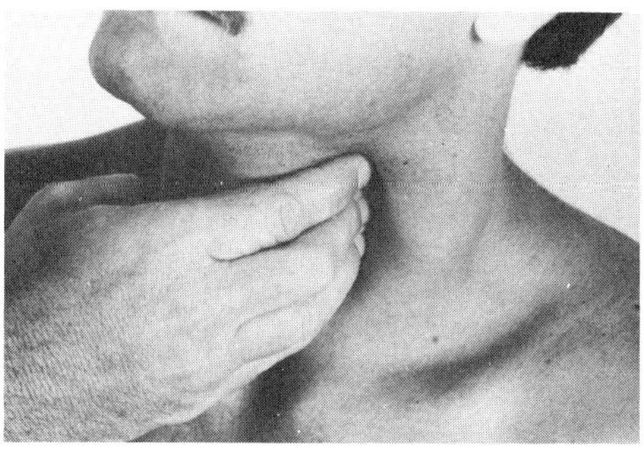

Figure 11-27.

NECK: AUSCULTATION

Introduction

Auscultation is performed with the bell of the stethoscope while the patient holds his or her breath.

Neck Bruits

- A bruit heard over the carotid artery may indicate narrowing of the lumen by, for example, atheromatous plaque.
- A continuous murmur may be heard if an arteriovenous fistula (which may occur as a result of vascular injury) is present.
- Certain tumors in the neck (carotid body tumor) are highly vascular, and an overlying bruit may be audible with the stethoscope.
- A bruit is often heard over the thyroid gland in patients with toxic goiter.

Sounds Originating From the Heart

A murmur originating from the heart may be heard in the lower part of the neck.

EXAMPLE: aortic valve stenosis

The site or origin of this type of murmur can usually be discerned by observing the gradual increase in intensity of the sound as the stethoscope is "inched" down the neck and over the anterior chest wall.

Stridor

Stridor is the noise that originates from the trachea if narrowing of the lumen of the larynx or cervical trachea has occurred.

NOTE: Stridor is an important sign because it indicates the dangerous narrowing of the upper airway that may precede complete obstruction and asphyxia.

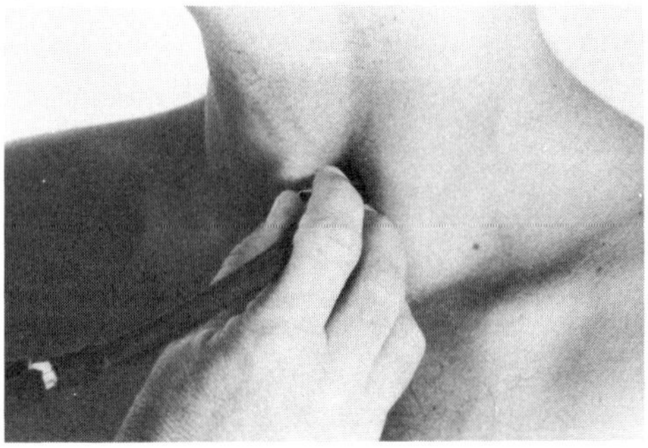

Figure 11-28.

NECK: THYROID GLAND

Introduction	The thyroid contains two lateral lobes and a median band of tissue, the isthmus. The thyroid gland lies at the level of the second and third tracheal rings.
Thyroglossal Ducts and Cysts	In some persons, a remnant of the connection between the thyroid and the embryonic pharynx (the pyramidal lobe) extends upward from the isthmus. The remnant of the connection between the posterior tongue and the thyroid may persist as the <u>thyroglossal duct</u>, which can extend from the <u>foramen caecum</u> of the tongue to the pyramidal lobe. In other instances, part of the duct may enlarge to form a <u>thyroglossal cyst</u>.

Examination

STEP	ACTION	NOTES
1	Inspection	
	a. With the patient seated, and the neck extended, inspect the neck.	a. The thyroid gland is <u>not</u> normally visible, but a goiter (enlarged thyroid) or thyroid nodule may be seen.
	b. Ask the patient to swallow.	b. The thyroid ascends with the trachea during swalling; any enlargement that moves upward is likely to be within or adherent to the thyroid.
2	Auscultation. Listen carefully with the bell of the stethoscope directly over the thyroid.	A <u>systolic bruit</u> almost always indicates diffuse toxic goiter. The sound is caused by increased blood flow to the thyroid. See Figure 11-28.
3	Palpation.	
	a. Stand behind the seated patient.	a. The patient must be relaxed and comfortable, with his or her chin lowered.
	b. Place your fingers anteriorly, with the tips over the thyroid and with the thumbs resting on the posterior portion of the neck.	

(Continued)

NECK: THYROID GLAND, Continued

STEP	ACTION	NOTES
	c. Identify the cricoid cartilage in the midline of the neck, just below the laryngeal cartilage, and find the superior border of the isthmus just inferiorly.	c. Thyroid tissue is almost always within 1 cm of the cricoid cartilage.
	d. With the fingertips of both hands resting on either side of the trachea, ask the patient to swallow.	d. Swallowing yields a general impression of the overall size and configuration of the isthmus and the medial aspects of the lateral lobes.
	e. To examine the right lobe and isthmus, tilt the head to the right, but keep the chin down.	
	f. Place the fingertips of your right hand behind the patient's right sternocleidomastoid muscle, while the fingertips of your left hand gently displace the trachea to the right.	
	g. Ask the patient to swallow, and assess the extreme right lateral border of the thyroid.	
	h. Repeat the previous maneuver while placing the fingertips of the right hand anterior to the right sternocleidomastoid muscle, and retracting it slightly posteriorly.	h. This permits evaluation of the main body of the lateral lobe.
	i. Examine the left lobe in a similar fashion.	i. The thyroid may also be palpated while the examiner is standing in front of the patient. An anterior approach is preferred by some examiners, but, in general, it is less satisfactory for beginners.

(Continued)

NECK: THYROID GLAND, Continued

Record Abnormal Nodules

The examiner should feel as much of the thyroid gland as possible, and should record the:
- size
- configuration
- consistency
- presence and number of abnormal nodules

Size Evaluated by Weight

Thyroid size is usually evaluated in comparison to a normal gland; a popular method is to estimate the weight of the thyroid in grams.

> NOTE: The normal thyroid gland weighs less than 25 g, with the right and left lobes weighing 10 g each and the isthmus weighing approximately 5 g.

If the right lobe is estimated to be two times normal size (20 g) and the left lobe and isthmus are normal (15 g), the overall estimated weight is about 35 g. This estimate is useful to the examiner who needs to determine whether the size of the thyroid gland changes with time.

Diffuse Goiter

The thyroid may become diffusely or focally enlarged: Diffuse goiter may be due to:
- diffuse toxic goiter (Graves' disease)
- iodine deficiency
- chronic lymphocytic thyroiditis (Hashimoto's thyroiditis)
- rare congenital thyroid enzyme defects

In most cases of diffuse goiter, the thyroid is smooth or slightly irregular (particularly with thyroiditis) and firm. It moves upward freely with swallowing, and its right lobe is often larger than the left.

Multinodular Goiter

Multinodular goiter (multiple palpable nodules) may result from:
- simple colloid nodular goiter
- thyroiditis
- neoplasms

(Continued)

NECK: THYROID GLAND, Continued

Single Thyroid Nodule

An isolated thyroid nodule may often be felt within an otherwise normal thyroid gland. Such a nodule may be:
- a cyst
- a benign or malignant neoplasm
- an area of hemorrhage

These nodules vary greatly in:
- consistency
- size
- configuration

Tender Nodule

A tender nodule indicates subacute thyroiditis or recent hemorrhage into an adenoma or carcinoma. If thyroid enlargement or a nodule is found, search for lymphadenopathy in the surrounding area.

Tracheal Deformity

Tracheal deformity or displacement can be caused by goiter. Stridor or hoarseness usually indicates invasion by malignant neoplasm.

Restricted Movement

Restriction of gland movement is a strong indication of malignant neoplasm.

Posterior Palpation

To use a posterior approach for palpation of the thyroid (Fig. 11-29):
- Palpate the body of the right lobe with the right second and third fingertips; repeat for the left lobe, using the left second and third fingers.
- Palpate the medial thyroid and the isthmus in the same manner.
- Palpate the lateral edges of each lobe.

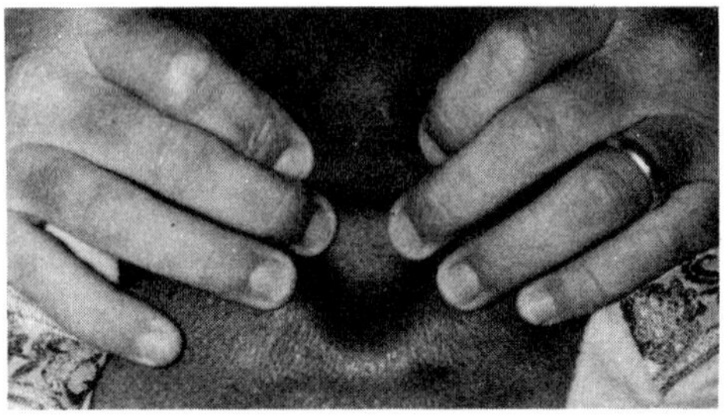

Figure 11-29.

NECK: EVALUATION OF A MASS

Introduction

The following characteristics of a neck mass should be determined:

- size
- site
- shape
- surface (smooth, lobulated)
- consistency
- mobility
- tenderness
- appearance of the overlying skin
- presence of pulsation or bruit

Site

The site of the mass gives some indication of the structure that is involved and of the area that is drained by the involved nodes.

EXAMPLES:

- Location in the submandibular triangle may indicate origin in the submandibular gland.
- Proximity to the thyroid lobe may indicate a thyroid tumor.
- Nodes high in the posterior triangle may indicate disease in the nasopharynx.
- Submandibular lymph node enlargement may indicate disease in the oral cavity.

Example of Submandibular Mass

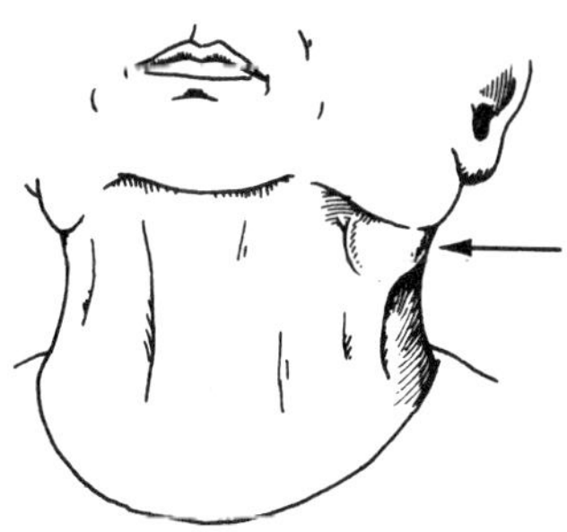

(Continued)

NECK: EVALUATION OF A MASS, Continued

Consistency	A solid mass usually indicates inflammation or neoplasm. Enlarged nodes secondary to metastatic carcinoma usually feel stony-hard. Firm or rubbery nodes usually indicate chronic inflammation or lymphoma.
Mobility	If a mass moves when the patient swallows, it is usually attached to or in the thyroid. Immobile lymph nodes indicate tumor invasion, one of the criteria for inoperable disease. Tumors of the carotid body usually move easily from side to side, but are restricted in upward and downward movement because they are attached to the carotid bulb.
Tenderness	Tenderness on palpation usually indicates acute inflammation.
Appearance of Overlying Skin	Erythema (redness) of the overlying skin indicates an inflammed lymph node or abscess. Fixation of the skin to the mass indicates malignant neoplasm.
Presence of Pulsation or Bruit	A pulsatile mass, or the presence of a bruit on auscultation, usually indicates: • vascular anomaly • aneurysm • vascular tumor • increased blood flow through the thyroid
Cystic Masses	Cystic masses are always benign. The presence of fluid within a mass may be determined by testing for fluctuance.

STEP	ACTION
1	Grasp the swelling between the thumb and middle fingers of one hand. See Figure 11-30.
2	Press the index finger of the opposite hand firmly on the surface of the mass.

(Continued)

NECK: EVALUATION OF A MASS, Continued

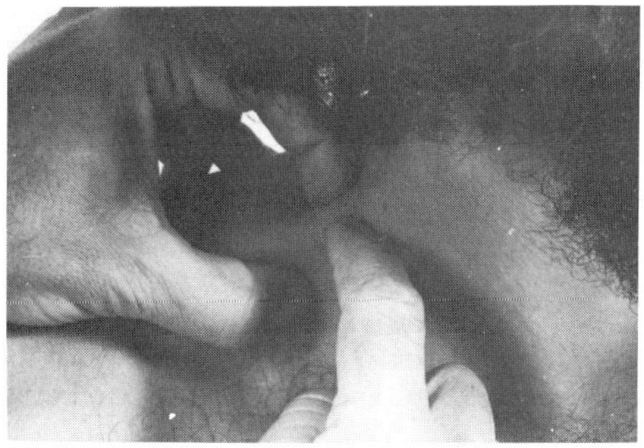

Figure 11-30.

If the mass is filled with fluid, the pressure with the index finger will cause the sides to expand, and the movement will be felt by the thumb and middle fingers of the opposite hand. Transillumination in a darkened room will sometimes reveal the presence of fluid.

Types of Cystic Masses

Cystic masses are usually:
- abscesses
- branchial cleft cysts
- thyroglossal duct cysts

TYPE OF CYSTIC MASS	DESCRIPTION
abscess	characterized by tenderness and erythema of the overlying skin
branchial cleft cyst	occurs in the lateral aspect of the neck, deep to the sternomastoid muscle
thyroglossal duct cyst	found near the midline of the anterior part of the neck along the path of descent of the thyroid gland from the base of the tongue (foramen caecum) to the neck

NOTE: Thyroglossal duct cysts move upward upon swallowing or protrusion of the tongue.

(Continued)

NECK: EVALUATION OF A MASS, Continued

Aneurysm

Aneurysm of the carotid artery usually occurs in the region of the bifurcation of the common carotid and can be recognized by its prominent pulsations that are synchronous with the systolic pulse.

Lipomas

Lipomas (fatty tumors) are occasionally found in the neck. These swellings are fluctuant because fat is in liquid form at body temperature. Lipomas in the neck are usually indiscrete, asymptomatic swellings.

Cervical Lymphadenopathy

Cervical lymph node enlargements may be acute or chronic.

Acute Cervical Lymphadenitis

Acute cervical lymphadenitis most often results from:

- bacterial infection (secondary to tonsillitis or dental disease)
- viral infection (measles, infectious mononucleosis,)
  On palpation, acutely inflamed nodes are tender and movable. After resolution of the infection, the nodes may remain palpable (up to approximately 1 cm in diameter). Some small nodes can be felt in the neck of healthy persons.

Chronic Cervical Lymphadenopathy

Chronic cervical lymphadenopathy may be caused by either chronic inflammation (as in tuberculosis or fungal infections) or malignancy. Progressive painless enlargement of cervical nodes is often the first symptom of malignant disease; therefore, it is best to assume that a malignancy is present until other evidence is gathered.

Sentinel Node

A sentinel node in the left supraclavicular area (Virchow's node) usually indicates that malignancy has spread from a primary cancer below the clavicle, usually:

- lung
- breast
- esophagus
- stomach

NECK: SALIVARY GLANDS

Parotid Gland

The parotid gland lies anterior to the external ear, overlying the ascending ramus of the mandible. The upper gland extends to the zygomatic arch. Inferiorly, the gland lies between the angle of the mandible and the mastoid tip. The facial nerve runs through the substance of the the gland dividing it arbitrarily into superficial and deep lobes. The parotid duct pierces the cheek to open in the upper buccal sulcus opposite the second molar tooth. Unless enlarged, the parotid gland is usually not palpable. See Figure 11-31.

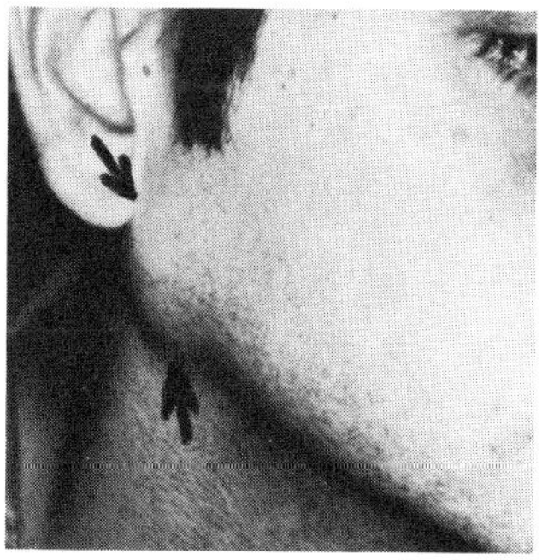

Figure 11-31.

Submandibular Gland

The submandibular gland lies in the submandibular triangle overlying the anterior and posterior bellies of the digastric muscle. Its deep lobe extends between the mylohyoid muscle and the floor of the mouth. The submandibular duct opens at the apex of a small papilla situated just lateral to the frenulum of the tongue. The gland may be best palpated by bimanual examination. See Figure 11-32.

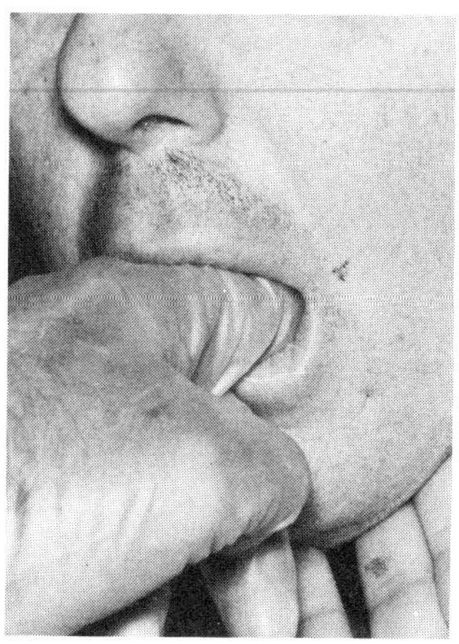

Figure 11-32.

NECK: SALIVARY GLANDS, Continued

Sublingual Gland	The sublingual gland can be observed as a fullness along the anterior floor of the mouth, immediately posterior to the opening of the submandibular duct.
Mumps	Salivary gland enlargement occurs most commonly as a result of mumps. The parotid is affected most often, and tender, diffuse enlargement of the gland results. The infection may be unilateral or bilateral, and occasionally the submandibular glands may be involved.
Calculi	Calculi (stones) may occur in the parotid or submandibular ducts and produce intermittent swelling of the gland (especially after meals), and a secondary bacterial infection in the gland may ensue.
Suppurative Parotitis	Suppurative infection may occur in dehydrated debilitated patients because of poor oral hygiene or ductal obstruction. The gland is swollen, painful, and tender, and pus may emerge from the ducts.
Tumors	Neoplasms may arise in the salivary glands, usually in the parotid. In general, they are firm, discrete, nontender, slowly growing masses. Tumors that originate in the minor salivary glands appear as firm submucosal swellings in the oral cavity or oropharynx.
Systemic Diseases	Diffuse enlargement of salivary glands may occur in a variety of systemic diseases: • sarcoidosis • Sjögren's syndrome • alcoholism • diabetes

SELF-ASSESSMENT

1. What is the normal position of the eyelids?

2. a. Name the extraocular muscles and their innervation.
   b. Diagram the cardinal movements of gaze with positions labeled for appropriate muscles.
   c. Name the muscle for lid movement and its innervation.
   d. Name the nerve responsible for forehead movement.

3. State the normal diameter ratio of retinal artery to vein.

4. Name six landmarks of the tympanic membrane.

5. State the innervation of pupillary constriction.

6. State the significance of the numerator and denominator in visual acuity 20/200.

7. Define anisocoria.

8. State the proper orientation of the pinnae for visualization of external ear canal in:
   a. adult
   b. child

9. Describe the location of the opening of the parotid duct.

10. Name the papillae that lie on the V-shaped row at the posterior two thirds of the tongue.

11. Name the cranial nerve responsible for sensory innervation of the:
    a. anterior two thirds of tongue
    b. posterior third of tongue

12. Describe the location for palpation of the carotid pulse.

13. State five characteristics used to describe lymph nodes.

14. State the upper limit of normal size for lymph nodes in the neck.

15. Name six areas in neck to examine for lymph nodes.

CHAPTER TWELVE

Thorax, Lungs, and Breasts

James C. Guckian, M.D.

INTRODUCTION

The Physical Examination and Chest Roetgenogram

Examination of the chest and lungs is mandatory for detection of various subclinical diseases and for formulation of an accurate diagnosis of symptomatic cardiorespiratory disease. Chest roentgenography may be essential, but it cannot supplant a physical examination. In fact, the findings on the x-ray film can be interpreted correctly only when correlated with findings from the history and physical examination; moreover, a physical examination may detect abnormalities that cannot be detected on the x-ray films.

THORAX: TOPOGRAPHICAL ANATOMY

Lines of Reference

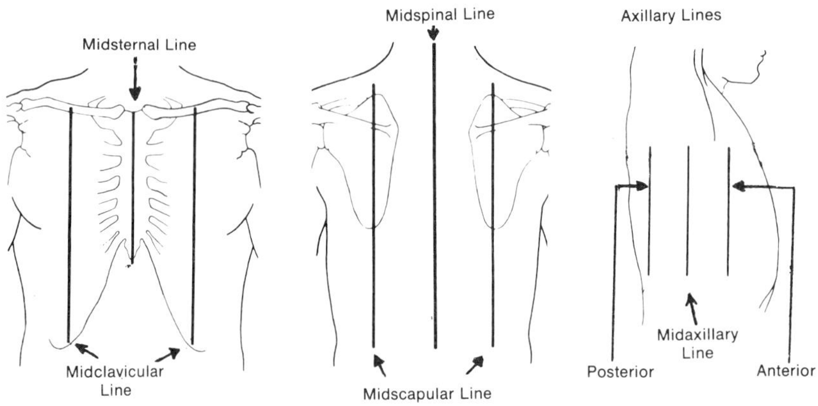

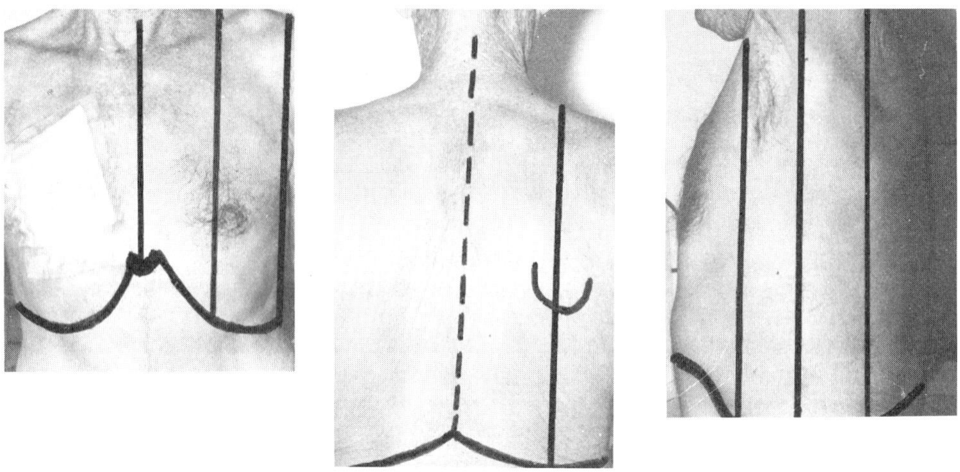

Location

Descriptions of the locations of abnormalities should include:

- the number of centimeters medial or lateral to the lines reference
- the specific interspaces between the lines of reference

  NOTE: Although anatomic regions of the thorax (e.g., scapular, interscapular) have been used to locate abnormalities, localization using lines of reference is more accurate.

(Continued)

THORAX: TOPOGRAPHICAL ANATOMY, Continued

WALL	REFERENCE LINE	LOCATION
anterior	• midsternal • midclavicular (right and left)	• middle of sternum • runs downward from the midpoint of each clavicle
	NOTE: The nipple is *not* a satisfactory landmark because its location varies, even in males.	
posterior	• midspinal (or vertebral) • scapular (right and left)	• runs down the posterior spinous processes of the vertebrae • runs parallel to the spine though the inferior angle of the scapula
	NOTE: Because the scapula is mobile, the scapular line should relate only to the position of the scapula when patients are erect, with their arms at their sides.	
lateral	• anterior axillary	• runs down from the origin of the anterior axillary fold along the anterolateral aspect of the chest
	• posterior axillary	• runs down along the posterolateral wall of the thorax (continues the posterior axillary fold)
	• midaxillary	• runs down from the apex of the axilla, midway between the above two lines

Manubriosternal Junction (Angle of Louis)	A useful additional landmark, the manubriosternal junction is an angulation of the sternum that corresponds to the anterior end of the second rib and is a good starting point for counting ribs and interspaces. In addition, it indicates the location of two other important structures that lie at the same level: • the bifurcation of the trachea • the upper level of the cardiac atria
Vertebra Prominens	The vertebra prominens (seventh cervical vertebra), found at the posterior base of the neck, is useful in identifying the thoracic vertebrae and posterior ribs.

THORAX: UNDERLYING ANATOMY

Lungs

Anatomical Relationships of Lungs

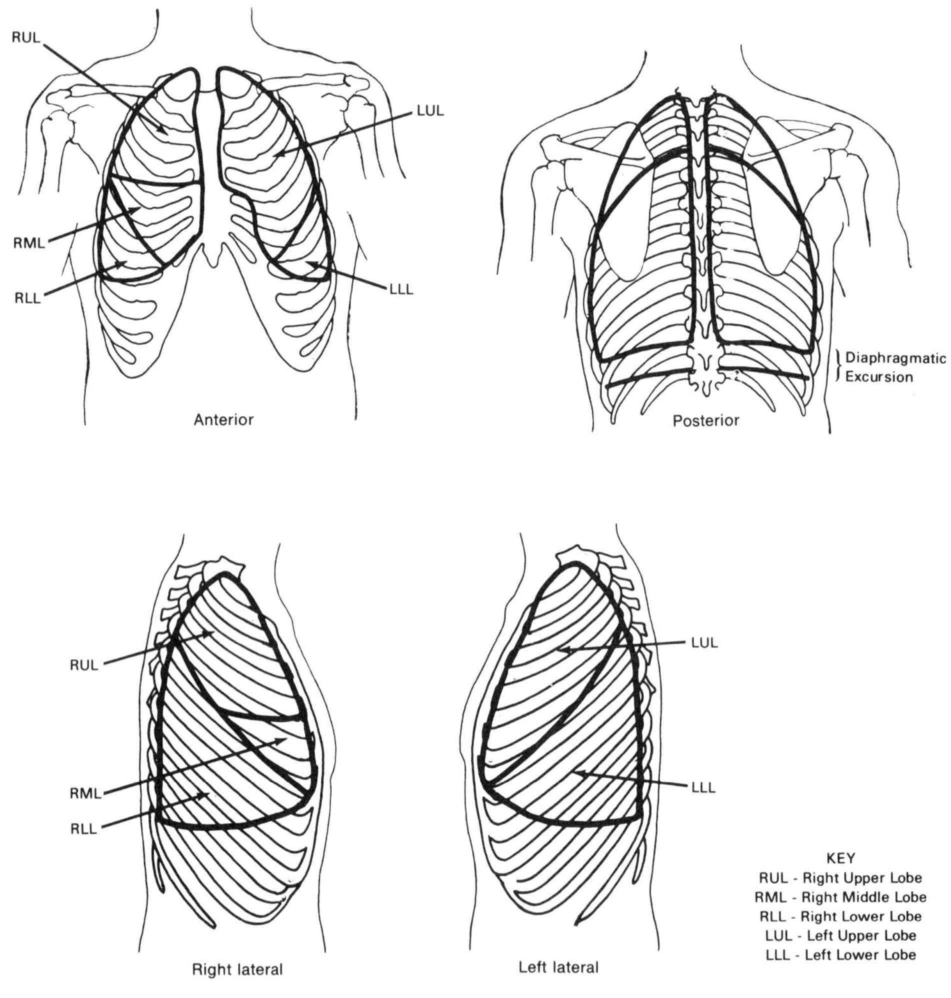

(Continued)

THORAX: UNDERLYING ANATOMY, Continued

Introduction

A physical examination of the chest requires knowledge of the location of the underlying thoracic structures and the structures in the upper abdomen.

Underlying Structures

STRUCTURES	LOCATION
apices of lungs	extend for about 3 cm above the clavicle on each side
right oblique fissure	extends from about the fourth thoracic vertebra downward and laterally; continues anteriorly and medially to the chondrocostal junction of the sixth rib; in the anterior half of the chest, the fissure separates the middle and lower lobes
middle lobe	lies between the upper and lower lobes, but is found only in the anterior half of the thorax
horizontal fissure	begins posterior to the midaxillary line at the fifth rib and then runs anteriorly in a horizontal plane to the third interspace
left oblique fissure	lies between the upper and lower lobes on the left and is located by a line drawn from the fourth thoracic vertebra, downward and laterally, which continues anteriorly and medially to the sixth chondrocostal junction

(Continued)

THORAX: UNDERLYING ANATOMY, Continued

Summary

- The anterior aspect of the right portion of the chest is composed of the upper and middle lobes; the upper lobe lies beneath the major portion of the left anterior hemithorax.
- The lower lobes represent only a small anterolateral and inferior portion of the hemithoraces.
- Posteriorly, a large proportion of the thorax is occupied by the lower lobes; only a small area of the upper lobes is located in the superior portion.

Warning!

In interpreting chest roentgenograms, inexperienced examiners often assume that any lesion seen in the upper part of the lung fields is located in the upper lobes; to avoid this error, recall the heights to which the superior segments of the lower lobes extend.

Dome of the Diaphragm

On the right, the dome of the diaphragm is about at the level of the fifth rib, in the midclavicular line. On the left, the dome of the diaphragm is about 2 cm to 3 cm lower.

THORAX: INSPECTION

Introduction

Inspection of the chest requires that:

- the patient be stripped to the waist
- the room be warm
- the lighting be good
- the examiner have a thorough knowledge of topographic anatomy

NOTE: Inspection should not be neglected, even though auscultation, palpation, and percussion are frequently more revealing.

Position of the Patient

Inspection is usually conducted with the patient seated. Differences in motility may be observed by looking from the side across the anterior and posterior aspect of the chest. The patient should be absolutely straight, even if supine.

Procedure

STEP	ACTION	NOTES
1	Observe the general condition and musculoskeletal development.	The size and shape of the normal thorax vary greatly. It may be difficult to differentiate normal variations from abnormal changes.
2	Observe the skin.	The skin of the thorax should be smooth, supple, and not excessively dry or oily. The adult male usually has a variable amount of hair; a complete lack of hair may indicate some disorder. Spider nevi on the chest and shoulders may indicate cirrhosis of the liver. Seborrheic dermititis often occurs on the anterior portion of the thorax.
3	Observe the anteroposterior diameter of the thorax. See Figure 12-1.	In patients with obstructive pulmonary disease, the anteroposterior diameter may be as great as (or even greater than) the transverse diameter. See Figure 12-2.
4	Observe the general slope of the ribs.	In normal subjects, the ribs are at about a 45° angle in relation to the spine; in patients with emphysema, the ribs are more nearly horizontal.

(Continued)

THORAX: INSPECTION, Continued

STEP	ACTION	NOTES
5	Observe the width of the costal angle.	The width is less than 90°and widens during inspiration because of lateral expansion of the thorax. In patients with emphysema, this angle is wider and does not vary much with respiration.
6	Look for asymmetry.	One side may be: • larger because of tension pneumothorax, pleural effusion, or partial (ball-valve) bronchial obstruction • smaller because of atelectasis or unilateral fibrosis If asymmetry is present, the abnormal side will move less than the other.

7	Look for retraction or bulging of interspaces.	• Retraction of the interspaces, which can be observed during inspiration, indicates obstruction of inflow of air into the airways.
		• Bulging of interspaces may result from a large pleural effusion or pneumothorax. It is often seen during the forced expiration of a patient with emphysema or asthma. Bulging may sometimes result from:
		  • tumor
		  • aortic aneurysm
		  • cardiac enlargement in infancy and childhood due to congenital heart disease
		• Normally, the two sides of the chest move synchronously and expand equally.
		• Asymmetry becomes much more obvious with forced inspiration; therefore, expansion should be observed during both quiet and deep breathing.

(Continued)

THORAX: INSPECTION, Continued

STEP	ACTION	NOTES
8	Examine the posterior part of the thorax.	Hair growth is usually less abundant than on the anterior aspect. Acne is often observed. The location of the scapulae and their range of motion should be observed. The spine should be straight, although when the patient is viewed from the side, a slight anterior concavity of the thoracic spine is normally seen.

Normal Findings

- One shoulder is often slightly lower than the other in normal persons.
- A depression of both the supraclavicular and infraclavicular areas is normal.
- The two hemithoraces are nearly symmetric. A right-handed person may have more muscular development on the right side than on the left; a left-handed person may have more on the left.
- The anterior hemithoraces, when viewed from above or from the side, project beyond the sternum, so that some depression exists in the midline between the sides of the chest wall.
- On inspiration, the anterior thoracic wall moves both upward and anteriorly as well as expanding outward and laterally.
- The scapular prominences are symmetrically located on the posterior thoracic wall. The scapulae are applied firmly to the underlying chest wall. Some depression exists between the medial scapular borders and the spine (the interscapular spaces).

Abnormal Findings

- Pectus carinatum: the sternum protrudes instead of being lower than the adjacent hemithoraces.
- Pectus excavatum: the sternum is abnormally depressed between each of the anterior hemithoraces.
  NOTE The sternum may be displaced so far posteriorly that it interferes with the function of the heart. See Figure 12-3.
- Kyphosis: an exaggerated anteroposterior curvature of the spine (hunchback, or humpback) (see Fig. 12-4)
- Scoliosis: a lateral curvature of the spine, causing widened intercostal spaces on the convex side and crowding of the ribs on the concave side; when

(Continued)

THORAX: INSPECTION, Continued

accompanied by kyphosis, it is called kyphoscoliosis. See Figure 12-5.

- Poker spine: an abnormally straight and stiff vertebral column, caused by ankylosing spondylitis

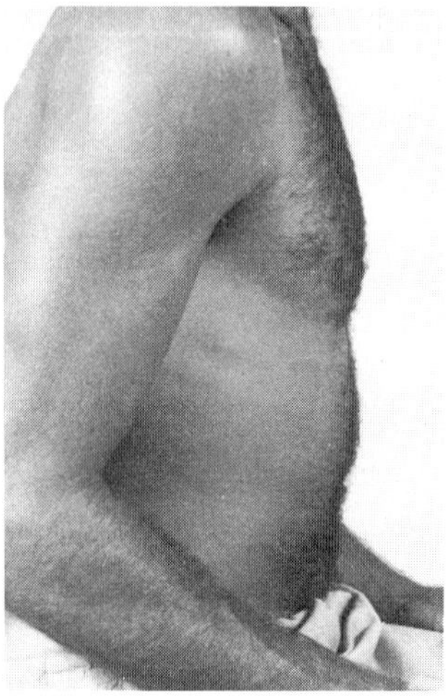

Figure 12-1.

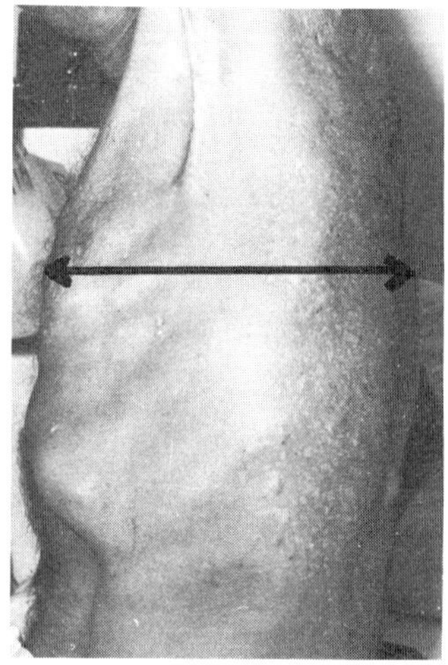

Figure 12-2.

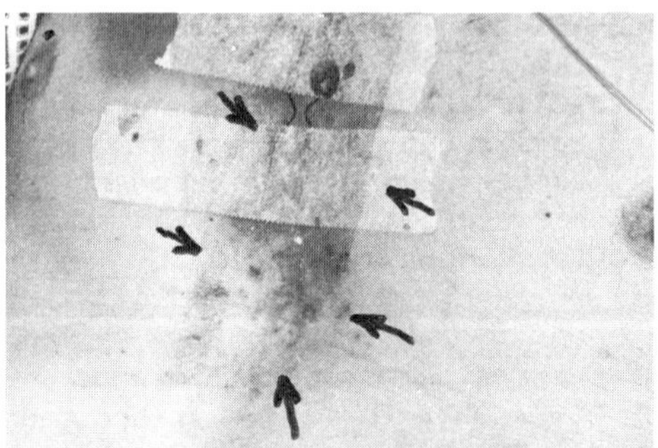

Figure 12-3.

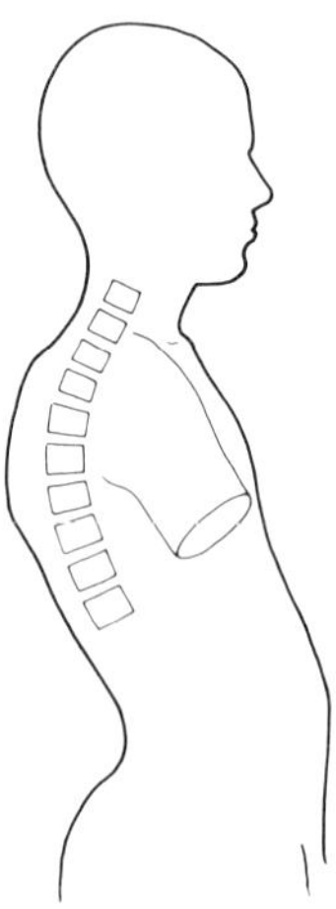

Kyphosis

Figure 12-4.

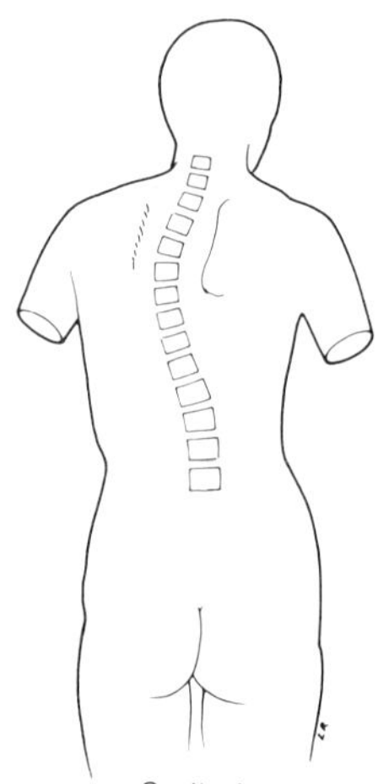

Figure 12-5.

Scoliosis

LUNGS: RESPIRATION

Introduction	Several abnormalities in breathing exist. To be more precise, examination detects abnormalities in ventilation, that is, the mechanical act of air exchange in inspiration and expiration.
Dyspnea	Dyspnea is not an abnormality of ventilation, but is a sensation of difficulty in breathing, often described as "shortness of breath" or "not getting enough air." Although dyspnea is a subjective symptom, examiners may observe tachypnea and hyperpnea (see below).
Inspiratory Stridor	Inspiratory stridor consists of low-pitched or crowing inspiratory sounds that occur when the trachea or major bronchi are obstructed because of: • tumor (intrinsic or extrinic) • foreign body • severe laryngotracheitis (for example diphtheria) • crushing injury The inward flow of air is impeded, and inspiratory retraction of the intercostal spaces may also occur.
Expiratory Stridor	Expiratory stridor, produced by obstruction in the bronchioles and smaller bronchi, may be due to: • asthma • bronchitis • bronchiolar edema • obstructive emphysema Expiration is prolonged because of the obstruction of the outflow of air.
Bradypnea	Bradypnea is abnormally slow ventilation.
Apnea	Apnea is temporary cessation of ventilation.
Tachypnea	Tachypnea is an abnormal increase in the rate of ventilation.

(Continued)

LUNGS: RESPIRATION, Continued

Hyperpnea	Hyperpnea is an increase in the depth, and perhaps the rate, of ventilation. The overall result is increased tidal volume and minute volume of ventilation.
Hyperventilation	Hyperventilation occurs when ventilation is greater than the body needs, and a low arterial carbon dioxide content results (diagnosis depends upon analysis of blood gases). It results from tachypnea and hyperpnea brought about by: • metabolic acidosis • vigorous exercise • some emotional states • lung disease This condition is not synonymous with hyperpnea, in which increased ventilation may be appropriate for body demands.
Periodic Respiration (Cheyne-Stokes Respiration)	In periodic respirations, periods of increasing (rate and depth) ventilation are followed immediately by shallower and shallower respiration until ventilation ceases. This period of apnea may last for several seconds. The patient often sleeps during the period of apnea, but becomes restless again as respiration resumes. Although periodic respiration sometimes occurs in normal persons when asleep, if usually indicates: • central nervous system disease • heart failure
Stertorous Respiration	Stertorous respiration (death rattle) often occurs in comatose patients just before they die. Rattling and gurgling sounds are produced by the passage of air through secretions in the main bronchi and trachea of patients so ill that their reflexes are no longer functional.
Sighing Respiration	Sighing respiration occurs when the normal ventilatory rhythm is interrupted often by a deep inspiration, followed by a prolonged expiration that is accompanied by audible sighing. A sign of anxiety or emotional distress, the disorder is almost never caused by organic disease. Sighing is a normal physiologic event, of course, so the diagnosis should be made only if more than two or three sighs per minute are observed.

(Continued)

LUNGS: RESPIRATION, Continued

Ataxic Respiration

Ataxic ventilation, a rare disorder, is characterized by a gross irregularity of:
- rate
- rhythm
- depth

It occurs most frequently in severe diseases of the central nervous system and indicates a poor prognosis.

Illustrative Spirograms

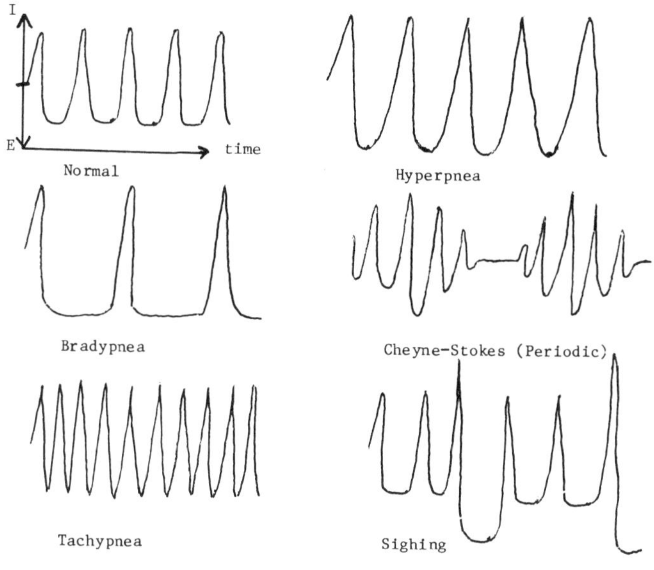

LUNGS: PALPATION

Introduction — Differences in expansion of the hemithoraces may be more easily discerned by palpation then by inspection.

Detecting Variations — Variations in expansion are detectable (on the anterior or posterior surface) when the examiner's hands are placed over the lower lateral aspect of the chest, with the thumbs along the costal margin pointing toward the xiphoid process anteriorly or meeting posteriorly in the midline. The expansion can be felt by the movement of the inverted "V" formed by the thumbs. See Figure 12-6.

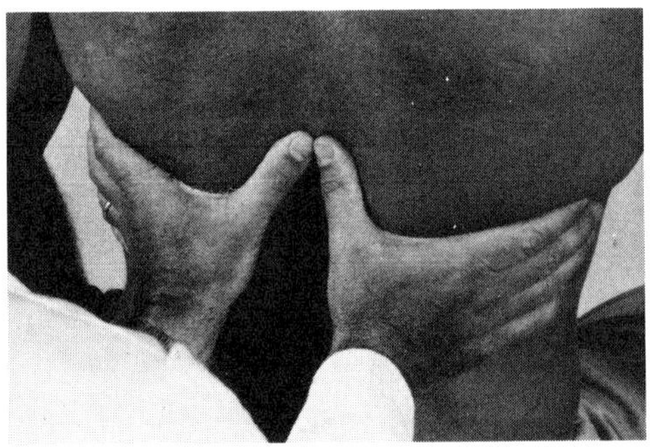

Figure 12-6.

Test Conditions — Expansion should be tested during both quiet and deep inspiration.

Asymmetric Expansion — The causes of asymmetric expansion were listed under Thorax: Inspection in this chapter.

LUNGS: VOCAL FREMITUS

Definition

Vocal fremitus, a palpable vibration of the throacic wall produced by phonation, should be evaluated carefully in patients with suspected respiratory problems. The vibrations are produced by air forced through partially open vocal cords, which set the chest wall in motion; the resulting vibrations are felt by the hand of the examiner.

Elicitation

The patient should be instructed to:

- repeat the following:
  - "ninety-nine"

  OR
  - "e-e-e"
- speak with uniform intensity, loud enough so that the fremitus can be felt

Detection

The examiner places his or her hand against the patient's chest wall.

BY USING	SOUND IS COMPARED
two hands	simultaneously, on both sides
one hand	alternately, by moving the hand from one side to the other

Various positions of the hands against the wall of the chest may be used:

- the palmar aspects of the fingers are placed against the chest wall: one hand or both hands (A).
- ulnar aspect of hand, with fingers extended (B)
- ulnar aspect of closed fist

(Continued)

LUNGS: VOCAL FREMITUS, Continued

A

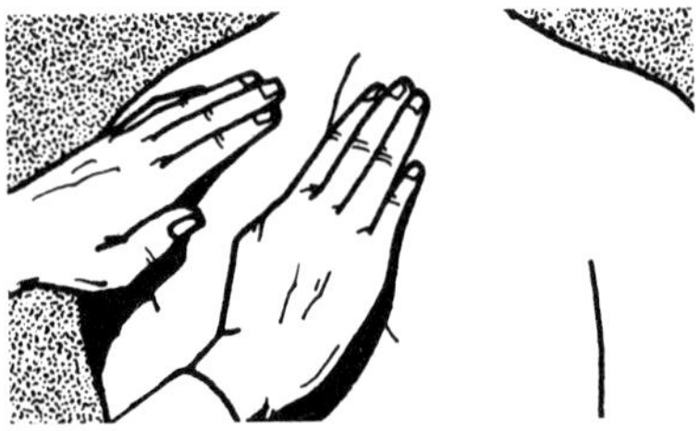

B

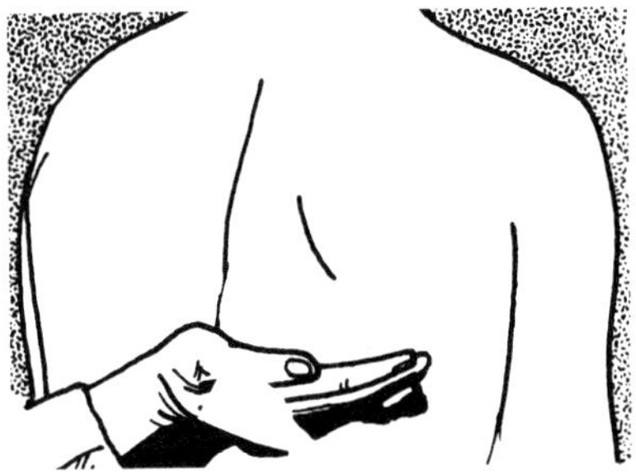

Intensity

In normal individuals, the intensity of vocal fremitus depends upon several factors:

FACTOR	PALPATION OF FREMITUS
nature of voice	• The intensity of fremitus increases with increased loudness of the spoken word. • Fremitus is more pronounced in subjects with deep voices (men) because the low tones, with their lower frequency and greater amplitude, produce greater vibrations of the chest wall.
thickness of thoracic wall	Subcutaneous tissue decreases the fremitus; thus, it will be more intense in a thin person than in an obese patient.

(Continued)

LUNGS: VOCAL FREMITUS, Continued

FACTOR	PALPATION OF FREMITUS
relation of bronchi to chest wall	Intensity is: • greatest in regions of the thorax in which large bronchi are closest to the thoracic wall; it becomes less intense as the distance from the major bronchi increases • maximal over the upper thorax anteriorly and along the course of the trachea and major bronchi posteriorly (between the scapulae and in the first and second interspaces just lateral to the sternum) • minimal at the bases

Abnormalities

Vocal fremitus, when abnormal, may be:

- increased
- decreased
- absent

CONDITION	FREMITUS	COMMENT
increased density of the lung because of consolidation (as in lobar pneumonia or hemorrhagic infarction)	increased, because liquid (pus, blood) conducts vibrations better than air	To produce an increase in fremitus, the area of consolidation must: • be connected with a patent bronchus • extend to the surface of the lung
solid or liquid medium between the lung and chest wall, as in: • fluid (effusion, pus, blood) in the pleural space • neoplasm in the pleural space	decreased or absent	The decrease or absence results from: • weaker transmission or production of vocal sounds • the presence of a poor conductor of vibrations through which the vibrations must pass
obstructed major bronchus	decreased or absent	Air flow through the bronchus is interrupted, so the chest wall does not vibrate.

LUNGS: OTHER TYPES OF FREMITUS

Pleural Friction	Pleural friction fremitus: • is producted when inflamed pleural surfaces rub together during respiration • produces a "grating" sensation that occurs with the respiratory excursion • may be palpable in both phases of respiration but can sometimes be felt only during inspiration
Rhoncal	Rhoncal fremitus is: • produced by passage of air through thick exudate, secretions, or an area of stenosis in the trachea or major bronchi • unlike friction fremitus, because rhonchal fremitus can be relieved by coughing or mechanical aspiration of the large airways, clearing the secretions from the tracheobronchial tree

LUNGS: PERCUSSION

Definition

Percussion involves "tapping" or "thumping" parts of the body to produce sounds.

Basis of Percussion

When the chest is percussed, all its contents are set into motion, and vibrations pass from the chest wall through the air to the examiner's ear. The nature of the sound produced depends chiefly upon the structures immediately underlying the area percussed. An air-filled structure (lung) will produce a tone that is different from that produced by a solid structure (heart or liver).

Limitations

Sound vibrations produced by percussion probably do not penetrate more than about 4 cm to 5 cm below the surface; therefore, solid masses deep in the chest cannot be outlined by percussion. In addition, since a lesion must be several centimeters in diameter to be detectable by percussion, only large abnormalities can be located.

Description

Percussion is done by striking the dorsal distal phalanx of the third finger of one hand that is held against the thorax with the distal tuft of the flexed middle finger of the other hand.

Procedure

STEP	ACTION
1	Press the distal phalanx of the middle finger of one hand (the left if the examiner is right-handed) firmly against the chest wall, with the palm and other fingers held off the skin.
2	With the tip of the flexed middle finger of the other hand, strike a short, quick blow at the base of the terminal phalanx of the finger held against the chest wall. NOTE: The action is at the wrist. Use the wrist, not the elbow or shoulder. Keep the elbow and shoulder rigid.

(Continued)

LUNGS: PERCUSSION, Continued

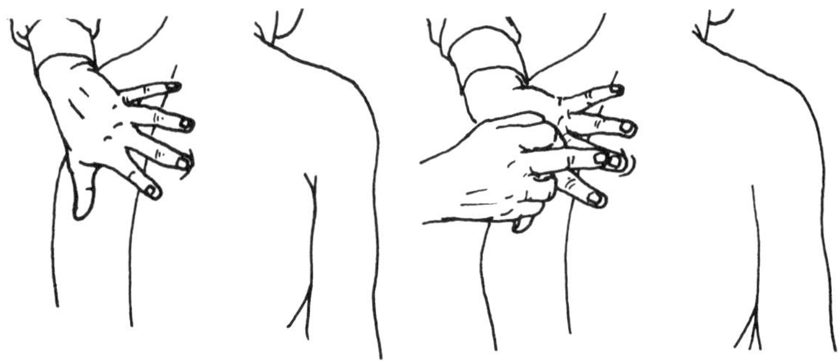

Practice Methods

When percussion is performed properly, the forearm is stationary, and all movement is executed from the wrist. The maneuver may be practiced in two ways.

Method I

STEP	ACTION
1	Place the right hand and forearm flat on a table.
2	Cock the hand back at the wrist.
3	Strike the table a quick blow with the tip of the flexed middle finger; return immediately to the position of the "cocked wrist," ready to strike again.

Method II

STEP	ACTION
1	Grasp the distal part of the right forearm with the left hand to prevent any movement of the right forearm.
2	Cock the wrist.
3	Strike a sharp, quick blow with the tip of the middle finger, and return to the "cocked wrist" position.

(Continued)

LUNGS: PERCUSSION, Continued

Important!

For percussion to be most effective:

- The distal phalanx of the finger must be pressed firmly on the chest wall to obtain a clear note.
- The striking finger must strike the other finger only instantaneously; it must be withdrawn immediately.
- The examiner must be sensitive to the vibratory sensations and sounds that are received from the chest wall.
- The examiner must compare one side of the thorax with the other side.

Use Light Percussion

The momentum of the striking finger determines the portion of lung that will vibrate. A light blow causes less vibration in the deeper and more distant portions and makes possible sharper localization of changes in the lung underlying the area being considered.

Posterior Wall

For percussion of the posterior wall, the patient's head should be inclined forward and the forearms rested on the thighs. This posture moves the scapulae laterally. The examination begins at the apices. This area is bounded medially by intrinsic neck muscles and laterally by the scapula. Percussion is continued downward to the bases, alternating side to side, where the location of each hemidiaphragm is ascertained. See Figure 12-7.

Anterior Wall

The anterior thoracic wall is examined with the patient supine. The upper, middle, and lower interspaces are percussed, with the two sides being compared. See Figure 12-8.

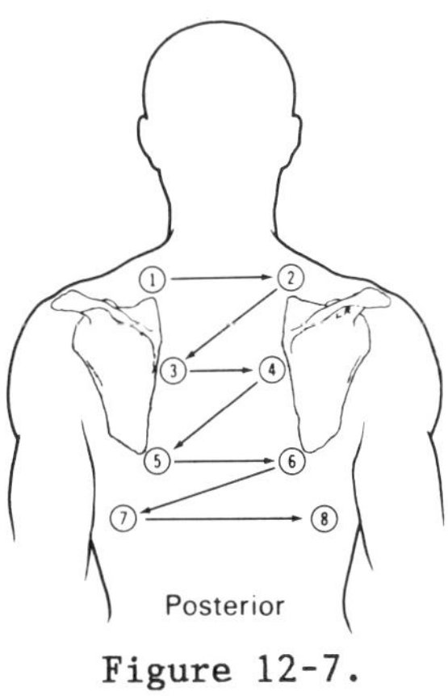

Figure 12-7.

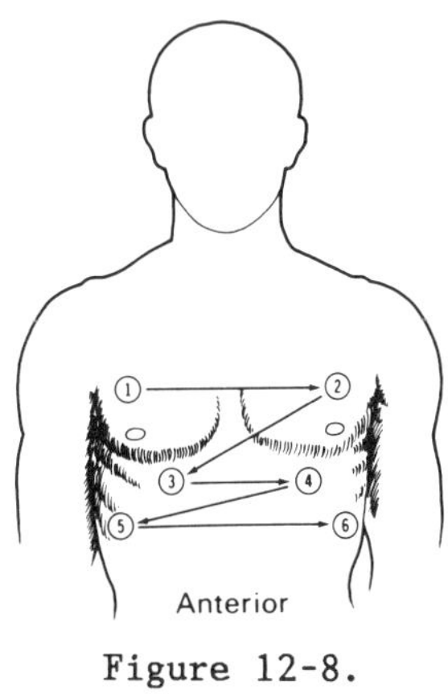

Figure 12-8.

LUNGS: PERCUSSION-- EXAMINATION

Classification The sounds produced by percussion are generally classified into the following categories.

SOUND	DESCRIPTION/EXPLANATION
resonance (normal condition over lungs)	• not loud • easy to hear • sustained • moderately low pitch The normal resonant note, which is the sound heard normally over the lungs, can be recognized only with experience.
hyper-resonance	• lower in pitch than normal resonance • well-sustained, with a "booming" character • relatively intense and easy to hear A hyperresonant note is found: • over the lungs of normal children • in adults with emphysema or pneumothroax
tympany	• relatively musical sound • usually higher pitch than that of normal resonance • only moderately well sustained • moderate or loud in intensity Tympany is produced by air in an enclosed chamber (stomach and bowel), and, in general, the greater the tension within the viscus, the higher the pitch. Tympany is heard anteriorly and laterally over the abdomen, except in the area of the liver. It does not occur in the normal chest, <u>except</u> below the dome of the left hemidiaphragm, where it is produced by underlying stomach or bowel.
dull-ness	• opposite of resonance and hyperresonance • short and not sustained • not loud (does not carry very far) • similar to a dull "thud" The finger perceives relatively little vibratory sensation; often, a sense of increased resistance is perceived (in contrast to hyperresonance). Dullness usually occurs when considerable solid or liquid medium is present in the underlying thorax (in proportion to the amount of air in the lung). Thus, dullness is found in consolidation of lung (as in pneumonia) or in cases in which fluid is present in the pleural space (transudate, pus, or blood).

(Continued)

LUNGS: PERCUSSION-- EXAMINATION, Continued

Normal Variations

Variations of the percussion note occur from patient to patient and in the same patient.

LOCATION	DESCRIPTION
apices and over the scapulae	Over these area, muscle and bone obscure resonant lung.
pectoral muscles and breasts	The percussion note is less resonant (more dull).
over the lower right ribs anteriorly	no resonance (dullness) because of the solid liver
over the lower left ribs anteriorly	a relatively tympanitic note, which results from the air-filled stomach or bowel under the hemidiaphragm

Zone of Transition

The change from resonance to dullness on the right anteriorly and from resonance to tympany on the left is not immediate; instead, there is a zone of transition. Dullness from the liver is usually observed at about the fifth interspace in the midclavicular line. The change from resonance to tympany over the left lower chest at about the sixth rib (in the midclavicular line) is also not an abrupt change. The dullness to the left of the sternum (caused by the heart) extends, in the left fifth interspace, to a point 1 cm to 2 cm medial to the midclavicular line.

(Continued)

LUNGS: PERCUSSION-- EXAMINATION, Continued

Percussion Notes

The diagram below illustrates normal percussion sounds elicited over the anterior thorax.

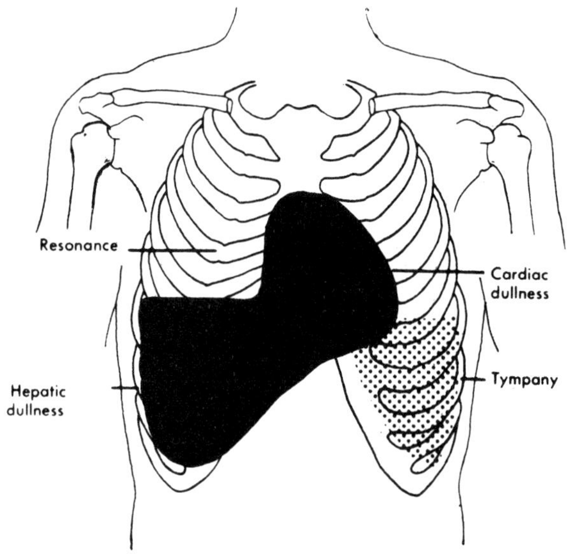

Diaphragmatic Excursion

The range of motion of the diaphragm may be estimated by percussion:

STEP	ACTION
1	Instruct the seated patient to take a deep breath and hold it.
2	Determine the lower margin of resonance-dullness (the level of the diaphragm) by percussing downward until a definite change in the percussion note is heard.
3	After instructing the patient to breath out as much as possible and to hold his or her breath, repeat the percussion.

(Continued)

LUNGS: PERCUSSION-- EXAMINATION, Continued

The distance between the levels at which the tone change occurs indicates the diaphragmatic excursion. Each hemidiaphragm is examined.

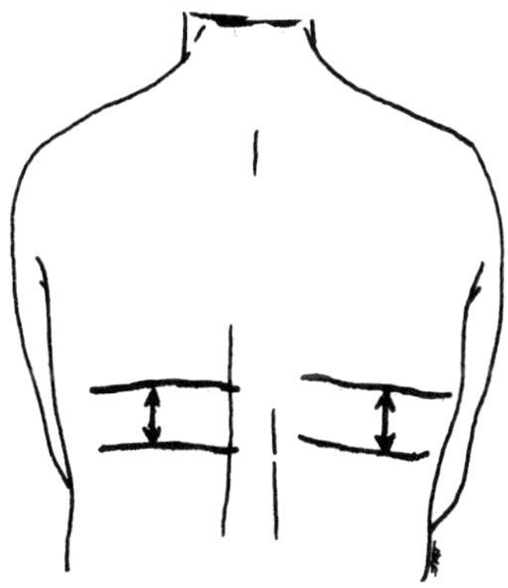

- The normal diaphragmatic excursion is about 3 cm to 4 cm.
- The diaphragm is usually high in any condition that:
  - causes an increased intra-abdominal pressure (ascites, pregnancy)
  - causes decreased thoracic volume (atelectasis)
- The diaphragm is fixed and lower than normal in pulmonary emphysema.
- It is difficult to distinguish between an elevated diaphragm and a disease in the thorax that causes dullness to percussion (for example, pleural fluid).

Definition	Auscultation is listening to sounds produced within the body.
Stethoscope	The usual stethoscope consists of a bell and diaphragm connected with rubber tubing to the earpieces.
Diaphragm and Bell	The diaphragm of the stethoscope is more sensitive to high-pitched tones than is the bell, whereas low-pitched sounds are heard better through the bell
Earpieces	Earpieces must fit properly so that the examiner can use the stethoscope for at least 5 minutes without causing discomfort. The earpieces must fit snugly to exclude extraneous sounds, but should not be so tight that they are uncomfortable. If earpieces are too small: • they can slip into the auditory canal, and all sounds will be occluded • they cause pain
Length and Tubing	The stethoscope should not be longer than 20 inches (the shorter, the better), and the thick plastic or rubber tubing should have an internal diameter of at least 1/4 inch. The optimal length of the stethoscope is about 12 to 14 inches.
Placement	The diaphragm of the stethoscope should be placed firmly against the chest wall to exclude extraneous sounds and to eliminate sounds that may result from light contact with the skin or hair.
Warning!	Confusing sounds may be produced by: • movement of the stethoscope on the skin or hair • breathing on the tubing • sliding fingers on the tubing or chest piece
Patient's Breathing	The patient should be asked to breath through the mouth a little deeper than usual. Breathing through the open mouth minimizes the sounds produced in the nose and throat. Deep forced inspiration should be avoided because confusing muscle sounds may be produced.
Sequence	Corresponding areas of each side are auscultated from the top of the thorax downward (alternating from side to side as in percussion).

LUNGS: AUSCULTATION-- FINDINGS

Analysis

Soft sounds produced by the movement of air in the bronchoalveolar system are called breath sounds. Breath sounds are analyzed according to certain criteria.

CRITERION	DESCRIPTION/EXPLANATION
pitch	Breath sounds may vary from high to low in pitch.
intensity	Breath sounds may be: • loud or soft • louder in one phase (inspiration or expiration) than the other
duration	The lengths of the expiratory and inspiratory phases are compared.

Vesicular Breath Sounds

Vesicular breath sound probably result from the movement of air in the bronchioles and alveoli. A gentle rustling sound, vesicular breathing is relatively low-pitched. Vesicular respiration seems longer in inspiration than in expiration because much of expiration is not audible. Inspiration is also higher in pitch and louder. Vesicular breath sounds are heard normally over most of the lungs.

Bronchovesicular Breath Sounds

Where the trachea and major bronchi are close to the chest wall, a mixture of tracheobronchial and vesicular sounds are heard-- the bronchovesicular breath sound. This sound is heard on each side of the sternum in the first and second interspaces, between the scapulae, and over the apices, anteriorly and posteriorly. In bronchovesicular breathing, the inspiratory phase is similar to that of vesicular breathing, except that it is slightly louder and higher in pitch. The expiratory phase is longer, higher in pitch, louder, and more tubular than the vesicular sound. In bronchovesicular breathing, the expiratory and inspiratory phases are very similar in:

- duration
- pitch
- intensity
- quality

A brief pause may be noted between inspiration and expiration.

(Continued)

LUNGS: AUSCULTATION-- FINDINGS, Continued

Breath Sounds

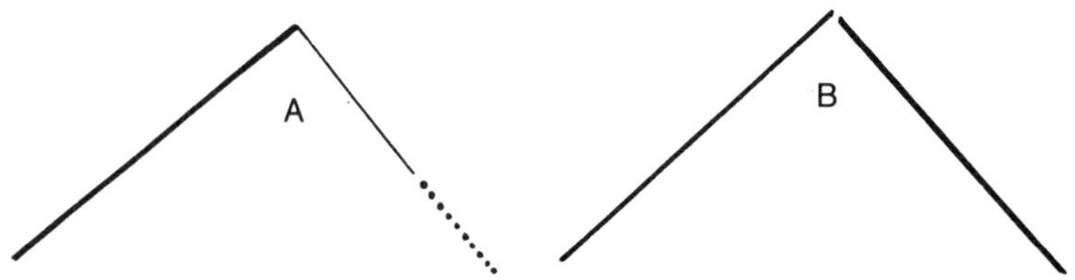

(A) Vesicular breath sounds. Inspiration (ascending arm) is louder, longer, and higher pitched than expiration (descending arm).

(B) Bronchovesicular breath sounds. Inspiration and expiration are similar in duration and intensity.

BREASTS: INSPECTION

Introduction

The breast is the most common site of cancer in women. Chronic cystic mastitis and other benign lesions must be differentiated from cancer. If any abnormality is detected or suspected, two types of breast examinations should be performed:
- with the patient sitting
- with the patient supine

Male

Breasts of men must also be examined because, although uncommon, carcinoma does occur there, with the same general characteristics as in female breasts. Men may also be afflicted with gynecomastia (enlargement of the male mammary gland). See Figure 12-9.

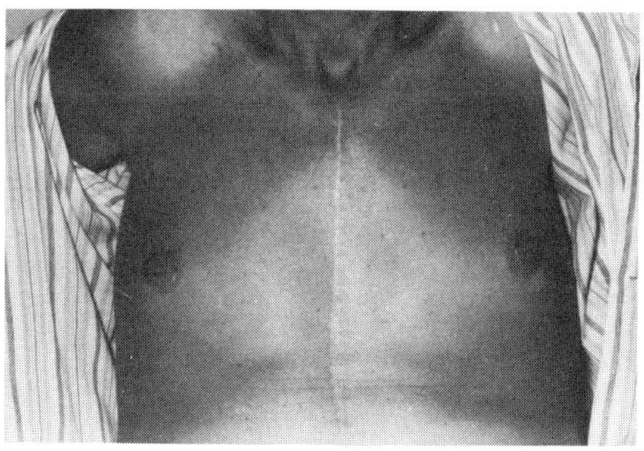

Figure 12-9.

Examination

To avoid embarrassment, the breasts should be covered until the actual examination. During the examination, the following characteristics should be inspected:
- symmetry
- skin changes
- nipples
- masses
- veins
- retraction of skin

Symmetry

Asymmetry of the breasts will be most obvious when the patient is sitting. Asymmetry usually results from normal differences in development of the breasts, but can also indicate:
- cysts
- inflammation
- neoplasm

(Continued)

BREASTS: INSPECTION, Continued

Erythema	Erythema may be produced by inflammation or an inflammatory neoplasm in the superficial lymphatics, in which case the redness is a local reaction to the cancer.
Edema	Edema makes the hair follicles and follicular openings more prominent. Edema may be caused by either inflammation or neoplasm, but if no pain, tenderness, or erythema is present, the edema is almost always due to cancer. Yet, the presence of any one of these three findings, along with edema, does not rule out cancer. "Orange peel" skin (or peau d'orange or "pigskin") is produced by lymphedema or extravasation of intravascular fluid into the interstitial space.

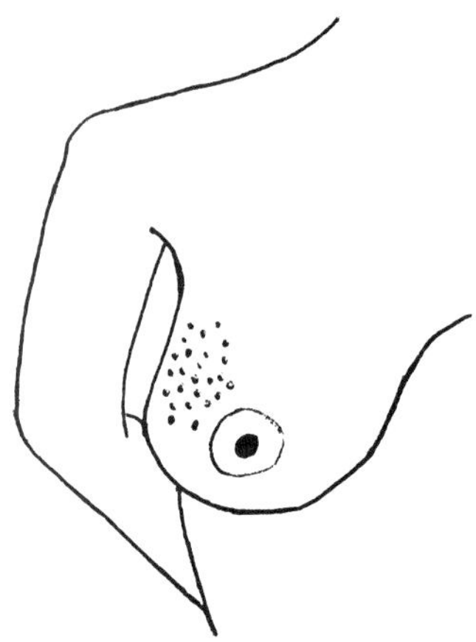

Pregnancy	During pregnancy: • the breasts become larger • the areolae become larger in diameter and darker • the axillae may look full and give the impression that a mass is present (axillary "tail" of breast). The increase in breast size is caused by glandular enlargement in preparation for lactation.

(Continued)

BREASTS: INSPECTION, Continued

Nipples

The following characteristics of the nipple should be observed:

- size
- shape
- discharge
- condition of skin

NOTE: Both men and women may have up to four accessory nipples along the mammary line that are about 2 mm to 4 mm in diameter, pigmented, and raised above the skin.

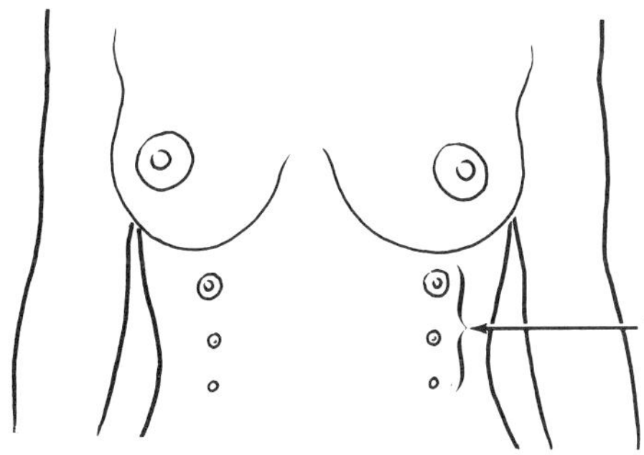

CONDITION	EXPLANATION/DESCRIPTION
inversion	is significant only if it has occurred recently (see Fig. 12-10)
ulceration	Ulceration of the nipple may indicate a malignancy (Paget's disease), especially if only one nipple is affected. If both are involved, the patient probably has a benign skin disorder.
discharge	Any discharge appearing at the nipple should be observed to be one of the following: • serous • blue • yellow • green • sanguineous Nipple discharges indicate a disease of the duct system, such as: • cystic mastitis • neoplasm

(Continued)

BREASTS: INSPECTION, Continued

CONDITION	EXPLANATION/DESCRIPTION
	NOTE: A blood discharge is usually caused by benign intraductal papilloma; bloody discharge occurs in only about 1% of patients with carcinoma.
pregnancy	During pregnancy, the nipples are larger and more mobile.

Skin Retraction

Skin retraction consists of dimpling of any part of the skin of the breast. It occurs when an infiltrating process exerts tension on the breast ligaments. If the involved ligaments supply the nipple, the nipple will point toward the site of the lesion. Several diseases may produce the retraction.

PROCESS	DESCRIPTION
fat necrosis	Necrosis, usually produced by trauma, leads to fibroblastic proliferation, which, in turn, produces a mass, scarring, and retraction of the ligamentous fibers.
acute inflammation	Inflammation may cause the same type of retraction as fat necrosis. The acute onset and signs of inflammation distinguish the process from cancer.
cancer	If the breast does not show evidence of acute inflammation, skin retraction usually indicates cancer. In early lesions and in patients with large breasts, skin retraction may be one of the earliest physical findings in carcinoma.

Advanced Cancer

In advanced carcinoma, other findings include:
- a fixed immobile mass
- fixation of the mass to skin
- ulceration

(Continued)

BREASTS: INSPECTION, Continued

Appearance of Retraction

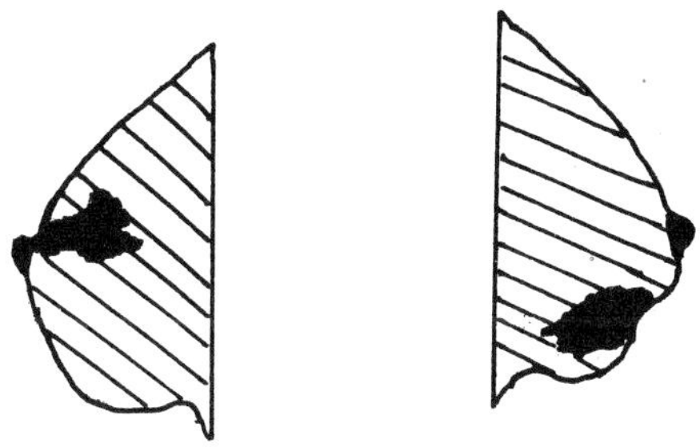

Detecting Retraction

Retraction is best detected with the patient sitting, with her arms extended over her head.

STEP	ACTION/DESCRIPTION
1	Ask the patient to raise her arms directly overhead; the breasts are usually elevated equally by this action. See Figure 12-11.
2	Observe the breasts for evidence of retraction. The retraction may vary from a small dimple to a flattening of an entire quadrant as the arms are raised.

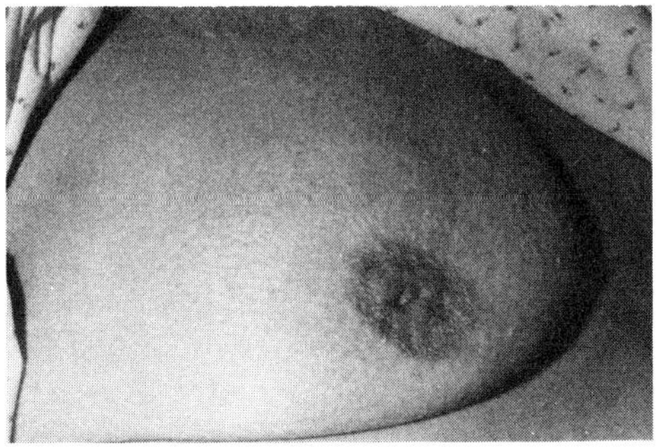

Figure 12-10.

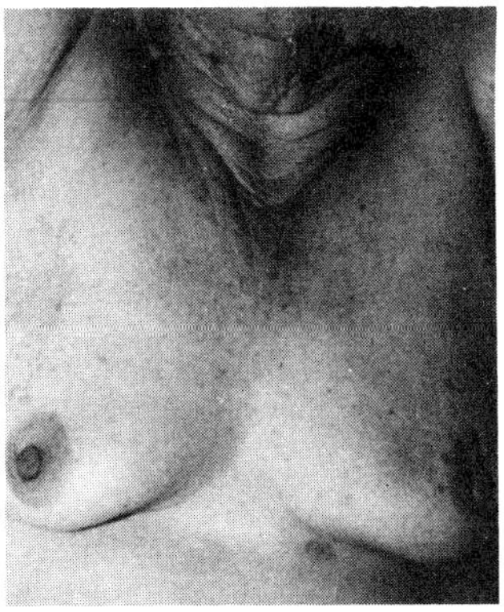

Figure 12-11.

BREASTS: PALPATION

Introduction	Palpation should first be done with the patient supine. Physical qualities that should be noted are: • consistency • elasticity • tenderness • masses
Consistency	The breasts of older women are usually stringy and nodular, whereas, in younger patients, they are softer and more homogeneous. Breasts consist of lobules that should <u>not</u> be mistaken for tumors.
Physiologic Changes	Cyclic, hormone-mediated physiologic changes occur in the breasts. The breasts become engorged, lobular, and sensitive before the menses begin and decompress after the menses start. Chronic cystic mastitis, which may result after years of these changes, produces nodules and cysts of various sizes (1 cm to several centimeters). The nodules are produced by cystic dilatations of the ducts.
Pregnancy	During pregnancy, the breasts become firmer and larger, and the lobulations become so distinct that they may be interpreted as tumors.

(Continued)

BREASTS: PALPATION, Continued

Procedure

Palpation should begin at the upper lateral aspect of each breast.

STEP	ACTION
1	Gently palpate the left breast, using the palmar aspect of the proximal and middle phalanges, with a rotary motion.
2	Palpate each quadrant again, more firmly. Proceed until the breast has been examined completely.
3	Observe any masses on the nipple. A subcutaneous mass in the areolar area may be a sebaceous cyst or an intraductal papilloma. Pressure over a papilloma may produce a serous or sanguineous discharge.
4	Examine the right breast in the same way.

Caution!

The examiner should not compress a portion of the breast between the thumb and fingers, because the breast between two folds of skin may feel like a mass. Instead, the breast should be compressed gently and firmly against the chest wall.

BREASTS: CHARACTERIZING MASSES

If a mass is found, its features should be observed.

FEATURE	NOTATIONS
location	A useful method for localizing tumor masses is to consider each breast as if it were the face of a clock with the nipple in the center. A lesion can then be observed to be along a specific (o'clock) axis. The distance between the mass and nipple should be estimated. 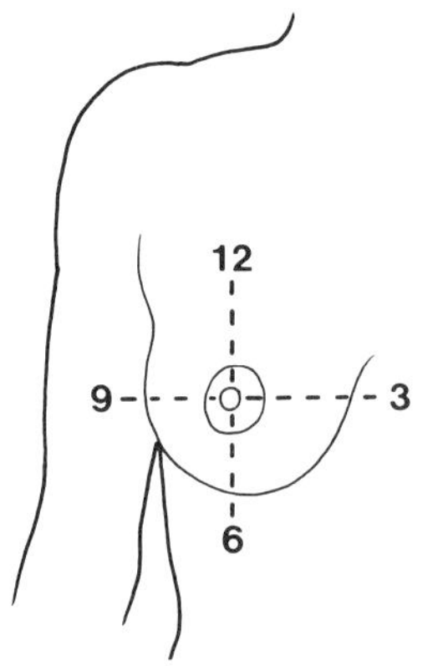
size	The size of the mass, in two planes, should be estimated in centimeters so that later changes in size can be identified.
contour	Contour of the surface of the mass should be described. • Benign neoplasms have a smooth, regular contour. • Malignant neoplasms may have irregular, hard margins. • Inflammatory lesions have irregular contours.
consistency	The consistency of the mass should be described as soft, cystic, firm, or stony hard. • A soft, cystic consistency denotes a benign lesion. • A firm mass that has an irregular surface usually indicates a malignant neoplasm. • A firm, tender area may be produced by an abscess.

(Continued)

BREASTS: CHARACTERIZING MASSES, Continued

FEATURE	NOTATIONS
tenderness	If the lesion is tender, the degree of tenderness should be determined. • An inflammatory process is usually very tender. • Mild tenderness occurs in cystic mastitis. • Most malignant lesions are not tender.
mobility	The examiner should determine whether the lesion is: • freely movable • movable only in certain directions • fixed If the mobility of the mass is curtailed, the examiner should determine whether the curtailment is produced by: • fixation to deep structures • fixation to the skin • fixation to the surrounding breast tissue. • Benign lesions are usually movable. • Inflammatory lesions may be fixed. • Early malignant lesions are movable. • Advanced malignant lesions become increasingly fixed.
discreteness	Discreteness indicates a benign process, whereas a lack of discreteness suggests inflammation or cancer. If the boundaries of the mass are difficult to determine, the mass is likely to be cancer.

Axillae

The axillae should be explored with one hand while the examiner's opposite hand holds the ipsilateral arm of the patient. By moving the patient's arm, enlarged lymph nodes that cannot be felt when the arm is at the side can be palpated. See Figure 12-12.

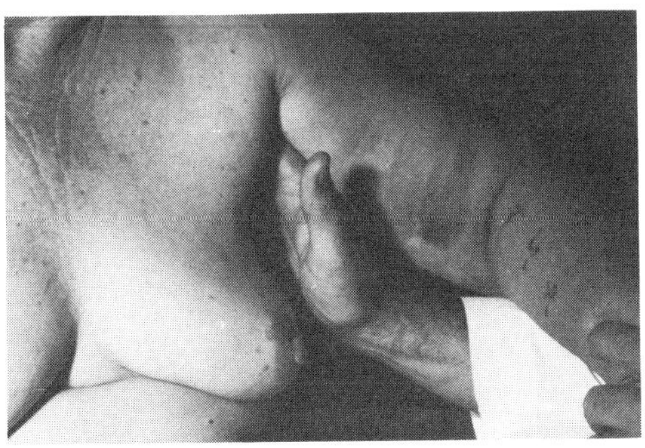

Figure 12-12.

SELF-ASSESSMENT

1. Name the pulmonary lobe associated with the following thoracic topography (male):
   a. right nipple
   b. left nipple
   c. the level of the sternal angle; the right midclavicular line
   d. the level of the sternal angle; the left midclavicular line
   e. the lower third of the medial scapular border, right side
   f. at the most inferior percussible extent of the lung posteriorly; the paraspinal area, left
   g. the right fifth intercostal space, midclavicular line

2. Define <u>bronchovesicular</u>.

3. Name three terms to describe percussion findings of the thorax.

4. Give examples of where each of the above percussion findings can normally be found.

5. Name two terms used to describe normal breath sounds.

6. Give examples of where each of the above auscultatory findings can normally be found.

7. State the normal topographical location of the major fissure.

8. State the normal topographical location of the horizontal fissure of the right lung.

9. State the approximate position of the inferior boundary of the lung at normal midinspiration (assuming that the left lung is somewhat lower than the right).

10. Which rib is directly opposite the sternomanubrial junction?

11. State several characteristics of benign breast lesions.

12. State several characteristics of malignant breast lesions.

13. What kind of breast lesion does tenderness usually signify?

14. Name several characteristics useful in describing a breast mass.

CHAPTER THIRTEEN

The Cardiovascular System

James C. Guckian, M.D.

THE CARDIAC CYCLE

Introduction

The pressure curves of the cardiac cycle must be known so that the various acoustical events in that cycle can be understood. In the diagram below, the left atrial pressure curve and the aortic pressure curve are superimposed on the left ventricular pressure curve. The source of heart sounds on the left side of the heart are indicated as they relate to pressure changes.

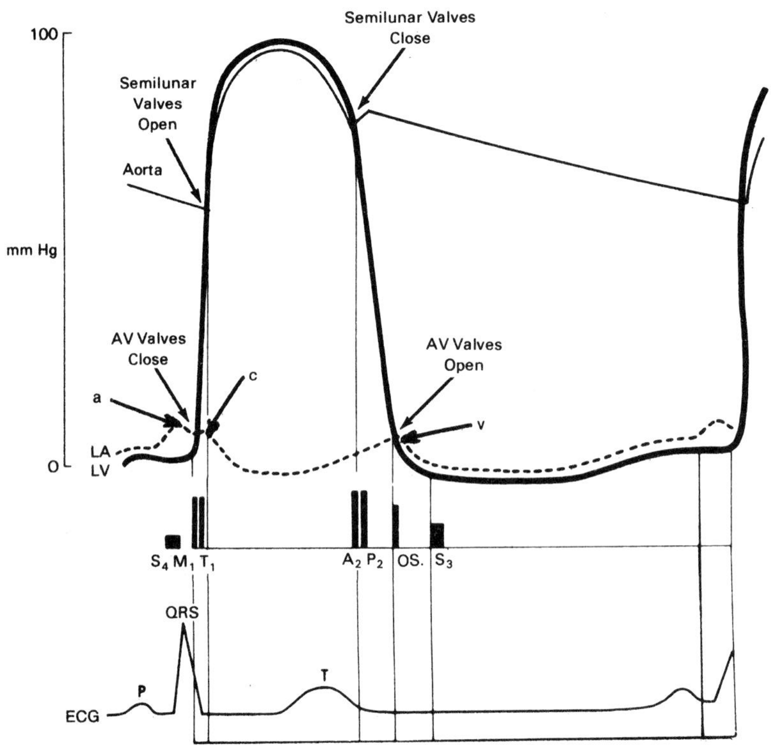

LV, left ventricle; LA, left atrium. M_1 and T_1, mitral and tricuspid components of the first heart sound. A_2 and P_2, aortic and pulmonary components of the second heart sound. S_3 and S_4, third and fourth heart sounds. OS, opening snap of atrioventricular (AV) valves (not heard normally)

(Continued)

THE CARDIAC CYCLE, Continued

Heart Sounds

- The left ventricular curve (LV) begins with an even, sharply rising limb, a rounded peak, and a descending limb that falls rapidly to the baseline.
- The left atrial curve (LA) is characterized by three positive waves that correspond to the three waves that may be observed in the cervical veins:
  - atrial contraction ("a" wave)
  - ventricular contraction ("c" wave)
  - rapid ventricular filling ("v" wave)
- The aortic pressure curve (aorta) follows the left ventricular curve closely from the first time they cross to their second crossing.
  - Because of a slight pressure gradient, the aortic curve is below the ventricular curve.
  - The aortic curve falls abruptly just before it crosses the ventricular curve for the second time.
  - Immediately after the second crossing is the dicrotic notch, which is produced by closure of the aortic valve and a gradual decline in pressure during diastole.

Heart Sounds, Pressure Curves, and ECG

When the electrocardiogram (ECG) and heart sounds are superimposed on the pressure curves, the acoustical events within the cardiac cycle can be correlated temporally.

- The P wave indicates atrial depolarization, followed by atrial systole.
- The QRS complex, which results from depolarization of ventricular myocardium, appears earlier than the mechanical contraction.
- Contraction of the ventricles begins at the peak of the R wave; right ventricular depolarization and contraction occur later than left ventricular contraction.

First Heart Sound

The first heart sound has two components:

- The mitral component (M_1), produced by closure of the mitral valve, results from a sudden increase in left ventricular pressure such that ventricular pressure exceeds left atrial pressure, causing closure of the mitral valve. M_1 coincides with the R wave on the electrocardiogram.
- The tricuspid component (T_1), which follows M_1, is caused by similar hemodynamic events in the right side of the heart and is produced by closure of the tricuspid valve.

  NOTE: When left ventricular pressure is greater than aortic pressure, seen on the ascending limb of the ventricular pressure curve, the aortic valve opens. The process does not produce any sound.

(Continued)

THE CARDIAC CYCLE, Continued

Isometric Contraction	The period between closure of the mitral valve and opening of the aortic valve is called isometric contraction; both valves are closed at this time, and blood does not traverse cardiac chambers.
Second Heart Sound	The second heart sound has two components: • The aortic component (A_2), is produced when the aortic pressure exceeds left ventricular pressure (descending limb of the ventricular pressure curve), causing closure of the aortic valve. • The pulmonary component (P_2), which is caused by similar events in the pulmonary artery and right ventricle and immediately follows A_2, is produced by closure of the pulmonic valve. Both components of the second heart sound normally coincide with the T wave on the electrocardiogram.
Opening Snap	After closure of the aortic valve, left ventricular pressure falls rapidly. Ultimately, aortic pressure is exceeded by atrial pressure. At this point, the mitral valve opens, normally without producing a sound. The subsequent rapid filling of the ventricle causes the atrial "V" wave. NOTE: In mitral stenosis, an opening snap (OS) is audible at this time.
Third Heart Sound	After opening of the mitral valve, blood flows rapidly from the left atrium into the left ventricle because of the pressure gradient between the two chambers-- the period of rapid ventricular filling. In this period, the examiner may hear: • the third heart sound (S_3) OR • the pathologic counterpart of the third heart sound, the ventricular gallop
Fourth Heart Sound	During presystole, or the late phase of diastole, the pressure gradient between the left ventricle and left atrium is much smaller than in the earlier phase. When the atrium contracts, corresponding to the P wave on the electrocardiogram, the examiner may hear the fourth sound (S_4) or the abnormal atrial gallop.

(Continued)

THE CARDIAC CYCLE, Continued

Right side of Heart	Pressure pulses similar to those that occur on the left side of the heart occur on the right side, but acoustical and mechanical events occur slightly later on the right than on the left.
Asynchrony of Sounds	• Mitral valve closure (M_1) precedes closure of the tricuspid valve (T_1). • Aortic valve closure (A_2) precedes pulmonary valve closure (P_2). • A_2 may be heard anywhere over the precordium. The best location is not necessarily the aortic valve area; often, it is heard best at the apex or over the pulmonary area, where it can be distinguished readily from P_2, which occurs later. • The second heart sound in the pulmonary area is split; A_2 occurs about 0.05 seconds before P_2. The split is most obvious at the end of inspiration, because inspiration increases right ventricular filling and prolongs right ventricular ejection. Prolonged ejection delays pulmonary valve closure. • Left ventricular filling is slightly <u>reduced</u> during inspiration, causing slightly earlier closure of the aortic valve. However, respiratory movements of A_2-P_2 are normally determined mainly by right ventricular events as noted above. Auscultation over the pulmonary area thus reveals split sounds on inspiration and a single sound or narrowing of the split on expiration as P_2 moves back toward A_2. NOTE: Splitting of the second sound is best heard during normal (not forced) inspiration.

VENOUS BLOOD PRESSURE

Introduction	Venous pressure can be measured in intensive care units by using a manometer or transducer connected to a catheter in a vein. Under most circumstances, however, venous pressure is estimated by inspection of neck veins.
Jugular Veins	Because the pressure in the jugular veins depends upon changes within the right atrium of the heart, an examination of these veins provides information about hemodynamic events in the right side of the heart and allows an estimate to be made of the venous pressure. The internal and external jugular veins are examined with the patient in a sitting position or with the patient reclining at an angle of about 45°. The vertical height (cm) of the jugular venous pulse above the manubrium is recorded. External jugular veins are valved and therefore less reliably reflect RA pressure than the nonvalved internal jugular veins.

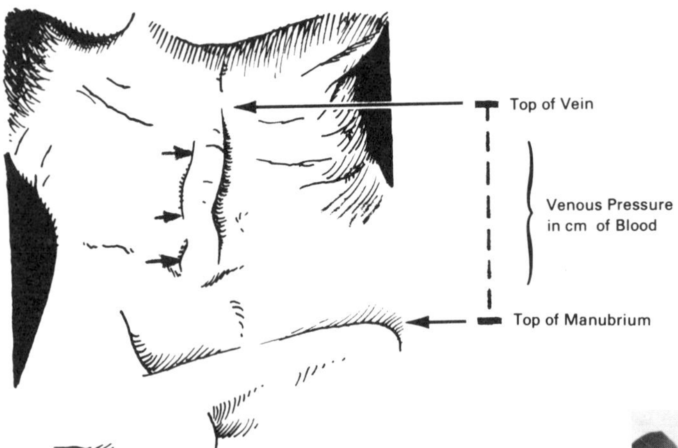

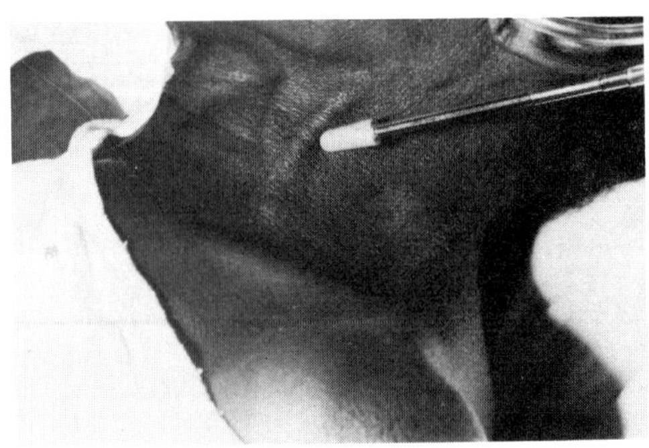

Distended external jugular vein in patient with severe right-sided heart failure.

(Continued)

VENOUS BLOOD PRESSURE, Continued

Evaluation of Venous Pressure

Elevated venous pressure can be interpreted as follows:

IF	THEN
venous pressure is substantially increased	• the jugular veins should be examined with patient sitting upright • the jugular veins may be distended as high as the mandible NOTE: The venous pressure is increased in: • right-sided heart failure • constrictive pericarditis • cardiac tamponade • tricuspid stenosis or insufficiency • obstruction of the superior vena cava • obstruction of the superior vena cava should be suspected if the jugular veins do not pulsate
venous pressure is slightly or moderately increased	• the jugular veins should be inspected with the patient reclining and his or her upper body raised 45 degrees from horizontal • clothing should be removed from around the neck • the neck should not be flexed. In this position, a normal jugular pulse should be visible about 2 cm above the manubrium. Distances over 4 cm indicate elevated venous pressure.

Right Jugular Pulses

Evaluation of the jugular pulses is performed by raising the patient's chin slightly and turning it to the left or right to expose the right supraclavicular fossa. The pulse waves of the internal jugular are visible over the sternomastoid muscle or adjacent to it. The waves of the external jugular pulse may be seen as the vein crosses the sternomastoid muscle. The timing, i.e., occurrence in systole or diastole, of venous waves can be evaluated by simultaneously palpating the opposite carotid artery or by listening to the heart.

(Continued)

VENOUS BLOOD PRESSURE, Continued

Differentiation of Pulses

Several differences between jugular pulsations and those of the carotid artery make it easy to avoid confusing the two:

- The level of pulsation in the jugular veins descends on inspiration and ascends on expiration. Respiration does not change the carotid pulse.
- Slight pressure just above the sternoclavicular joint or directly over the pulsation will eliminate the jugular pulse. Eliminating the carotid pulse requires a great deal of pressure (DON'T TRY!).
- Normally, the carotid pulse has only one phase. The jugular venous pulse normally has two or three positive waves.
- The pulse in the cervical veins becomes more prominent when the patient reclines and less prominent when he or she sits upright. Carotid artery pulsations are not affected by changes in position.
- In cases of right-sided heart failure and constrictive pericarditis, pressing the right upper abdomen for about 30 seconds will increase the venous pressure. The jugular pulses will increase, and distention of the neck veins will rise to higher levels. This rise in jugular venous pressure is the <u>hepatojugular reflux</u>.

Demonstration of Hepatojugular Reflux

The method for demonstrating hepatojugular reflux is outlined below.

STEP	ACTION
1	Elevate the patient's head so that the veins are distended halfway up the neck.
2	Exert firm pressure with the palm of the hand for 30 seconds over the right upper quadrant of the abdomen. <u>NOTE</u>: Since the patient must breathe normally during the procedure, the examiner should not exert pressure that will cause pain. Any abnormal breathing will produce a Valsalva maneuver, which causes the veins to distend.
3	Determine whether the neck veins distend more or rise to higher levels.

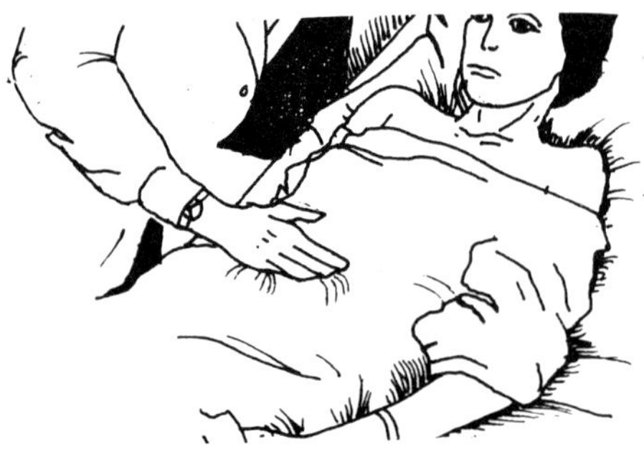

HEART: LANDMARKS AND TOPOGRAPHIC ANATOMY

Introduction	The heart is examined by: • inspection • palpation • auscultation • percussion (which has only limited usefulness)
Surface Landmarks	The anatomic landmarks that are used to locate and describe the heart, valve areas, and great vessls are the: • midsternal line • midclavicular lines • anterior, middle, and posterior axillary lines • suprasternal notch • manubriosternal junction (sternal angle; for counting ribs and interspaces) • precordium (area of the anterior thorax that overlies the heart)
Anatomy	The base of the heart is upward; the apex is downward and toward the left. The left and right borders of the heart may be located by examination. The largest portion of the anterior aspect of the heart is made up of: • the right atrium, occupying a small area beneath the lower sternum • the right ventricle, occupying most of the area beneath the sternum and to the left of the sternum • the left ventricle, which occupies a small area at the apex of the heart. NOTE: Thus, most of the anterior surface of the precordium is occupied by right ventricle.

(Continued)

HEART: LANDMARKS AND TOPOGRAPHIC ANATOMY, Continued

Topographic Anatomy of the Heart

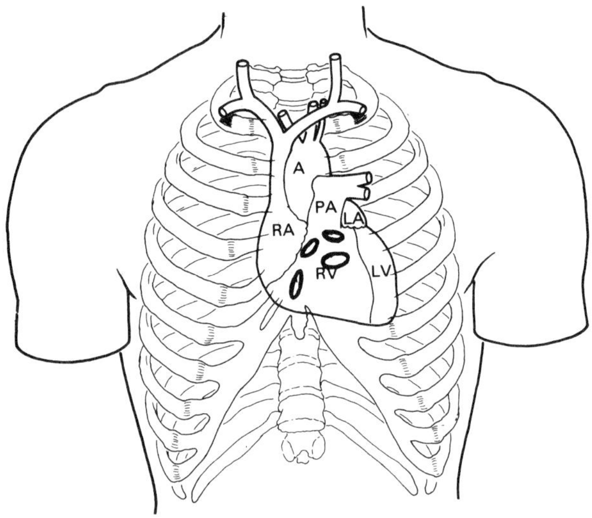

Abbreviations:
RA - right atrium
RV - right ventricle
LA - left atrium
LV - left ventricle
A - aorta
PA - pulmonary artery

Circles = Valve locations

(Continued)

HEART: LANDMARKS AND TOPOGRAPHIC ANATOMY, Continued

Cardiac Valves

The cardiac valves lie within a relatively small area. The following areas are the anatomic sites of the valves; these are not the areas in which the valve sounds are best heard.

VALVE	LOCATION
pulmonary	behind the third left chondrosternal joint
aortic	behind the sternum, to the right of the pulmonary valve
mitral	behind the fourth left chondrosternal joint
tricuspid	behind the sternum, to the right of the mitral valve

Valve Areas

Anatomic valve sites are indicated by closed circles. Areas where the valve sounds are heard best are indicated by open circles.

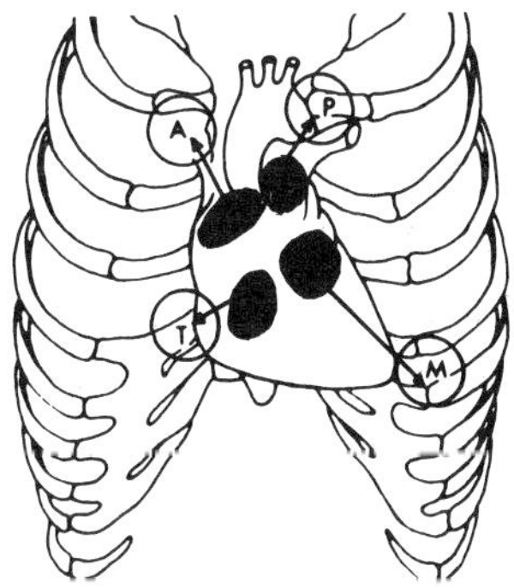

Describing Findings

The landmarks and anatomic relationships enable an examiner to describe and locate cardiac findings. Descriptions and exact localizations are extremely important in a cardiac examination.

Position of the Heart

The position of the normal heart varies according to the the person's build and the configuration of the chest. In most people, the heart occupies an oblique position, with approximately one third lying to the right of the midline and two thirds lying to the left (sthenic persons). In subjects who are short and stocky (hypersthenic), the heart occupies a more transverse position. In asthenic persons, the heart takes a vertical position in the midline.

INSPECTION AND PALPATION

Introduction

The pulsations that are seen on the anterior chest can be palpated, although the corollary may not be true. In general, the outward movements over the precordium can be detected by palpation.

Position of Patient

For inspection and palpation of the anterior part of the chest, the patient should be supine or with the upper body elevated about 45°.

Deformities

The following deformities in shape and contour of the chest may change the shape and position of the heart:

- depression of the sternum (pectus excavatum)
- pectus carinatum
- kyphosis of the dorsal spine
- scoliosis

In some disorders (Marfan syndrome), deformities of the chest suggest the presence of specific abnormalities of the heart.

Tangential View

Vascular and cardiac pulsations are seen best from a tangential view. See Figure 13-1.

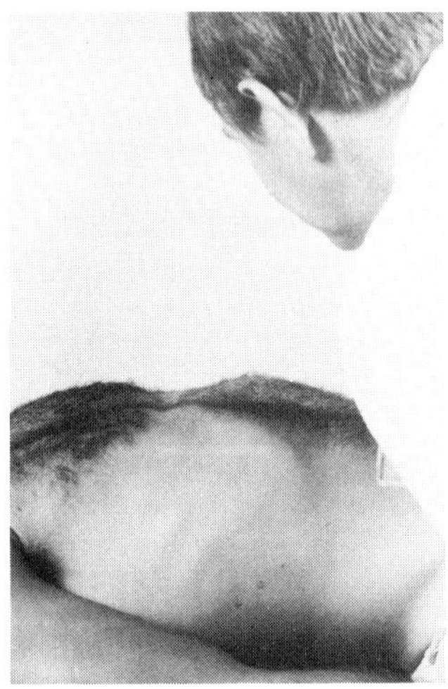

Figure 13-1.

Timing of Pulsation

The timing, that is, whether in ventricular systole or diastole, of pulsations must be determined. Thus, after pulsations are detected by inspection or palpation, the examiner determines their time in the cardiac cycle by simultaneous auscultation of the heart or palpation of the carotid artery. The pulsations are then evaluated in terms of whether they occur during systole, diastole, or both.

INSPECTION AND PALPATION, Continued

Dual Purpose of Palpation	Palpation is used to confirm the observations of inspection and to detect pulsations that are not visible.
Point of Maximal Impulse (PMI)	With each ventricular systole, the heart rotates abruptly to the right. This movement thrusts the apex of the heart against the chest wall and produces an impulse. The apex of the heart is the left ventricle; thus, the impulse is produced by the left ventricle. The point at which the left ventricle strikes the chest wall can be palpated in normal persons. In thin persons, the impulse may be seen also. This impulse is termed the point of maximal impulse or PMI.
Palpating the PMI	To palpate pulsations, the examiner may either place the fingertips (A, below) over the apical area of the precordium or place the fingers and the palm of the hand over the apical precordium (B, below).

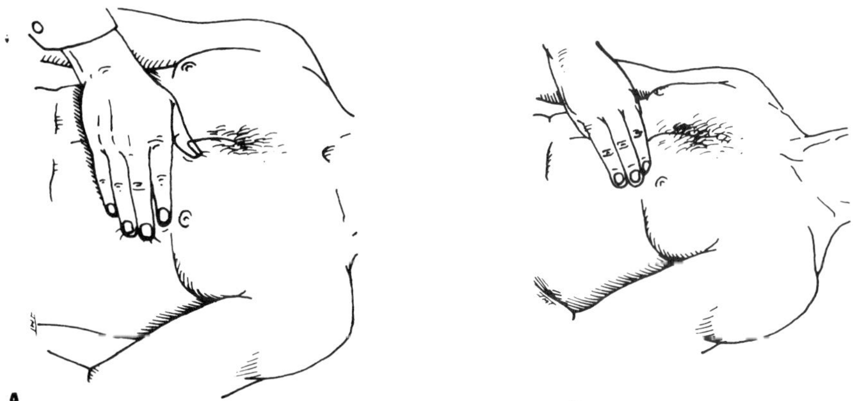

A B

Definition of Thrills	Thrills are palpable vibrations produced by: • abnormal flow of blood from one chamber of the heart to another through a restricted channel (e.g., ventricular septal defect) • turbulent flow of blood across an abnormal valve (e.g., pulmonary valve stenosis). Palpating a thrill is similar to the sensation of touching the back of a purring cat.

(Continued)

INSPECTION AND PALPATION, Continued

Production of Thrills

STAGE	DESCRIPTION
A	Blood flows through a stenotic valve, great vessel, or ventricular septal defect.
B	Turbulent currents develop on the other side of the narrow area.
C	The currents cause the wall of the chamber to vibrate.

Description of Thrills

Thrills should be described in terms of:
- location
- time in the cardiac cycle

Thrills may occur:
- in systole
- in diastole
- in a continuous manner

The intensity of the thrill increases with an increase in the:
- velocity of the blood (increased cardiac output)
- degree of narrowing of the channel involved
- difference in pressure across the narrowed segment

Six Areas of Examination

Inspection and palpation during a cardiac examination focuses on six areas:
- suprasternal area
- aortic valve area
- pulmonary valve area
- parasternal area (right ventricular)
- apex of precordium (left ventricle)
- epigastric area

Suprasternal

Pulsations are observed, and the area is palpated for thrills.

Aortic

Because this area is located in the right second intercostal space (adjacent to the sternum), pulsations that result from aortic aneurysms may be discovered here. In aortic stenosis, a systolic thrill that radiates into the neck may be palpated.

(Continued)

Pulmonary

In the pulmonary area, located in the left second intercostal space (adjacent to the sternum), a systolic thrill may be palpated in patients with pulmonary stenosis. Pulsations in this area may be caused by:

- pulmonary hypertension, due to:
  - mitral stenosis or insufficiency
  - left-to-right intracardiac shunts
  - primary pulmonary hypertension
  - cor pulmonale
  - multiple pulmonary emboli
- aneurysmal dilation of the pulmonary artery

Parasternal (Right Ventricular)

In the parasternal area, the lower half of the sternum and the adjacent intercostal spaces (left and right), slight pulsations may occur in children or thin-chested adults, which are aggravated by an increase in cardiac output such as with:

- fever
- hyperthyroidism
- anemia

Abnormal pulsations in this area are usually produced by right ventricular hypertrophy. In right ventricular hypertrophy, the pulsations have a lift and are well sustained. An increase in right ventricular pressure usually results from:

- pulmonary stenosis
- pulmonary arterial hypertension (see list of causes under Pulmonary, above).

Apical Area

The detection and evaluation of the point of maximal impulse (PMI) is one of the most important parts of the cardiac examination. The examiner should pay particular attention to its:

- location
- size
- duration
- elevation

PMI Location

In normal adults, the PMI is located in the fifth left intercostal space at (or slightly medial to) the midclavicular line. In conditions in which the heart is displaced to the left (pregnancy, ascites, paralyzed diaphragm) the PMI may be located slightly lateral to the midclavicular line. A disease that displaces the mediastinum may also displace the PMI.

<u>EXAMPLES</u>:

- A large right pleural effusion may displace the impulse to the left.
- Massive atelectasis on the right will displace the PMI toward the right.

(Continued)

INSPECTION AND PALPATION, Continued

PMI Size	The diameter of the PMI is normally less than 2 cm.
PMI Duration	The first systolic outward movement of the left ventricle begins with the first heart sound. This outward movement lasts only through the first third of systole. Toward the end of the first third of systole, the movement shifts inward. Thus, the outward thrust of the PMI normally lasts no longer than one third of systole. The PMI has increased duration, but is not displaced, in persons with: • a thin chest • anemia • fever • hyperthyroidism
PMI Elevation	The height of the lift of the chest wall by the left ventricular impulse is dependent on: • thickness of the chest wall • left ventricular stroke volume • thickness of the left ventricular myocardium
Abnormalities of the PMI	The PMI is changed by: • left ventricular hypertrophy or dilatation • left ventricular stroke volume In left ventricular hypertrophy or dilatation the PMI may be: • forceful • lifting • enlarged • sustained throughout most of systole • displaced downward and laterally
Epigastric Area	Pulsations of the aorta or right ventricle may occur in the epigastrium. Pulsations in normal individuals may be due to: • fever • anemia • hyperthyroidism Large pulsations of the aorta may be produced by aortic aneurysms or aortic valvular regurgitation. In thin individuals with right venticular hypertrophy, pulsations of the right ventricle may be seen and felt in this area. Hepatic pulsations may also occur in this region, especially if tricuspid regurgitation is present.

AUSCULTATION: METHOD

The Setting

Because heart sounds are low-pitched and close to the limit of the range of human hearing, auscultation requires:

- concentration by the examiner
- a relaxed patient
- quiet surroundings with no conversation

Instruments Required

Both the bell and the diaphragm of the stethoscope should be used:

- The bell makes it easier to hear low-pitched sounds
- The diaphragm facilitates hearing of high-pitched sounds.

Procedure

The examination by auscultation must be systematic. With the diaphragm of the stethoscope, the examiner should start at the apex and move along the left sternal border to the pulmonary and aortic area, inching the stethoscope from one area to the other until the entire cardiac area has been covered.

- Auscultate with the diaphragm at the:
  - apex
  - left lower sternal border
  - tricuspid area
  - left sternal border in the third interspace
  - pulmonic area
  - aortic area
  - suprasternal notch
- Auscultate at the apex with the bell.

VALVE AREA	AREA FOR AUSCULTATION
aortic	second right intercostal space, just lateral to the sternum
pulmonary	second left intercostal space, just lateral to the sternum
mitral	fifth left intercostal space, 1 cm to 2 cm medial to the midclavicular line (apex)
tricuspid	junction of the xiphoid process and the sternum

(Continued)

AUSCULTATION: METHOD, Continued

Listening to Heart Cycle Components

In learning auscultation, a student must listen to various specific components of the cardiac cycle in turn, and <u>not</u> try to listen to everything at once.

LISTEN FOR	PROCEDURE
the first heart sound	• Identify it. • Evaluate its intensity. • Determine whether it is split, caused by mitral and tricuspid valve closure. • Evaluate variations in intensity with cardiac cycle.
the second heart sound	• Identify it. • Evaluate its intensity. • Assess the type and degree of splitting caused by inspiration and expiration.
sounds in systole	• Note any sounds.
sounds in diastole	• Note any sounds.

Additional Auscultatory Positions

If the patient has had symptoms of a cardiac disorder, <u>or</u> if the examiner hears abnormal cardiac sounds, the examiner should:

- listen to the apex with the bell, with the patient in the left lateral decubitus position (See Fig. 13-2)
- listen in the aortic and pulmonic valve areas with the diaphragm, with the patient sitting and leaning forward (See Fig 13-3)

Rate and Rhythm

Common disturbances of rhythm (arrhythmias) should be detected by palpating the pulse. Many alterations of rhythm, however, can be diagnosed best by palpating the pulse and simultaneously listening to the apex of the heart. Diagnosis of the more complex arrhythmias can be made only by electrocardiography.

(Continued)

AUSCULTATION: METHOD, Continued

Sinus Arrhythmia	In sinus arrhythmia, irregularity in the pulse in children, young adults, and occasionally older persons, the pulse rate increases with inspiration and decreases with expiration. Deep respiration can enhance the irregularity. Sinus arrhythmia is the most common alteration of rhythm, and it is not clinically important except that it must be differentiated from other arrhythmias.
Premature Contraction	This arrhythmia is caused by a premature beat (extrasystole), which arises in the ventricle, atrium, or atrioventricular node.
Arrhythmias With Pulse Deficit	Some arrhythmias may involve a discrepancy between the rate of the palpable pulse and the rate heard over the heart. In these cases, the apical pulse rate may be greater (perhaps 140 per minute) than the radial pulse rate (100 per minute, a pulse deficit of 40 per minute).
Percussion of Heart--Note!	Percussion is generally only useful in the cardiac examination if: • the apical impulse is difficult to detect. Percussion may locate the the left border of cardiac dullness. Usually the right border of the heart cannot be detected by percussion. Cardiac dullness may be absent in pulmonary emphysema because of increased retrosternal air. • pericardial effusion is present. Percussion may outline the increased area of cardiac dullness caused by pericardial effusion.

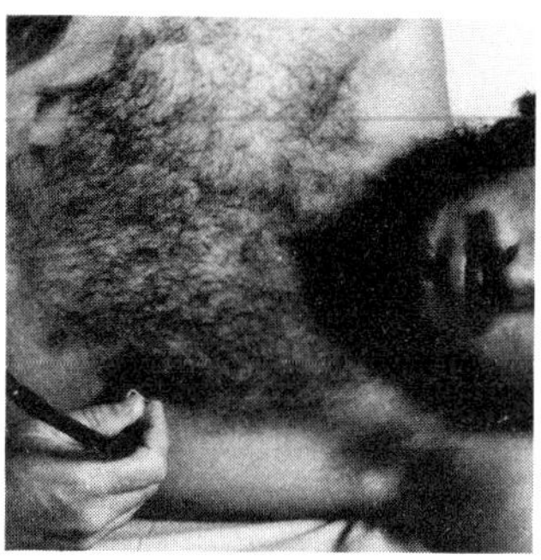

Figure 13-2.

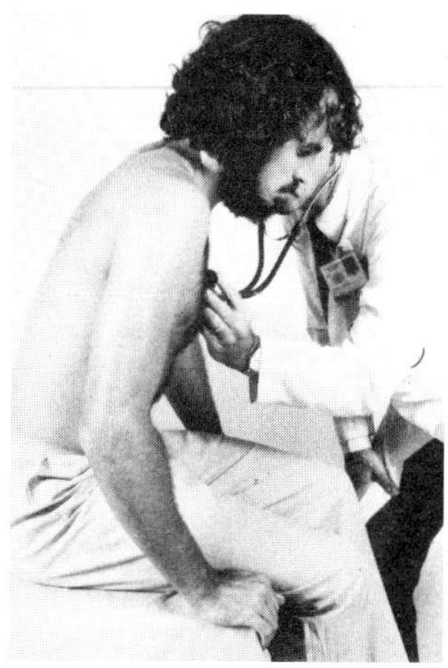

Figure 13-3.

(Continued)

AUSCULTATION: HEART SOUNDS

Introduction

In normal adults, the first and second heart sounds are audible, whereas the third and fourth sounds are usually inaudible. Unless an examiner identifies the first and second heart sound properly, he or she will be unable to locate abnormal sounds in the cardiac cycle.

Characteristics of Heart Sounds

The first and second heart sounds sound like "lubb dup." When the heart is beating slowly and regularly, these two "syllables" can be differentiated easily. A longer pause (ventricular diastole) occurs between the second sound and the next first sound than between the first and second sound (ventricular systole). As the heart rate increases, the diastolic interval decreases, and distinguishing the first from the second heart sound may be difficult. The first sound can then be identfied by palpation of the carotid artery but <u>not</u> of the radial pulse.

The Heart Sounds

The following table describes the four heart sounds

SOUND	TIMING	ACOUSTICAL PROPERTIES
first heart sound (S_1)	occurs synchronous with apical impulse; corresponds with beginning of ventricular systole and arterial pulse	sounds like "lubb"
second heart sound (S_2)	occurs at end of systole; corresponds with onset of ventricular diastole	sounds like "dup"
third heart sound (S_3)	occurs in early diastole, approximately 0.12-0.14 seconds after the second heart sound	heard in normal children and young adults, usually at the apex with the bell of the stethoscope
fourth heart sound (S_4)	occurs late in diastole or just before the first sound at the time of atrial contraction	low-pitched sound heard at the apex

(Continued)

AUSCULTATION: HEART SOUNDS, Continued

Recording of Heart Sounds

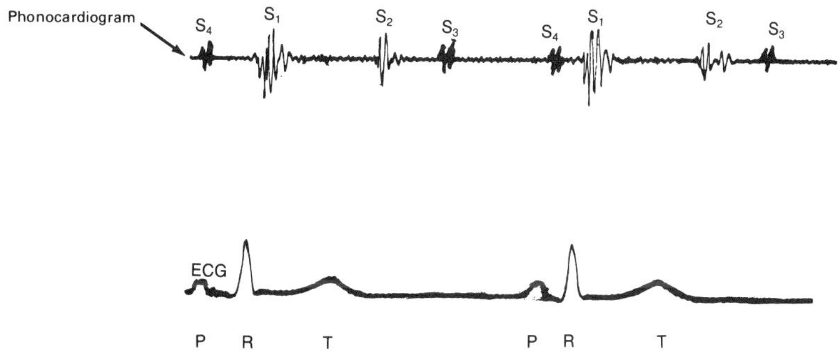

Third and Fourth Sounds

The third and fourth sounds indicate abnormalities in the following situations:

- When an adult with heart disease develops a third sound not heard previously, it indicates ventricular failure with elevated ventricular diastolic pressure and volume.
- When the fourth sound is heard at all (since it is rarely heard under normal conditions), it indicates atrial systolic strain or elevated atrial pressure as a result of increased ventricular end-diastolic pressure or resistance.

SELF-ASSESSMENT

1. Characterize the normal point of maximal intensity (PMI) or the apical impulse of the heart.

2. Name the areas for examination of cardiac sounds.

3. Locate each of these areas (question 2) with respect to thoracic topography.

4. Which valve closes when the aortic pressure exceeds left ventricular pressure?

5. Which three body positions are helpful when auscultating the heart?

6. State an order or routine for listening to cardiac auscultatory findings.

7. What is the R wave (ECG)? What causes it?

8. State the differentiating characteristics between venous and arterial neck waves.

9. What is the normal venous pressure?

10. State the anatomic origin of the first and second sounds.

11. State the physiologic origin of third and fourth sounds.

12. Which sound is heard normally with greater intensity at the base of heart?

13. Which sound is heard normally with greater intensity at the apex?

14. When the second sound splits normally, (a) In which phase of respiration is the splitting greatest? (b) Which sound comes first?

15. Explain the cause of splitting of the second sound.

CHAPTER FOURTEEN

Abdomen and Lower Extremities

J. Marc Shabot, M.D.

GENERAL INFORMATION: ABDOMINAL EXAMINATION

Position of Patient

The patient should be in a relaxed supine position, with the head elevated on a pillow and the arms along the sides. Since the structures to be investigated are beneath the abdominal wall, relaxation of the abdomen is essential.

Abdominal Quadrants

The anterior surface is divided into quadrants by two intersecting lines:

- One extends horizontally across the abdomen at the level of the umbilicus.
- The other extends vertically from the xiphoid to the symphysis pubis.

The important structures found in each quadrant are listed below.

NOTE: The medial halves of the right and left upper quadrants are often called the epigastrium.

Topographic Anterior Anatomy

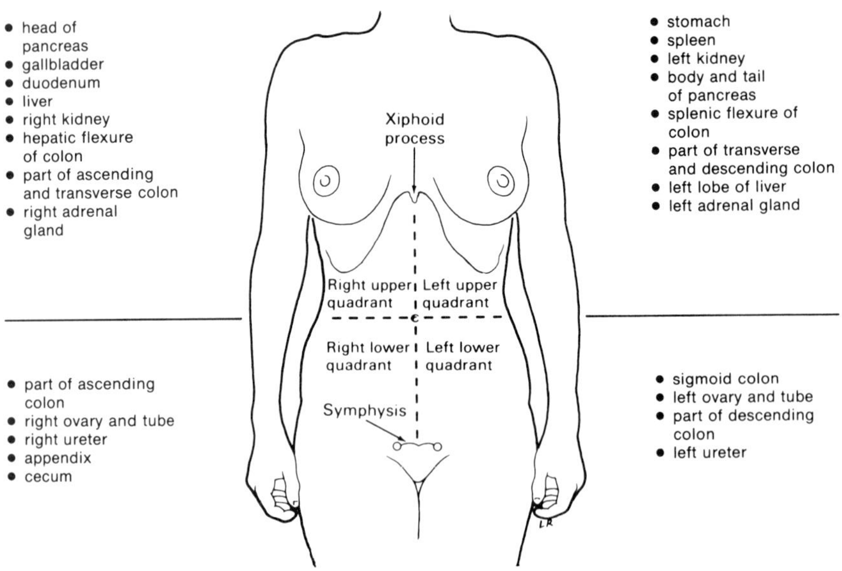

INSPECTION: SURFACE

Preparation

- The patient should be draped, but skin from the sternum to the pubis must be exposed.
- The room should have good lighting (oblique lighting will sometimes reveal features not otherwise visible).

Inspect Surface

The surface of the abdomen should be inspected for:

- condition of skin
- symmetry
- masses
- contour

Indications

IF THE FOLLOWING ARE OBSERVED	THEN THE EXAMINER MAY SUSPECT
blue or silver striae (vertical, wrinkled streaks) (See Fig. 14-1)	• prolonged stretching of skin due to: ascites, obesity, pregnancy, tumor, adrenocortical hyper-function (Cushing's syndrome)
tight, glistening skin (See Fig. 14-2)	• ascites • edema of the abdominal wall
small nodules	metastatic neoplasm
scars (note locations)	prior surgery
pulsations	• aortic aneurysm • tortuous aorta in slender person

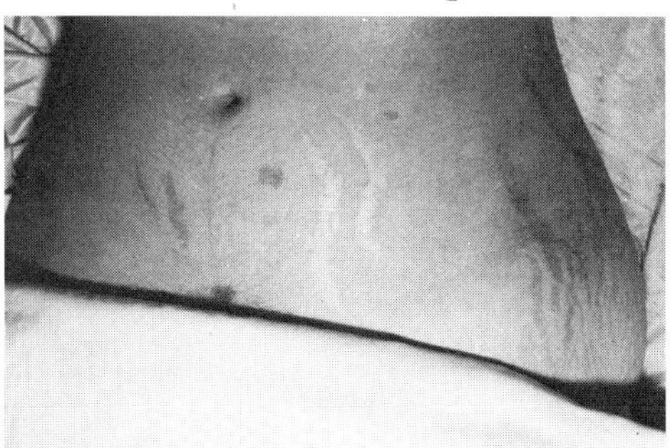

Figure 14-1.

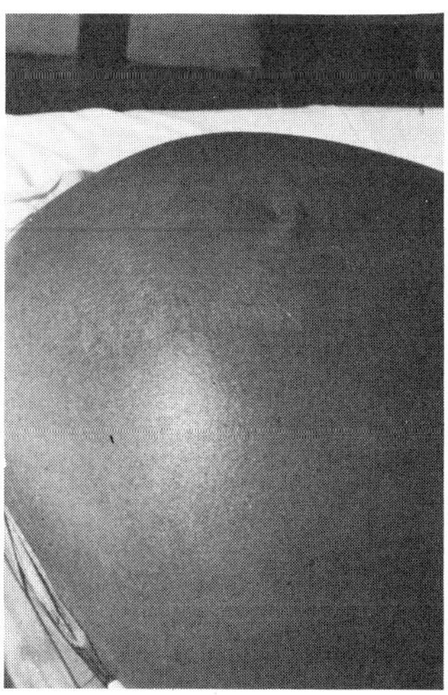

Figure 14-2.

NOTE: Visible (and palpable) pulsations may be transmitted to the abdominal wall by a tumor that overlies the aorta.

INSPECTION: FULLNESS

Inspection — To determine the degree of fullness, the abdomen is observed from the side.

Normal Patients

IF THE	THEN PATIENT LIKELY
abdomen is flat from xiphoid to symphysis pubis (scaphoid) (See Fig. 14-3)	is normal
abdomen is symmetrically protuberant (rounded) (See Fig. 14-4)	• is obese OR • has ascites OR • has intestinal obstruction

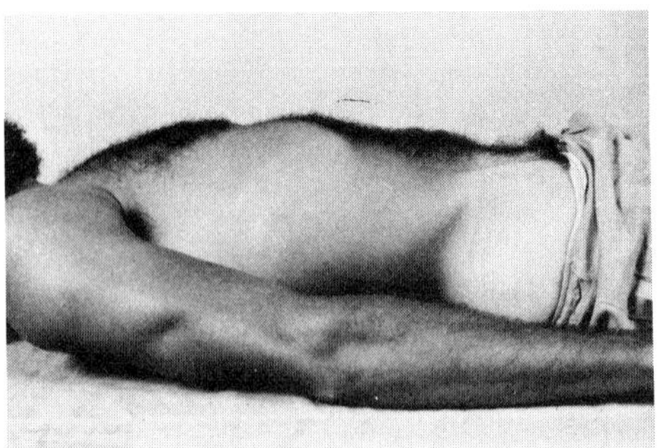

Figure 14-3.

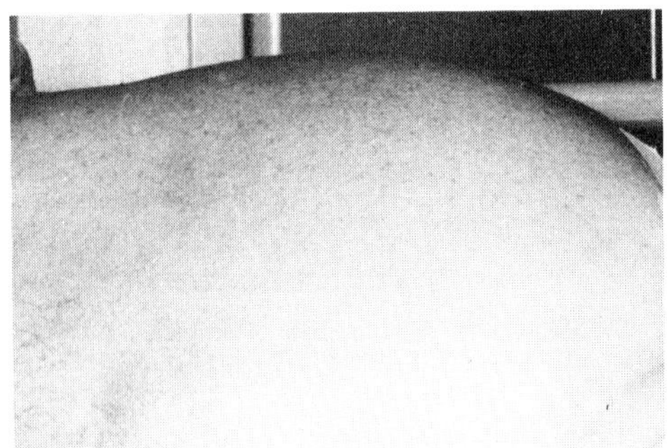

Figure 14-4.

(Continued)

INSPECTION: FULLNESS, Continued

Abdomen Distended

IF FULLNESS IS OBSERVED	THEN EXAMINER SHOULD SUSPECT
in the epigastric area	a mass originating in the upper abdominal structures: • liver • pancreas • stomach • transverse colon
in lower abdomen	• bladder distention • pregnancy • masses arising from: ovaries uterus colon
in the flanks	• ascites • cystic disease of the kidneys

NOTE: The cause of fullness or abdominal distention can be determined from the history and other physical findings.

Umbilicus

IF THE UMBILICUS IS	THE CAUSE IS USUALLY
inverted	obesity
everted or herniated	ascites

Peristaltic Contractions

When abdominal distention is accompanied by visible peristaltic movements, it almost always indicates mechanical intestinal obstruction.

INSPECTION: VEINS

Inspect Veins	In normal persons, the veins in the abdominal wall are hardly visible; distention of these veins indicates increased collateral circulation as a result of obstruction in the: • portal venous system OR • vena cava

Test for Flow Direction in Collateral Venous System

STEP	PROCEDURE
1	Empty 4 cm to 5 cm of a vein by "stripping" and compressing it between two fingers. See Figure 14-5.
2	Allow the vein to refill from one direction by removing one finger (See Fig. 14-6). Observe the rate of filling.
3	Empty the vein again as in Step 1 and allow to fill from the other direction by removing the other finger. Observe the rate of filling.
4	Compare the two rates of filling. The faster rate indicates the direction of flow.

Blood Flow in Abdominal Veins

WHEN FLOW OF BLOOD IN THE ABDOMINAL WALL IS	THE EXAMINER SUSPECTS
away from the umbilicus	the normal situation OR portal hypertension
toward the umbilicus	vena cava obstruction

See Figure 14-7.

Vena Cava Obstruction

WHEN THE FLOW DIRECTION IS REVERSED IN THE	AND THE DIRECTION IS	THE EXAMINER SUSPECTS OBSTRUCTION IN THE
upper abdominal veins	downward	superior vena cava
lower abdominal veins	upward	inferior vena cava

(Continued)

INSPECTION: VEINS, Continued

Liver Disease	In chronic liver disease, vascular cutaneous angiomas appear on the upper extremities, face, neck, and chest.
Cutaneous Angiomas (Spider Nevi)	"Spider nevi" can be differentiated from other lesions in that: • they blanch with gentle pressure on the central arteriole (see below) • they fill from the central arteriole out to the vascular branches

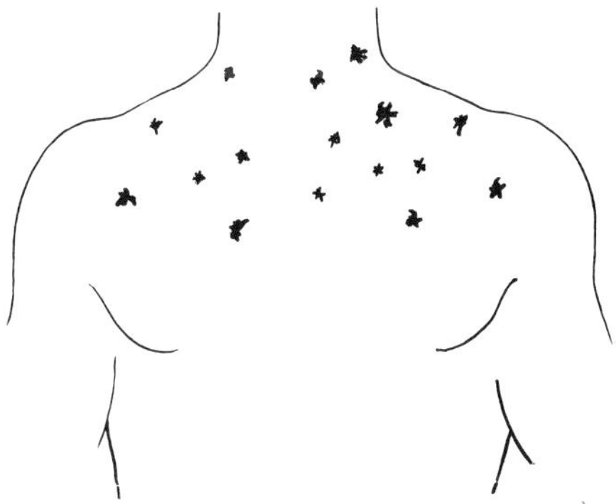

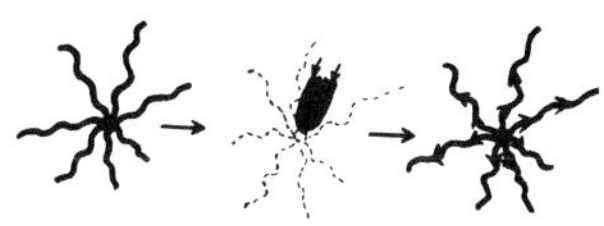

See Figures 14-8 and 14-9.

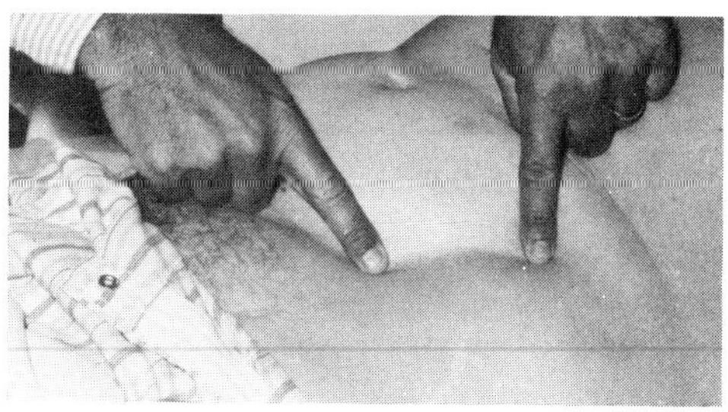

Figure 14-5.

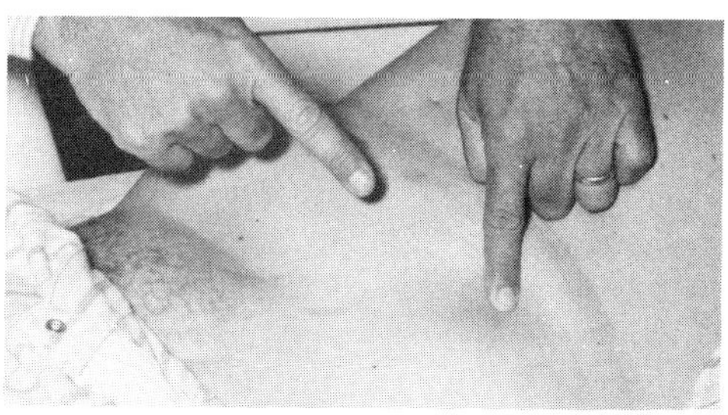

Figure 14-6.

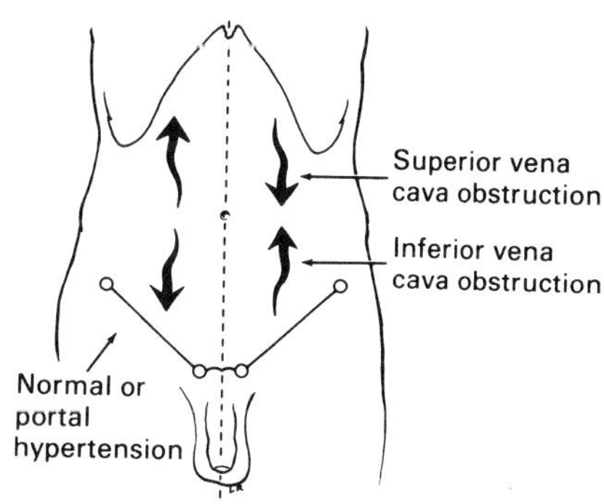

Figure 14-7.

Figure 14-8.

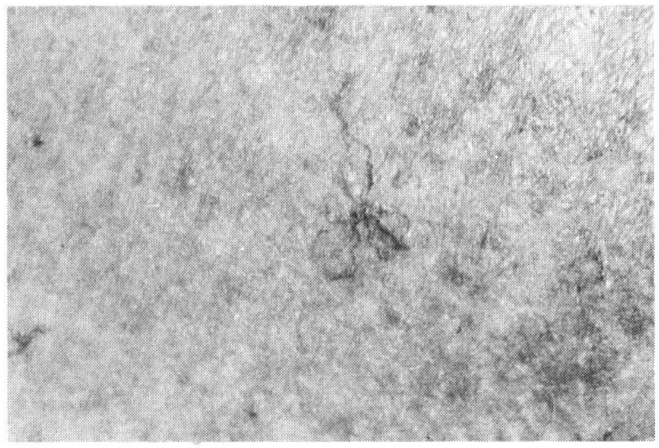

Figure 14-9.

INSPECTION: PIGMENTATION AND HAIR

Inspect Pigmentation

Abnormal pigmentation should be characterized in terms of whether it is:

- localized or diffuse
- increased or decreased

Hyperpigmentation from systemic disorders may be more noticeable on the skin of the abdomen, because changes in the color of the skin there are not as likely to be the result of exposure to sunlight. Since some systemic disorders cause increased pigmentation in areas of trauma, the abnormal coloring may be most obvious at the belt line or on recent scars.

Intra-abdominal Hemorrhage

Intra-abdominal hemorrhage sometimes causes a bluish pigmentation. A major intraperitoneal hemorrhage should be suspected if the umbilicus is bluish. Bluish flanks indicate extravasation of blood from intra-abdominal organs into extraperitoneal sites (as in hemorrhagic pancreatitis).

Inspect Hair

The distribution of pubic hair, termed the escutcheon, normally varies according to sex:

- Female distribution is a triangle with the base above the symphysis.
- Male distribution is a diamond with the upper vertex often extending to the umbilicus.
  See Figures 14-10 and 14-11.

The escutcheon may be changed by:

- chronic liver disease
- endocrine disorders

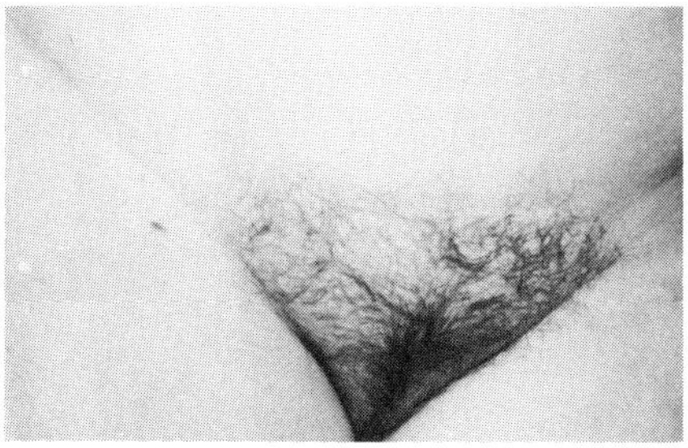

Figure 14-10.

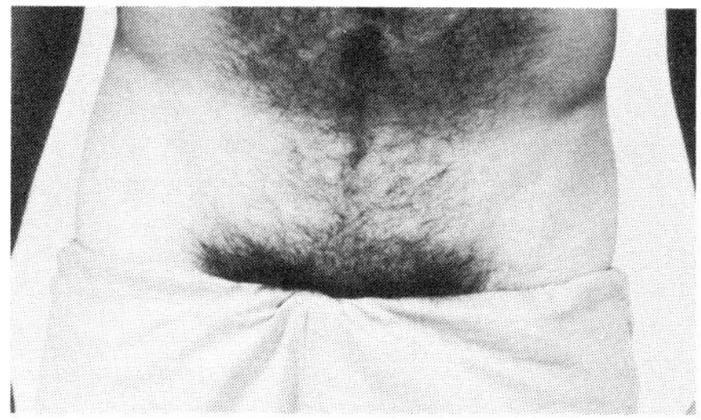

Figure 14-11.

AUSCULTATION: BOWEL SOUNDS

Varied Sequence — Auscultation is performed after inspection in the abdominal examination (unlike examinations of other body systems), because auscultatory findings may be affected by palpation of the abdomen. Enhanced peristaltic sounds may obscure other sounds, such as bruits and friction rubs.

Normal Bowel Sounds — Bowel sounds produced by intestinal peristalsis are present in the abdomen of normal persons. Thus, one goal of auscultation of the abdomen is to differentiate between normal and abnormal bowel sounds.

Differences in Bowel Sounds — Intestinal peristalsis produces gurgling noises that vary a great deal in:

- frequency
- intensity
- location
- pitch

The variations are caused by the constant changes in bowel contents and motility.

Examination Procedure

STEP	ACTION	COMMENT
1	Place the diaphragm of the stethoscope lightly against the abdominal wall.	Light pressure helps to eliminate extraneous sounds and sounds from movement of the diaphragm.
2	Listen for peristaltic sounds.	A wide range of bubbling or gurgling sounds may be heard.
3	Listen for two abnormalities.	• peristaltic silence • rush (see below)

(Continued)

AUSCULTATION: BOWEL SOUNDS, Continued

Abnormalities

ABNORMALITY	DESCRIPTION	PROBABLE CAUSE
silence	near-total absence of peristaltic sounds for minutes	immobile bowel or adynamic ileus caused by: • peritonitis • reflex paralysis (postoperative) • severe hypokalemia
	short, but frequent peristaltic sounds	increased intestinal motility (hyperperistalsis) caused by: • anxiety • infectious diarrhea • irritation of the intestinal mucosa (for example, blood)
rush; loud gurgling sounds	frequent, loud, high-pitched, tinkling, rushes, accentuated during peristaltic waves and cramping pain	Hyperperistalsis also may be caused by the intestine's attempt to squeeze contents through an obstructed area, that is, intestinal obstruction.

AUSCULTATION: BRUIT

Importance

As mentioned in the previous chapter, a bruit indicates vascular disease if it is heard consistently in an area with the patient in several positions.

Types of Bruit

LOCATION	PROBABLE CAUSE
over abdominal aorta	• atherosclerotic plaques • aneurysm • aortic compression by a tumor
over renal arteries	renal artery stenosis
right upper quadrant	vascular tumor involving the liver (hepatoma, hemangioma)

AUSCULTATION: FRICTION RUBS

Indications

Friction rubs are grating sounds produced by movement of roughened serous membranes over one another. Because movement is required to produce the sound, the patient should be instructed to breath deeply. Friction rubs may be heard over the abdomen, as indicated below.

LOCATION	PROBABLE CAUSE
over spleen	• abscess • infarction
over liver	• primary or metastatic neoplasm • abscess

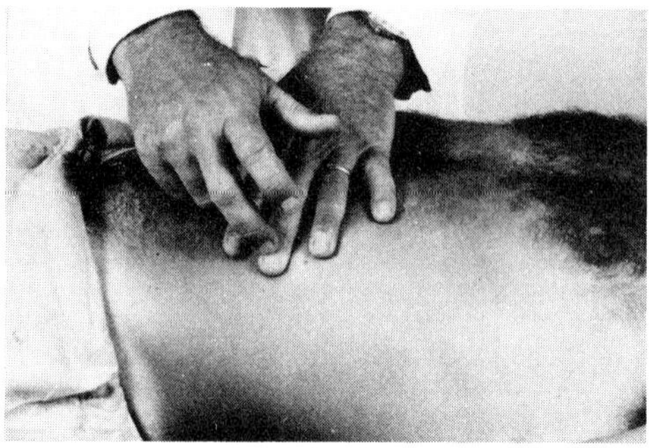

Figure 14-12.

PERCUSSION: OVERVIEW

Introduction

The objective of percussion of the abdomen is to determine whether the abdomen contains:

- intestinal distention
- free fluid
- abnormal solid masses
- hepatomegaly
- splenomegaly

Procedure

A systematic procedure for percussion should be used. The patient should be supine, and the examiner should stand at the patient's right.

STEP	ACTION	COMMENTS
1	Percuss downward over the lower left chest wall in the anterior axillary and mid-axillary lines.	A resonant note will normally be produced over the underlying lung, and a tympanitic note over the underlying stomach or colon. See Figure 14-12.
2	Listen for dullness in the gastric area.	Dullness could be caused by: • consolidation of the left lower lung • pleural effusion • splenomegaly
3	Percuss downward over the right lower chest wall in the anterior axillary and mid-clavicular lines.	Liver dullness should be appreciated.
4	Percuss at least one area in the right upper, left upper, right lower, and left lower quandrants.	A tympanitic note is heard, depending on amount of gas in the intestine.
5	Percuss in supra-pubic area.	Dullness caused by distention of the bladder may be heard.
6	Percuss the flanks for shifting dullness in the abdominal cavity.	Shifting dullness may be caused by free fluid (ascites).

PERCUSSION: LIVER DULLNESS

Variation	The normal upper border of liver dullness in the midclavicular line is the fifth or sixth interspace. Determination of the span of liver dullness is more important than pinpointing its upper border. The span of liver dullness is about 10 cm (upper limit of normal is about 12 cm) in the adult.
Determination of Liver Span	The span of liver dullness is evaluated by percussing downward from the fourth interspace in the midclavicular line until the upper border of dullness is determined. Percussion then proceeds downward over the liver until the lower border of liver dullness is located. A change to tympany marks the lower border of the liver. The normal lower limit of liver dullness is at or just below the costal margin. Dullness that extends into the normally tympanitic right upper quadrant indicates one or more of the following: • hepatic enlargement • downward displacement of the liver (e.g., by emphysematous lungs) • a mass adjacent to the liver
Absence of Liver Dullness	Absence of liver dullness can indicate: • perforation of a hollow viscus (e.g., duodenal ulcer), which allows air to enter the abdominal cavity • interposition of the hepatic flexure of the colon between the diaphragm and the liver • small, atrophic cirrhotic liver

PERCUSSION: SHIFTING DULLNESS

Action

When patients are lying supine, any ascitic fluid that is present will migrate into the flanks and produce dullness on both sides of the abdomen. The midabdomen is tympanitic, however, because of the bowel. When dullness is found in the flanks, a mark is made on the skin at the junction of dullness and tympany. Percussion from the flank to the midline is then repeated with the patient lying on his or her side. A mark is again made at the junction of dullness and tympany (see Figs. 14-13 and 14-14). The procedure is repeated after turning the patient to the other side.

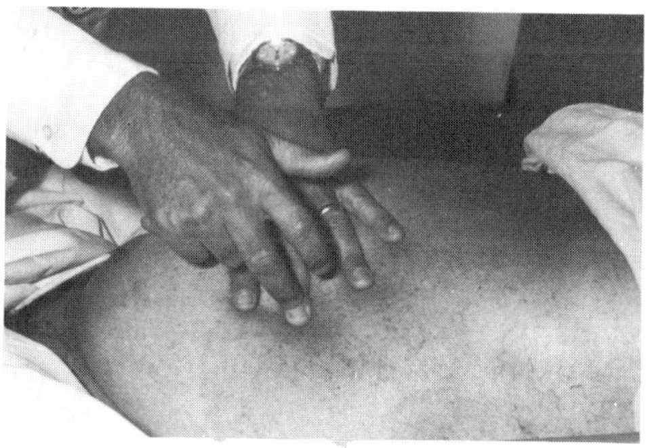

Figure 14-13.

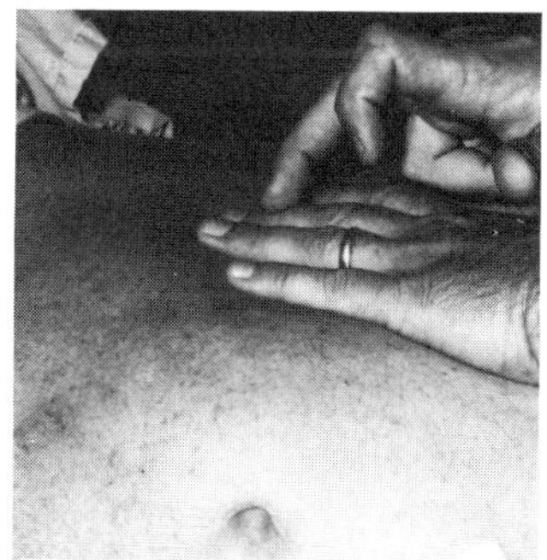

Figure 14-14.

Result

Since ascitic fluid will flow downward, the level of dullness will move toward the midline; that is, the level of dullness shifts. The bowel, which will have been displaced upward by the fluid, will produce a tympanitic note in the upper flank. This procedure can be repeated, turning the patient to the opposite side.

Shifting Dullness on Right Side

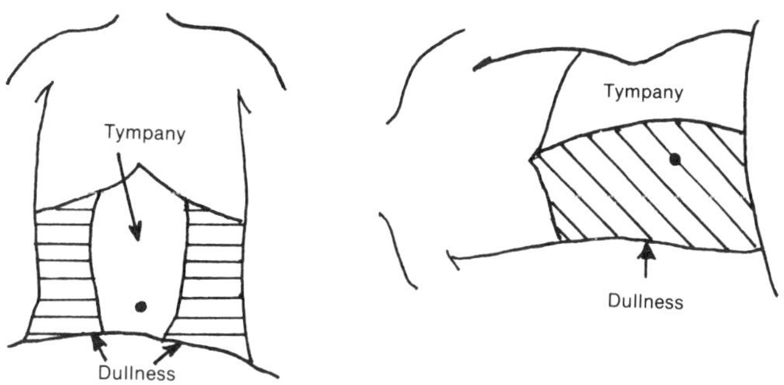

PALPATION: OVERVIEW

Introduction

Palpation, the final step in the abdominal examination, requires a great deal of skill and practice. The patient should be supine with the arms at the sides. The examiner's hands should be warm.

Types of Information

Several types of findings helpful to diagnosis may be yielded by palpation:
- pain from pressure applied to the abdomen
- contraction of the abdominal muscles (a finding related to pain and caused by intra-abdominal inflammation)
- tumors
- organ enlargement

Procedure

STEP	ACTION	COMMENT
1	Palpate gently over the entire abdomen at first.	• Do not attempt to elicit pain or to palpate deeply for tumors or enlarged organs. • Estimate muscle tone in various quadrants.
2	Ask the patient to flex the thighs and knees, if necessary, to achieve muscle relaxation.	This may be necessary for patients who are tense or who have muscular abdominal walls.
3	Palpate to locate painful areas.	Evaluate the constancy and severity of tenderness.
4	Palpate for enlargement of: • the spleen • the bladder • the liver	
5	Palpate deeply for: • masses • tenderness	Masses may be: • neoplasms • cysts • aneurysms • feces-filled bowel

(Continued)

PALPATION: OVERVIEW, Continued

Ticklishness	If the patient is ticklish, the examiner may first try to ignore this and continue. If that does not work, the patient's own hand can be placed on the abdomen. The examiner may then exert pressure on the abdomen through the patient's own hand. When the patient is relaxed, the examiner places his or her own hand on the abdomen and allows the patient to maintain contact with the abdomen with that hand.
Beginning Palpation	Palpation must begin with gentle exploration. The patient may be asked to breathe slowly and deeply, and questions may be asked about the history. If the patient stays tense or if the abdominal wall is very muscular, flexion of the thighs and knees may help. No attempt should be made either to elicit tenderness or to palpate for a tumor or enlarged organ at this time.

PALPATION: MUSCLE RESISTANCE

Involuntary and Voluntary Muscle Resistance

Muscle rigidity or resistance can be estimated during light palpation; if present, the examiner should determine whether it is voluntary or involuntary.

TYPE	CHARACTER	CAUSE
involuntary rigidity	reflexive, uncontrollable increase in tone	inflammatory lesions that involve the peritoneum
voluntary rigidity (tightening)	conscious or unconscious tensing	fear or nervousness; will disappear when patient relaxes

Test for Voluntary Tightening

To confirm that rigidity is caused by voluntary tension, an examiner may use the stethoscope for palpation. Because patients do not associate the instrument with pain or pressure, they will usually not react to it with voluntary muscle guarding. The examiner should apply the stethoscope lightly at first and then with increasing pressure. If rigidity is voluntary, the examiner can apply considerable pressure in this way and the abdominal wall will probably become more relaxed eventually. In involuntary rigidity, however, the response will be the same as that produced by manual palpation. See Figure 14-15.

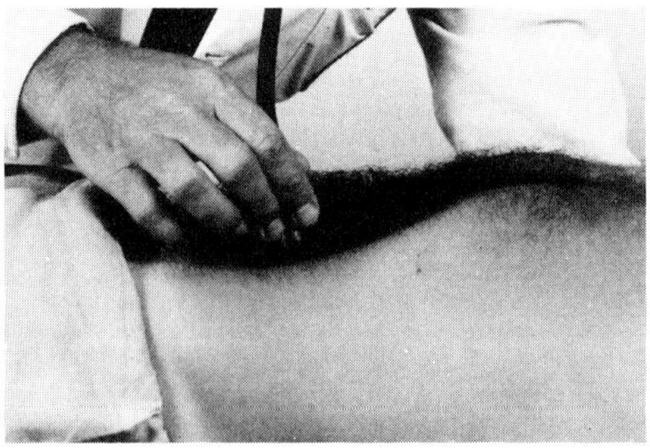

Figure 14-15.

PALPATION: EVALUATING PAIN

Locating Pain

After light general palpation, any painful areas within the abdomen are located and evaluated.

Types of Pain

Pain may be:

- visceral
- parietal (or somatic)
- both visceral and parietal

TYPE	CAUSE/LOCATION	CHARACTER	EXAMPLE
visceral	arises from within an abdominal organ	dull, poorly localized, difficult for patient to characterize	• distention of intestine from obstruction • pancreatic tumor
parietal (somatic)	inflammation of structure innervated by somatic sensory nerves	sharp, well-localized	inflammation of: • parietal peritoneum from peritonitis • ruptured appendix
combined	inflammation originating within a viscus and extending to the peritoneum	begins as visceral and becomes somatic as different areas are involved	appendicitis in which visceral pain becomes parietal in the right lower quadrant

(Continued)

PALPATION: EVALUATING PAIN, Continued

Rebound Tenderness

When pain has been elicited, the examiner should test for rebound tenderness, an indication of peritonitis that is found only when the parietal peritoneum becomes inflamed. The tenderness is usually substantial. The examiner may use two techniques to determine rebound tenderness:

- Press firmly over a region far from the tender area, and then release the pressure suddenly. The patient with rebound tenderness will feel a sharp pain in the area of disease and frequently will grimace.
- Rebound tenderness may be elicited by applying gentle pressure over the tender area and having the patient cough.

  NOTES:
  - If the area involved is small, rebound tenderness may be elicited only over the area.
  - Parietal (somatic) pain and rebound tenderness may be elicited by having the patient cough.

Constancy of Pain

After a painful area is located, the examiner should assess the constancy of the pain by palpating the area again.

IF PAIN	THEN THE CAUSE IS
is constant or increases with deeper palpation	inflammation
tends to disappear, even though pressure is continued	• visceral OR • psychogenic

PALPATION: SPLEEN

Introduction	An abdominal examination includes palpation for enlargement of the spleen, bladder, and liver.

Palpating for Splenic Enlargement

STEP	ACTION	COMMENT
1	Stand at the patient's right.	Patient is supine.
2	Place your left hand under the patient's left costovertebral angle, exerting pressure aimed to move the spleen anteriorly.	Steps 2 and 3 are done at about the same time.
3	Work the fingers of your right hand gently upward until they are beneath the patient's left anterior costal margin.	See the figure on the next page.
4	Keeping the hands stationary in this position, ask the patient to take a deep breath.	Enlargement of the spleen will be felt as a mass that slides out from under the ribs and bumps against the examiner's right hand.
5	Roll the patient toward the right (see the figure on the next page).	This is done if splenic enlargement is suspected but the spleen cannot be felt in step 4.
6	Place the hands as described in steps 2 and 3 and repeat step 4.	A spleen that cannot be felt with the patient supine may sometimes be palpated in this position.

<u>NOTE:</u> Because the spleen is not normally palpable in adults, it must be considered to be enlarged if it is felt at all.

(Continued)

PALPATION: SPLEEN, Continued

Palpation of Spleen: Supine Position

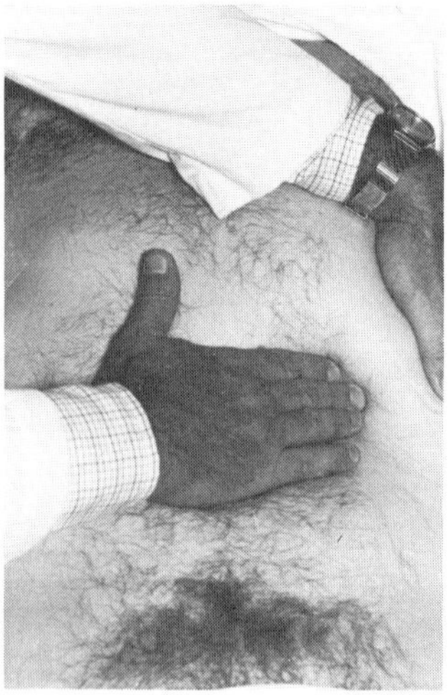

Palpation of Spleen: Right Lateral Decubitus Position

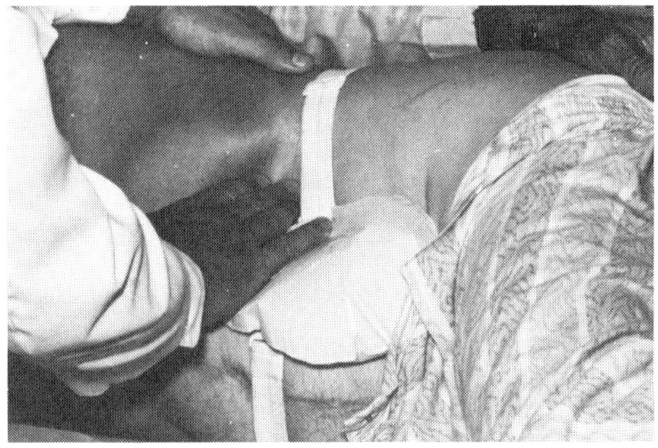

Examiner's left hand presses spleen anteriorly.

Extra-large Spleen

An inexperienced examiner may miss a spleen that is so large that its edge is far below the costal margin. Percussion of the left upper quadrant should prevent this error. If the spleen is not felt under the left costal margin, but enlargement is still suspected, the examiner should palpate more medially and inferiorly.

PALPATION: BLADDER

Palpating for Bladder Enlargement

An abnormally distended bladder may be palpated in the suprapubic region, whereas a normal bladder filled with urine cannot be felt. An abnormally distended bladder caused by obstruction of the urethra or by paralysis of the detrusor will feel the same before and after urination. Such an enlargement is often easier to detect by percussion than by palpation. See Figure 14-16. Proof that the mass is distended bladder may be obtained by inserting a urinary catheter through the urethra into the bladder.

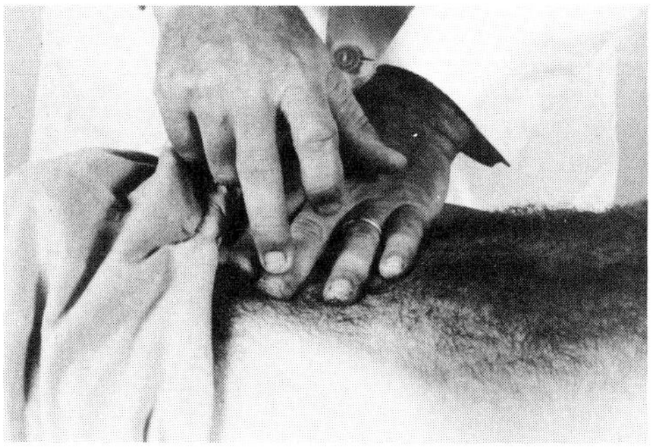

Figure 14-16.

PALPATION: LIVER AND NORMAL STRUCTURES

Palpating for Hepatic Enlargement

Ordinarily, the liver is not palpable, although it can sometimes be felt with the following procedure.

STEP	ACTION	COMMENT
1	Hold the right hand either parallel or perpendicular to the patient's long axis, at the level of the umbilicus.	See the photographs on the next page.
2	Work the fingers gently upward into the right upper quadrant.	
3	Holding the fingers in place, ask the patient to take a deep breath.	Sometimes the edge of a normal liver can be felt at, or slightly below, the right costal margin.

Palpation of the Liver

When the liver is palpated, a firm edge will strike the fingers when the patient inspires. When the edge is more than 2 cm below the costal margin, the liver:

- is abnormally large

OR

- is pushed downward by a low hemidiaphragm

OR

- has a congenitally large right lobe

Thus, in two circumstances, the liver can easily be palpated, but is not considered to be abnormally large (its total mass is normal). In emphysema, the diaphragm is depressed by the enlarged lung, which displaces the liver caudally.

(Continued)

PALPATION: LIVER AND NORMAL STRUCTURES, Continued

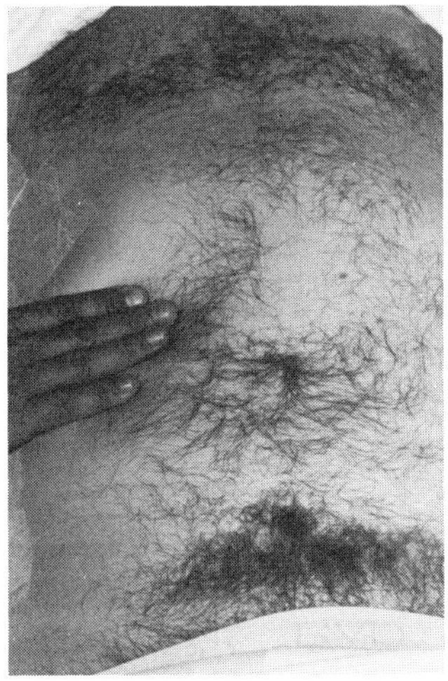

Examiner's fingers perpendicular to the patient's long axis.

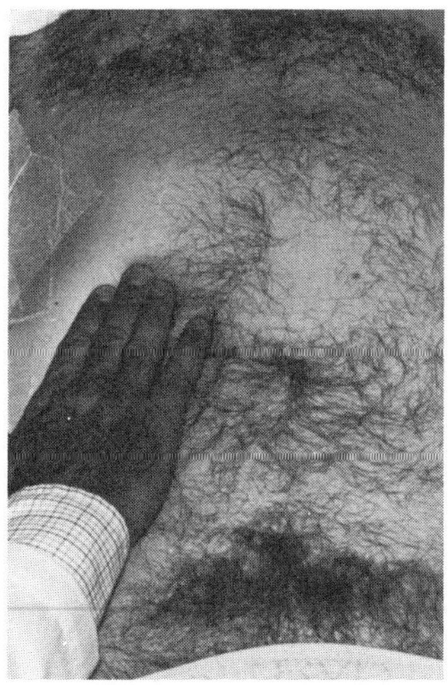

Examiner's fingers parallel to the patient's long axis.

Consistency

The surface and edge of the liver should be described in terms of whether they are:

- nodular
- soft
- smooth
- tender
- granular
- asymmetric

(Continued)

PALPATION: LIVER AND NORMAL STRUCTURES, Continued

Left Lobe of the Liver

The left lobe may be enlarged in the epigastrium, detected by percussion and palpation. Sometimes, an enlarged left lobe may extend below the umbilicus.

Other Normal Structures

Other normal organs may be felt in the abdomen:

STRUCTURE	LOCATION	COMMENT
inferior pole of kidneys	in either flank (with deep palpation of thin persons)	Normal kidneys descend slightly with inspiration and may be felt only in children and thin persons.
the cecum	in the right lower quadrant (see Fig. 14-17)	This soft, feces-filled intestine may frequently be palpated.
the sigmoid	in the left lower quadrant (see Fig. 14-18)	This sausage-shaped, feces-filled intestine is movable.

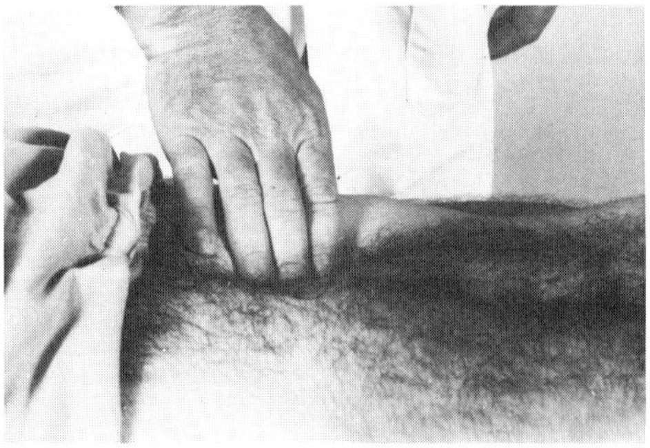

Figure 14-17.

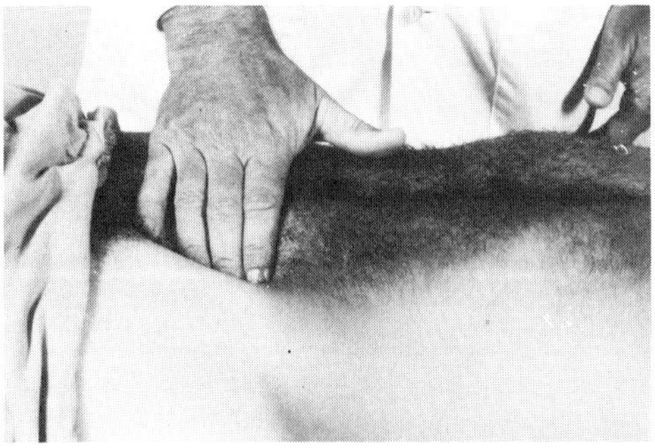

Figure 14-18.

PALPATION: ABNORMAL ABDOMINAL STRUCTURES

Introduction

The following abnormal structures may be palpated in the abdomen:

- neoplasms
- aneurysms of the abdominal aorta
- the gallbladders of patients with jaundice who have cancer of the head of the pancreas
- gallbladders that are inflamed because of obstruction of the cystic ducts by gallstones

Aneurysms

In thin patients, the normal aorta may be felt as a pulsatile structure in the mid-abdomen that extends down to the pelvic brim. Aneurysms are sausage-like enlargements of a segment of the abdominal aorta and are frequently felt as pulsatile and expansile masses. They often produce pain in the abdomen or back.

Distinguishing Aneurysms from Other Pulsatile Masses

The examiner must decide whether a pulsation is transmitted through an overlying structure from a normal or tortuous aorta or whether it is an aortic aneurysm. Aneurysmal pulsations are expansile. If the aorta is the site of an enlargement, then the examiner should palpate it to test for expansibility. Differentiating an aneurysm from an overlying mass with transmitted pulsations may be aided by demonstrating that the pulsations not only are felt directly over the mass, but that they also displace the examining fingers laterally.

Gallbladder

In normal persons, the gallbaldder cannot be palpated. In some patients with extrahepatic biliary tract obstruction, however, it may be felt in the right upper quadrant as a soft, cystic mass. A distended gallbladder (6 cm to 8 cm in diameter) appears to be attached to the liver and moves with respiration.

Differentiating Cancer from Gallstones

A palpable gallbladder helps to distinguish jaundice caused by cancer of the head of the pancreas or the common bile duct from jaundice caused by obstruction of the duct by gallstones. If a tumor is present in the common bile duct or head of the pancreas, the wall of the gallbladder is usually normal, and the organ can distend until it is palpable. In obstruction caused by gallstones, however, the gallbladder wall is inflamed or fibrotic, and the organ is not capable of distention and thus not likely to be palpable.

NOTE: The presence of a palpable gallbladder in a jaundiced patient is called Courvoisier's sign.

(Continued)

PALPATION: ABNORMAL ABDOMINAL STRUCTURES, Continued

Exception

In patients with obstruction of the cystic duct and cholecystitis, the gallbladder may be palpable as a very tender right upper quadrant mass (empyema of the gallbladder).

Abdominal Masses

Abdominal masses that are not an enlarged organ should be characterized in terms of their:

- size
- location
- consistency
- contour
- mobility
- tenderness

Masses in the abdominal wall may be distinguished from intra-abdominal masses or enlarged organs by palpation during voluntary tensing of the muscles. The patient should be asked to lift his or her head from the examining table. Abdominal wall masses will remain palpable during this action and may even become more obvious as they are elevated by the tensed muscle. In contrast, intra-abdominal organs or masses are more difficult to discern and may not be palpable when the muscles of the wall are tensed.

Umbilical Masses

The umbilicus should be palpated for signs of nodularity or a mass. Umbilical masses may be caused by metastasis of an intra-abdominal neoplasm through the peritoneum.

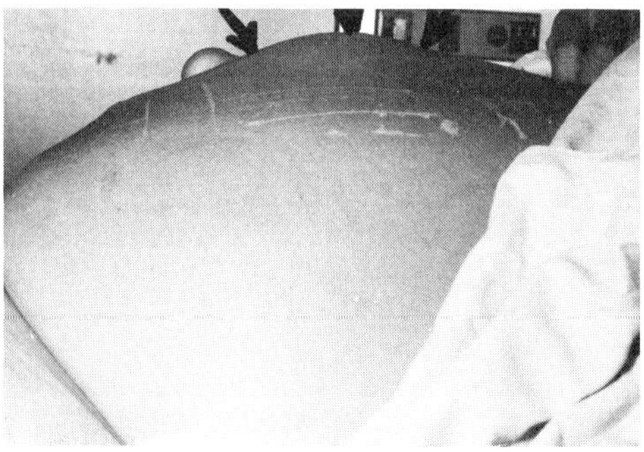

Figure 14-19.

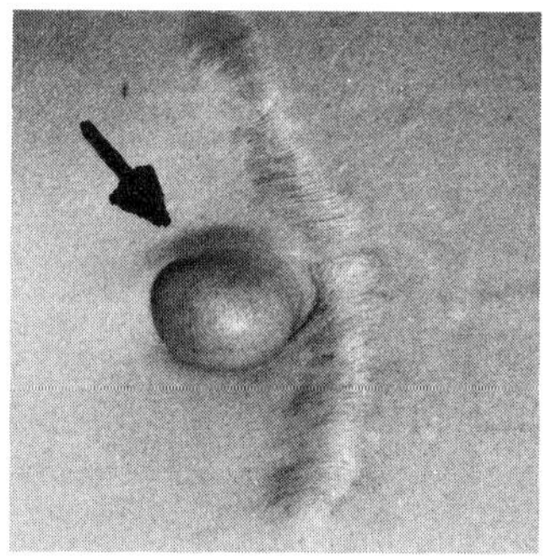

Figure 14-20.

PALPATION: HERNIAS

Hernias

Hernias are abnormal protusions of intraperitoneal organs through defects in the peritoneum.

TYPE	DESCRIPTION	COMMENTS
ventral	soft masses that protrude into the anterior abdominal wall (see Fig. 14-19)	usually occur in defects of abdominal muscles (surgical scars)
umbilical	a congenital defect in the base of the umbilicus (see Fig. 14-20)	usually large enough for insertion of finger; most obvious when patient coughs or strains
inguinal	a protrusion of peritoneum through the inguinal canal (see Fig. 14-21.	most common hernia; may contain bowel and/or mesentery

Diastasis Recti

Diastasis recti is a defect in the abdominal wall in the midline above the umbilicus in which there is herniation of omentum or intestine between the rectus sheaths. This condition, which is seen most often in obese persons or multiparous women, is not clinically important. See Figure 14-22.

(Continued)

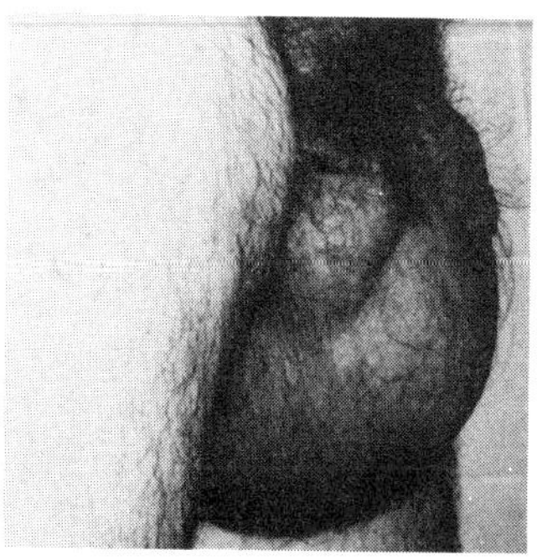

Figure 14-21.

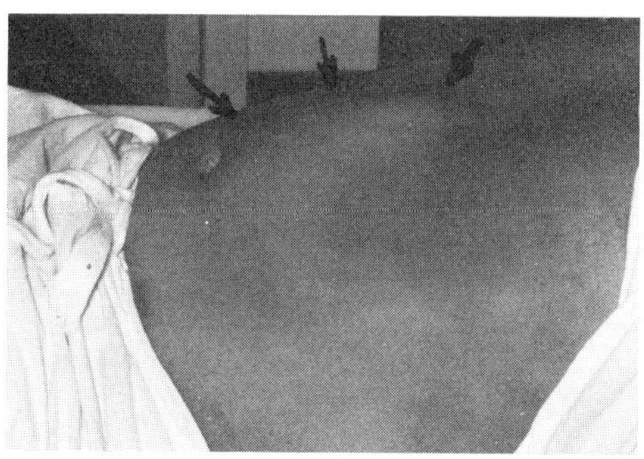

Figure 14-22.

PALPATION: HERNIAS, Continued

Palpating for Inguinal Hernias

The patient should be standing with the ipsilateral leg slightly flexed. The examiner, seated in front of the patient, should first observe both inguinal areas for of bulges. After inspection, an index finger should be inserted into both inguinal rings.

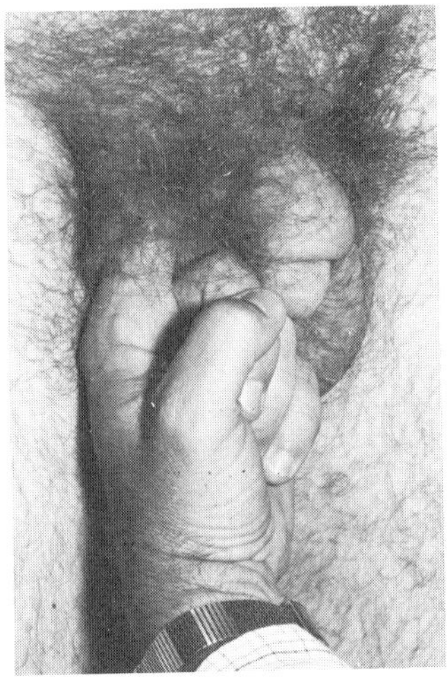

The loose skin on the side of the scrotum should be picked up and pushed ahead, following the spermatic cord, until the external inguinal ring is palpated. The examiners then determines whether the ring is normally tight or abnormally large and relaxed.

- Normally, the inguinal ring can be felt as a firm, sharp ring no larger than the tip of the index finger. The patient then is asked to "bear down" or to cough, which tenses the abdominal muscles. An impulse against the finger may be felt, but a mass does not protrude through the ring.
- An inguinal hernia is a soft, sausage-shaped mass that pushes against the tip of the examining finger. Some hernias consist of large loops of intestine. See Figure 14-21.

RECTAL EXAMINATION

Overview

The rectal examination, an essential part of every general physical examination, need not cause undue discomfort if proper procedures are followed.

Equipment

The required equipment for this examination includes:
- a good light source, e.g., a "gooseneck" lamp
- lubricating jelly
- glove

Patient Positioning

Four positions facilitate the rectal examination; each position has a specific utility.

PATIENT POSITION	POSITION UTILITY
left lateral decubitus: patient lies on the left side with the thighs and knees flexed (A, next page)	Best position for unconscious patients
knee-chest: patient rests on the knees with the shoulders and head on a bed (B, next page).	good position for assessing the prostate gland
bending over a table: patient bends at the waist over a table (C, next page)	usual position for assessing the rectum and the prostate gland of ambulatory men
dorsal lithotomy: patient lies supine with the knees flexed and the feet in the stirrups of the examining table	usual position for women so that the rectal examination is part of the pelvic examination

(Continued)

RECTAL EXAMINATION, Continued

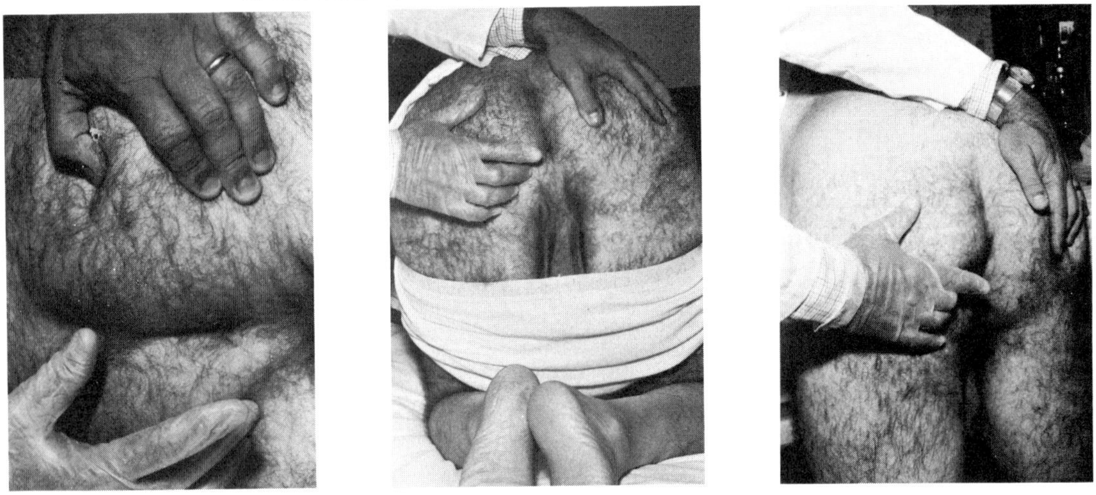

A B C

Procedure

STEP	ACTION
Position the patient suitably.	
Inspect the anal area.	Look for skin lesions, hemorrhoids, fissures, and fistulas. NOTE: Fissures or fistulas may produce pain when the buttocks are spread.
Lubricate the gloved index finger; insert the finger gently through the anus.	Apply the lubricated index finger to the anal sphincter using steady pressure; in a few seconds, the finger will painlessly enter the anal canal and rectum. Observe the: • anal sphincter tone as it contracts around the finger • presence or absence of stricture NOTE: Internal hemorrhoids can be felt only if thrombosed.
Palpate the mucosa of all walls of the rectum.	Feel for tumors.

(Continued)

RECTAL EXAMINATION, Continued

STEP	ACTION
Turn the examining finger anteriorly.	In men, evaluate the size, shape, tenderness, and consistency of the prostate gland.
Instruct the patient to bear down.	Feel for tumors that may descend and made palpable by the Valsalva maneuver.
Withdraw the finger; inspect any stool on the glove.	Observe the color: • If the stool is tarry black, upper gastrointestinal tract bleeding may be present. • If dark or red blood is observed, a sigmoidoscopic examination must be performed.
Test the feces for occult blood.	Place a small amount of stool on a card for chemical detection of blood (stool guaiac).

Notes on Procedure

- Cancer of the intra-abdominal organs often spreads to the peritoneum anterior to the rectum. The malignant deposits ("rectal shelf lesions") may be palpated as hard nodules just above the prostate or in the cul-de-sac in women.
- In the rectal examination of women, the cervix will be felt as a firm round mass in the anterior wall.

Sigmoidoscopy

In a digital rectal examination, about 6 cm to 8 cm of the rectum can be felt. A roentgenographic evaluation is valuable only above 15 cm to 20 cm in the rectosigmoid. Thus, 8 cm to 10 cm in the upper portion of the rectum can be examined only by sigmoidoscopy. Since benign and malignant lesions develop in this area, sigmoidoscopy is mandatory if patients (especially those over 40) have:

- rectal bleeding
- recent change in bowel habits
- lower abdominal pain

LOWER EXTREMITIES: GENERAL EXAMINATION

Overview

The characteristics of the lower extremities that should be observed are:
- condition of skin, hair, and nails
- symmetry
- presence of edema
- shape
- muscles and joints
- veins and arteries
- lymph nodes

The skin, bones, and joints of the lower extremities are subject to the same disorders that can affect the upper extremities, but because of the upright posture of humans and the attendant elevated hydrostatic pressure, the legs are subject to additional disorders.

Skin, Hair, and Nails

Some dermatologic diseases that affect the arms also affect the legs. The toenails may have the same diseases that affect the fingernails. Loss of hair on the foot and lower leg, dystrophic changes in the nails, and ulceration of the skin may reflect ischemia. Raynaud's phenomenon is sometimes observed in the toes.

Symmetry

Asymmetry of the legs may be caused by:
- unilateral edema
- atrophy
- trauma
- congenital defects

If the examiner suspects that a part of a leg is larger than in the other, the circumference of both legs should be measured at the same level, by using the following method:
- Instruct the patient to lie relaxed in a supine position.
- Make a mark at a chosen number of centimeters below (for calf) or above (for thigh) the inferior border of the patella.
- Measure and record the circumferences of both legs at this level.

If the examiner suspects that one leg is longer than the other:
- Instruct the patient to stand with his or her weight evenly distributed on the feet.
- Palpate and mark both posterior superior iliac spines.
- Measure and record the distance from the iliac spine to the floor.

(Continued)

LOWER EXTREMITIES: GENERAL EXAMINATION, Continued

Examining for Edema

Enlargement of the legs is often caused by edema. Edematous tissues will indent if an examiner presses them. Pitting edema may be observed by exerting gentle constant pressure with a finger. See Figure 14-23.

Causes of Edema

Edema usually begins in the most dependent areas, namely the feet or ankles. As edema worsens, it may extend to the knees, thighs, buttocks, and sacrum.

- Bilateral edema may result from:
  - heart failure
  - chronic liver disease
  - nephrotic syndrome
  - obstruction of the inferior vena cava caused by
    - tumors
    - thrombosis
    - gravid uterus
  - bilateral varicose veins
- Unilateral edema may result from:
  - unilateral varicose veins (see Fig. 14-24)
  - thrombophlebitis
  - lymphangitis or lymphatic obstruction
  - obstruction of the iliac or femoral veins by enlarged lymph nodes or tumors
  - stasis from disuse (in patients with hemiplegia).

Alterations in Shape of Leg

CAUSE OF ALTERATION	APPEARANCE
osteitis deformans (Paget's disease)	legs bowed; anterior tibial surface convex
syphilitic periostitis (caused by congenital syphilis)	tibial surfaces bowed anteriorly (saber shins)
poorly aligned fractures	various deformities
deformities resulting from tumor (see Fig. 14-25)	deformed tumorous enlargement

(Continued)

LOWER EXTREMITIES: GENERAL EXAMINATION, Continued

Condition of Muscles

Inspect muscles for development and palpate for tenderness. Muscle atrophy in the legs:

- may be unilateral or bilateral
- usually results from neuropathic paralysis (see Fig. 14-26)
- may occasionally be caused by disuse that results from previous musculoskeletal injury

Muscle tenderness is usually due to:

- excessive exertion in an unconditioned person
- myositis
- inflammation of adjacent structures, as in thrombophlebitis

Joints

Examine the joints for:

- deformity
- range of movement

Deformities usually result from arthritis, but tumors in or adjacent to joints may cause a deformity. The range of movement, done by the patient (active) and by the examiner (passive) should be assessed. This should be done with the hips, knees, and ankles.

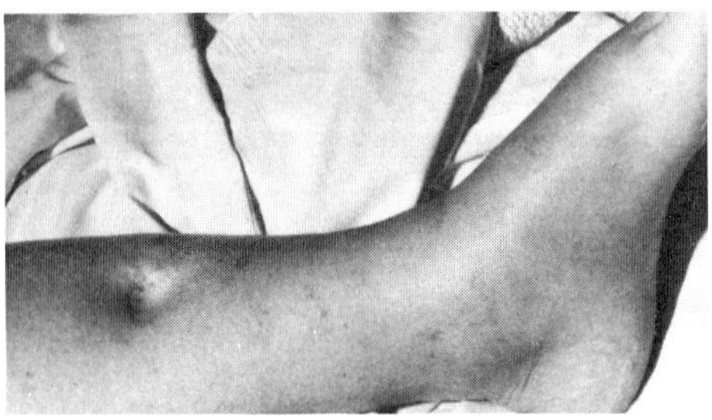

Figure 14-23.

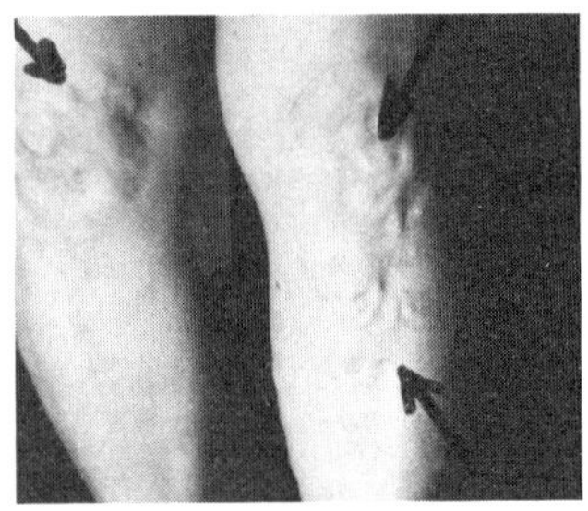

Figure 14-24.

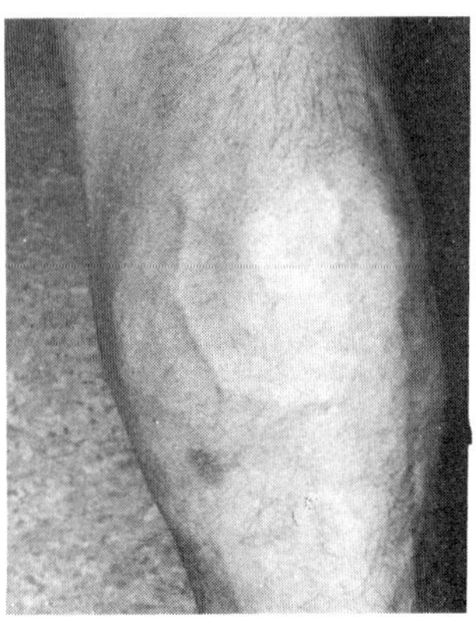

Figure 14-25.

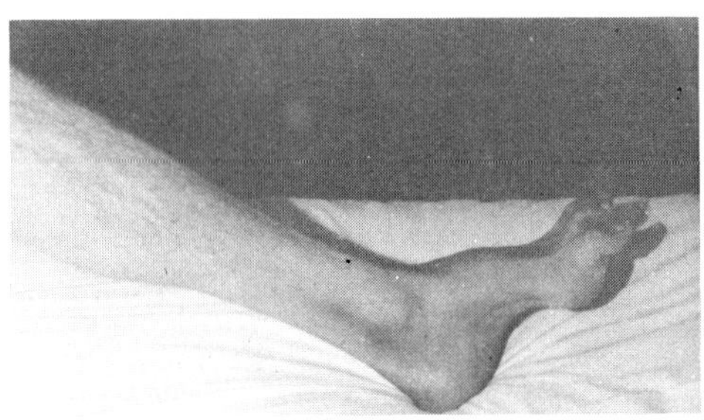

Figure 14-26.

LOWER EXTREMITIES: VEINS AND ARTERIES

Diseases of the Veins	Diseases of the leg veins that are more common than in the arms include: • varicosities • superficial thrombophlebitis • deep thrombophlebitis
Varicose Veins	Varicose veins are tortuous, dilated, and elongated veins that are often observed in adults, especially women. Deep varicose veins, due to incompetent venous valves, may be invisible. Varicose veins may cause: • stasis ulcers (see Fig. 14-27) • a bronze pigmentation ("stasis dermatitis"), which is hemosiderin from extravasated erythrocytes
Superficial Thrombophlebitis	In superficial thrombophlebitis, the veins are red, edematous, and tender, and the surrounding tissue may be similarly affected. The involved vein may be palpated as a cord in the subcutaneous tissues. Regional inguinal and femoral lymph nodes may be enlarged and tender. Pulmonary embolism occurs only rarely from superficial thrombophlebitis.
Deep Venous Thrombophlebitis	Deep thrombophlebitis may occur in the thigh, calf, or both. Venous stasis predisposes to thrombosis in patients: • who have recently had surgery or given birth • with congestive heart failure • with any chronic debilitating disease that keeps the patient in bed Because venous thrombosis generally produces little reaction in the vein wall, the thrombus has a tendency to dislodge and embolize to the pulmonary arteries. Thrombosis that causes enough inflammation of the vein to be detected is termed thrombophlebitis. Symptoms include fever, pain, particularly with walking or standing, and tenderness in the calf or thigh. The leg may be swollen (visibly or measurably) and warmer than usual, and its superficial (collateral) veins may be distended. Deep palpation or squeezing pressure usually elicits tenderness. Dorsiflexion at the ankle may elicit pain in the calf (Homan's sign; see Fig. 14-28)

(Continued)

LOWER EXTREMITIES: VEINS AND ARTERIES, Continued

Palpation of Arterial Pulses

An examination of the lower extremities must include palpation of the pulses.

PULSE	LOCATION FOR PALPATION
femoral	femoral triangle
popliteal	popliteal fossa (with the patient lying on the back with the knee and hip flexed about 45° (see Fig. 14-29)
posterior tibial	posterior to the internal malleolus (see Fig. 14-30 and figure A, below)
dorsalis pedis	between the first and second metatarsal bones (see figure B, below)

NOTE: About 10% of normal people do not have one or both dorsalis pedis arteries, or their arteries are located where they are not palpable. Thus, the absence of dorsalis pedis pulsations alone does not prove the existence of arterial disease.

A. Palpating the posterior tibial artery. B. Palpating the dorsalis pedis artery.

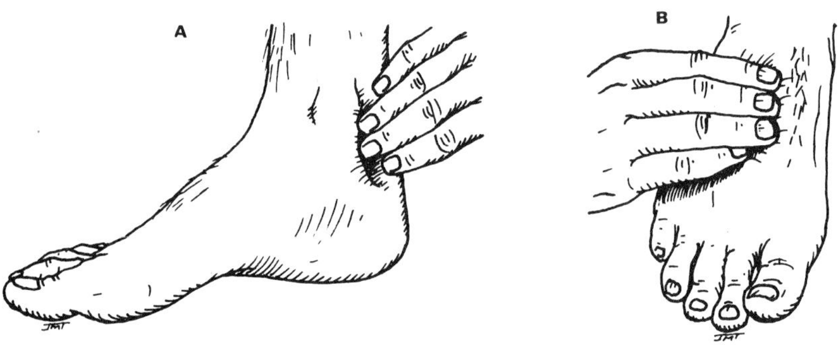

(Continued)

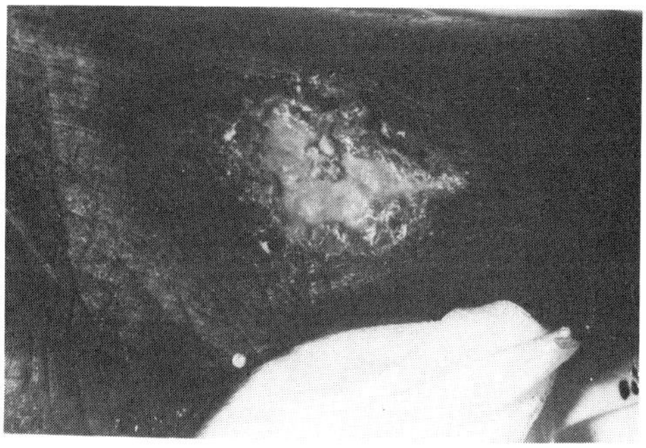

Figure 14-27.

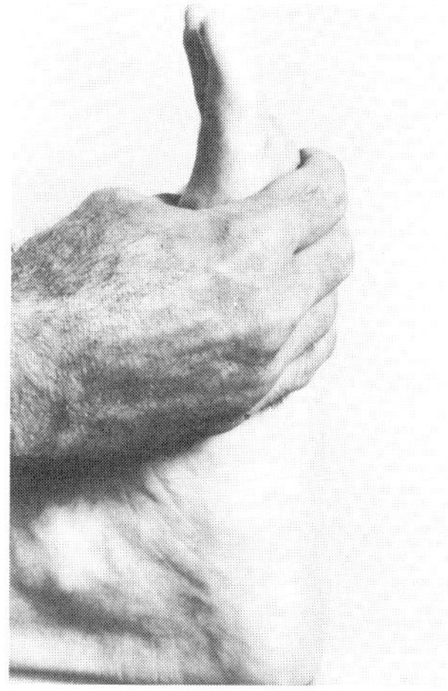

Figure 14-28.

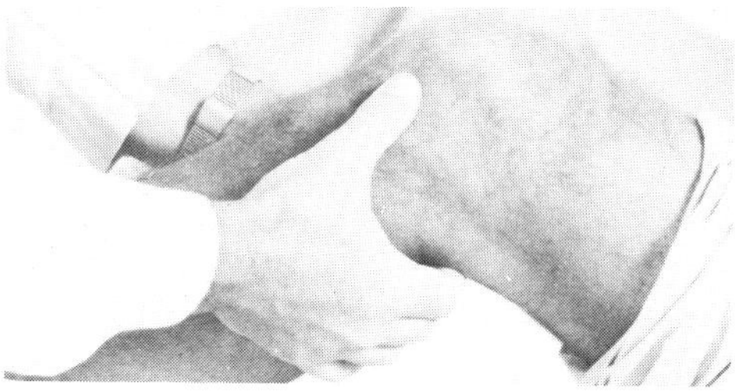

Figure 14-29.

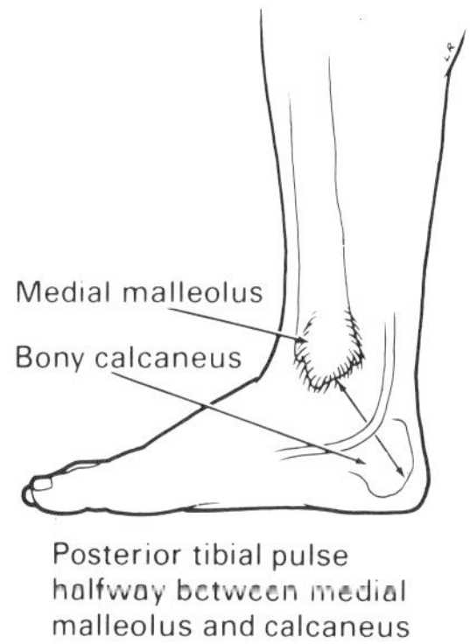

Figure 14-30.

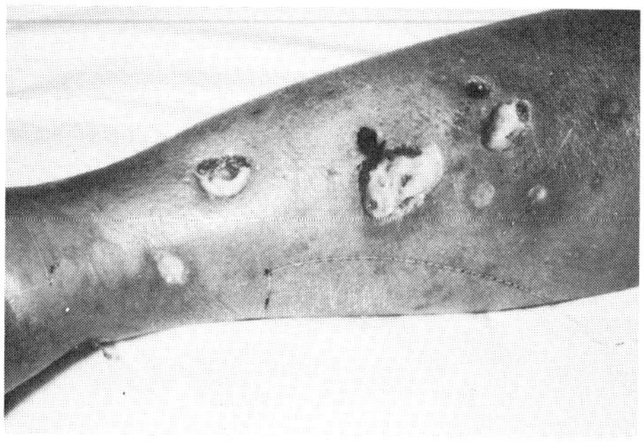

Figure 14-31.

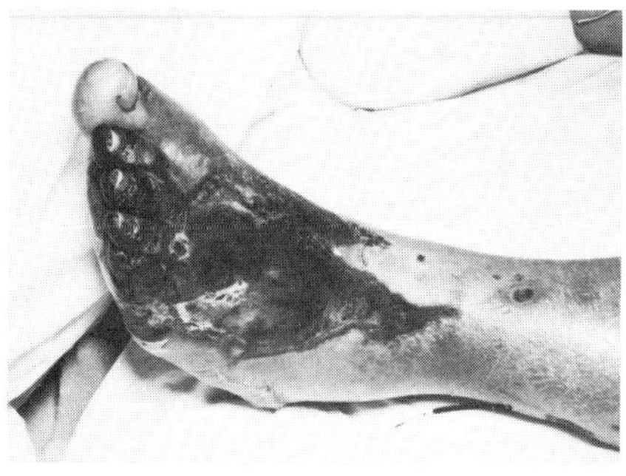

Figure 14-32.

LOWER EXTREMITIES: VEINS AND ARTERIES, Continued

Obstruction of Arteries	With obstruction of a major artery, pulses distal to the obstruction cannot be palpated. If the obstruction involves the common or external iliac artery, the femoral and all distal pulses may not be palpated.
Effects of Arteriosclerotic Ischemia	In patients with arteriosclerosis, any or all of the arterial pulses may not be detected, and the feet and distal legs: • are cold • blanch when the leg is raised • become red or cyanotic (reddish purple) when the leg is dependent Ulceration or gangrene of the toes may result. See Figures 14-31 and 14-32.
Arterial Bruits	Arteriosclerotic stenosis of the iliac, femoral, or popliteal arteries may produce a bruit upon auscultation. The bruit can be heard when the stethoscope is placed over the involved artery.

LOWER EXTREMITIES: LYMPH NODES

Regional Lymph Nodes

An examination of the lower extremities must include inspection and palpation of the lymph nodes. The groin contains two groups of lymph nodes:

- Inguinal lymph nodes are located in the region of the inguinal ligament and drain the genitalia, perineum, lower abdomen, buttocks, and parts of the thighs (see figure below).
- Femoral lymph nodes are located in the femoral triangle and drain the lower thighs, legs, and feet (see figure below).

Either or both groups of nodes may be enlarged because of:

- infections distant from the nodes, but in the area drained by the lymphatics (lymphangitis and lymphadenitis)
- systemic infections (for example syphilis and infectious mononucleosis)
- neoplasms
  - primary (lymphomas)
  - metastatic

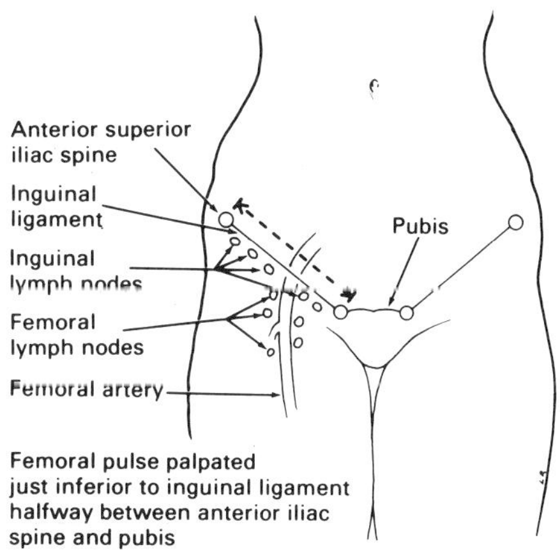

SELF-ASSESSMENT

1. Name the organs associated with each of the four abdominal quadrants.
2. State the normal size (span) of the liver in adults.
3. Describe the sequence of steps in a systematic examination of the abdomen.
4. List six general objectives of the examination of the abdomen.
5. Describe how to elicit shifting dullness, and explain its significance.
6. List the characteristics of visceral and somatic abdominal pain.
7. State six characteristics of an abdominal mass that should be described.
8. Name the two groups of lymph nodes in the groin and list the areas drained by each.

CHAPTER FIFTEEN

The Neurological Examination

Harold H. Morris III, M.D.

OVERVIEW

Introduction	The neurological examination may be conducted as a screening procedure or as a rigourous and detailed evaluation. The type of examination which is administered should be adapted to the individual problem of the patient. It is not necessary to perform a complete and detailed examination on every patient when it is irrelevant to the problem under consideration.
Medical History	The patient's history is the best indicator in the planning of the examination. If the history suggests neurological disease or if a neurological deficit is revealed, the examination must be extended to provide a complete study of the problem.
Examples	• In the case of a middle-aged businessman complaining of forgetfulness, it would be essential that a complete mental status examination be accomplished. • In an individual complaining of progressive weakness in his legs, a thorough evaluation of muscle strength and motor system is required.
Screening Procedure	When no neurological disorder has been indicated on the history, a satisfactory screening examination, to detect any abnormalities, can be accomplished within 5 minutes.
Interview	The experienced physician can obtain important neurological information during the interview. Observation of the patient during this time can uncover abnormalities in several areas: • speech • language function • memory • emotional status • judgment
Section Content	This section will discuss the major parts of the neurological exam that must be done when the history or screening examination suggests neurological disease. Parts of this exam are included in the screening examination (i.e., gait, cranial nerves, and tendon reflexes).

(Continued)

OVERVIEW, Continued

Note	This section is not intended to list all components of a detailed examination.

Outline for Neurological Examination	• mental status-- covered briefly in this book
	  • general behavior and appearance
	  • affect (mood)
	  • intellectual function, orientation to environment, and memory
	  • thought processes
	  • judgment, reliability, and insight
	• cranial nerves II-XII
	• motor function
	• gait/stance
	• coordination
	• tendon reflexes
	• abnormal reflexes
	• sensory function

CRANIAL NERVE I: OLFACTORY

Olfactory Nerve

The olfactory nerve is usually tested only if the patient has complaints of:
- anosmia
- a history of head injury

or if the examiner suspects a frontal lobe neoplasm

Testing Procedure

To test the olfactory sense:

STEP	ACTION
1	occlude one nostril
2	Patient sniffs and identifies an unknown substance. Use available and nonpungent substances such as soap, tobacco, or coffee.

Note

Unilateral loss is significant because it may indicate:
- olfactory groove meningioma
- laceration of the olfactory nerve from trauma to the head

CRANIAL NERVE II: OPTIC

Testing Visual Acuity

- Visual acuity can be measured at the bedside using a reading card.
- For neurological purposes, corrected visual acuity is most helpful; therefore, if the patient wears glasses, check acuity with them.

Visual Field

Visual field testing can be accomplished by using the confrontation test.

Fundus Examination

On fundus examination note the:

- color and outline of the optic disk
- presence or absence of spontaneous venous pulsations
- configuration, color, and size of arteries and veins
- presence or absence of macular abnormalities

Diagram of Major Lesions of Optic Pathways

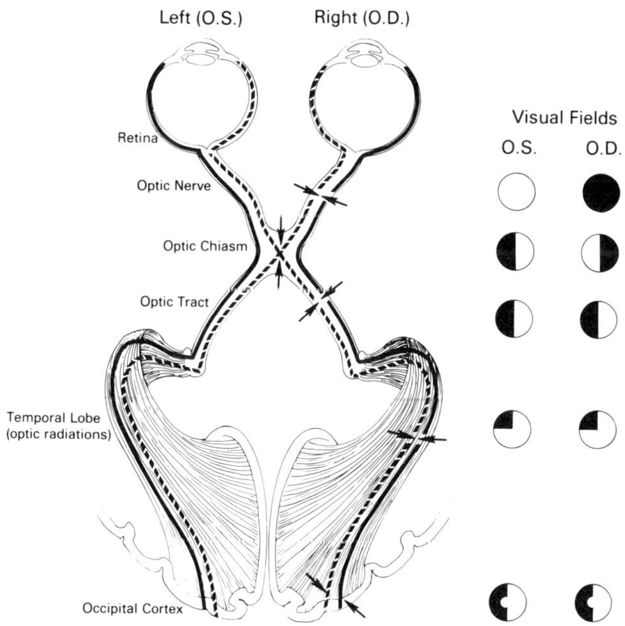

CRANIAL NERVES III, IV, VI: OCULOMOTOR, TROCHLEAR, ABDUCENS

Testing of Nerves

The testing of these three nerves can be accomplished by observing eye movements. Have the patient follow your finger with his eyes, while keeping his head stationary. Use the cardinal positions of gaze of the extraocular muscles.

Pupillary Light Reflex

Retinal nerve fibers subserving the pupillary light reflex:

- course posteriorly in the optic nerve and both optic tracts
- enter the pretectal area as they leave the tract and innervate the Edinger-Westphal nucleus of either side. Consequently, the illumination of one retina normally induces constriction of both pupils.

Unilateral Loss of Pupillary Light Reflex

In the unilateral loss of the pupillary light reflex, the consensual reactions are of diagnostic importance.

Disorders

If a disorder is caused by a unilateral loss of function of the right optic nerve then:

LIGHT DIRECTED INTO THE	WILL RESULT IN
right eye	no direct or consensual reaction
left eye	bilateral constriction

If there is damage to the pupillomotor fibers of the right oculomotor nerve, then:

LIGHT DIRECTED INTO THE	WILL RESULT IN
right eye	no direct reaction but a consensual reaction in the left
left eye	a direct reaction but no consensual reaction

(Continued)

CRANIAL NERVES III, IV, VI: OCULOMOTOR, TROCHLEAR, ABDUCENS, Continued

---

Convergence

If a patient is asked to focus on an object held about 6 inches away from the patient, there will normally be:

- convergence of the eyes upon the object
- accommodation
- pupillary constriction

Argyll Robertson Pupil

Argyll Robertson pupils (usually bilateral):

- are typically small and irregular
- may occur in tertiary syphilis
- have lost the ability to converge
- have lost the ability to react to light

Complete Third Nerve Lesion

In a complete third nerve lesion with loss of parasympathetic pupillomotor fibers, pupillary dilation results from unopposed action of the sympathetic nerves.

Interruption of Sympathetic Pathways

With interruption of the sympathetic pathways to the eye (Horner's syndrome), there is found:

- constricted pupil
- enophthalmos
- ptosis

These signs are sometimes accompanied by loss of sweating (anhydrosis) on the same side of the face. See Figure 15-1.

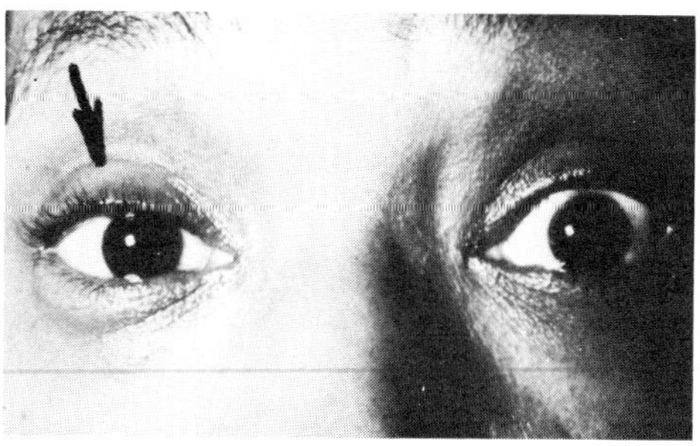

Figure 15-1.

Lesions of the Medial Longitudinal Fasciculus

Lesions of the medial longitudinal fasciculus produce an important and common sign called internuclear ophthalmoplegia, in which the medial rectus component of horizontal gaze is defective.

With a lesion of the left medial longitudinal fasciculus, attempted gaze to the right is characterized by:

- failure of the left eye to adduct
- satisfactory adduction of the right eye but with coarse monocular nystagmus

(Continued)

CRANIAL NERVES III, IV, VI: OCULOMOTOR, TROCHLEAR, ABDUCENS, Continued

The opposite is true of a lesion of the right medial longitudinal fasiculus. Convergence utilizes a different pathway, so this response is usually normal and demonstrates that both the third nerve and the medial rectus muscle are intact. Bilateral involvement of the fasciculi, most commonly a result of multiple sclerosis, is manifested by a combination of the above abnormalities.

Nystagmus

Nystagmus is a rhythmic and involuntary movement of the eyes. There are two types:

- pendular nystagmus
  - hereditary or associated with defective vision of early onset
  - present in the primary position and lateral gaze
- jerk nystagmus
  - slow drift from the point of fixation, with a rapid correcting movement
  - may be horizontal, vertical, or rotary

Labyrinthine Nystagmus

In acute labyrinth destruction, indications may include:

- nystagmus with a slow component toward the side of the lesion
- vertigo
- nausea
- falling to the same side

Brain Stem Lesions with Nystagmus

In medullary and pontine lesions, nystagmus:

- is more prominent in one direction
- may be horizontal, vertical, or rotary
- persists in the absence of vertigo or nausea

Nystagmus of Cerebellar Origin

Nystagmus of cerebellar origin:

- is most pronounced upon looking to the side of the lesion
- is associated with ipsilateral cerebellar motor signs

Toxic Nystagmus

Toxic nystagmus is caused by phenytoin or sedatives; abnormal movements are often present in all directions of gaze.

CRANIAL NERVE V: TRIGEMINAL

Motor Fibers

The motor fibers of the fifth nerve innervate:
- the masseter
- the temporalis
- the pterygoid

Testing Muscle Strength

MUSCLE	TEST
masseter temporalis See Figure 15-2.	Have the patient close his or her jaw against resistance of your hand. Palpate the muscles and note any asymmetry of contraction.
pterygoid See Figure 15-3.	Have the patient move the jaw contralaterally to the side and resist your attempt to push to other side. NOTE: In pterygoid weakness the opened jaw tends to deviate to the side of the weak muscles.

Sensory Division

The three sensory divisions of the trigeminal nerve are the:
- ophthalmic
- maxillary
- mandibular

Corneal Reflex

The corneal reflex is mediated through the ophthalmic division. Reflex is tested by touching the cornea with a wisp of cotton. Cerebellopontine angle tumors will frequently reduce the corneal reflex on the same side.

Other Sensory Divisions

The remaining sensory divisions, the maxillary and mandibular, supply sensation for the following areas:

MAXILLARY	MANDIBULAR
• upper teeth and jaw • mucosal surfaces of the uvula, hard palate • nasopharynx • lower parts of the nasal cavity	• tongue • lower teeth • gums • floor of the mouth • buccal surface of the cheek

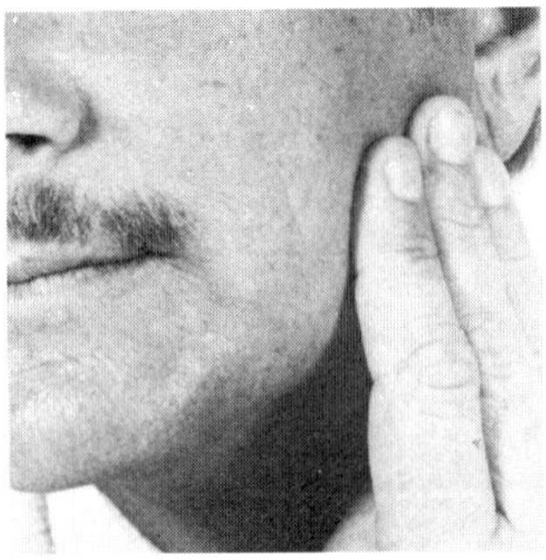

Figure 15-2.

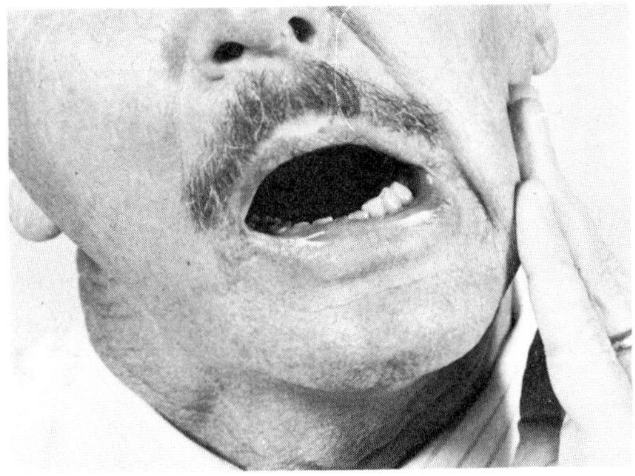

Figure 15-3.

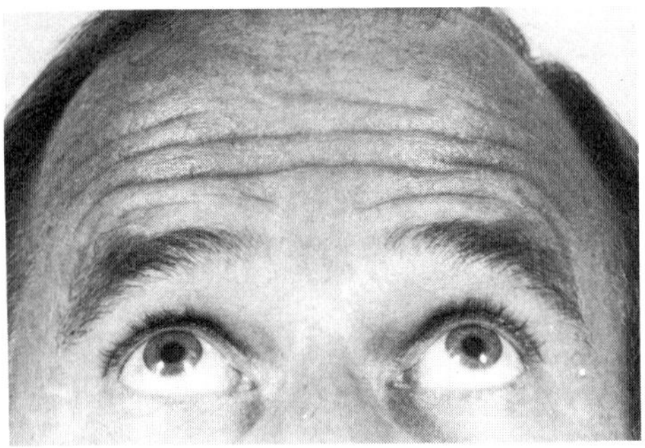

Figure 15-4.

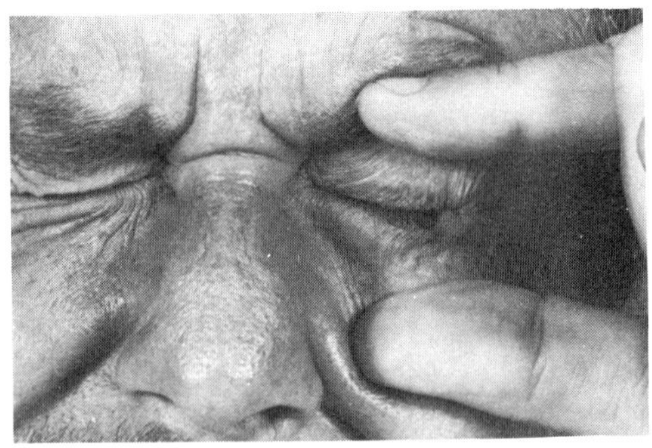

Figure 15-5.

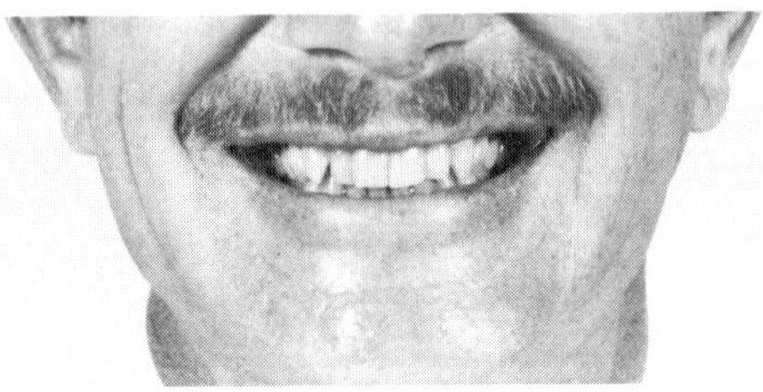

Figure 15-6.

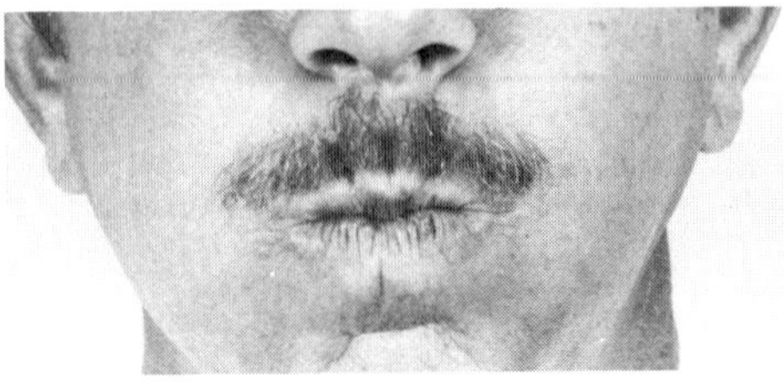

Figure 15-7.

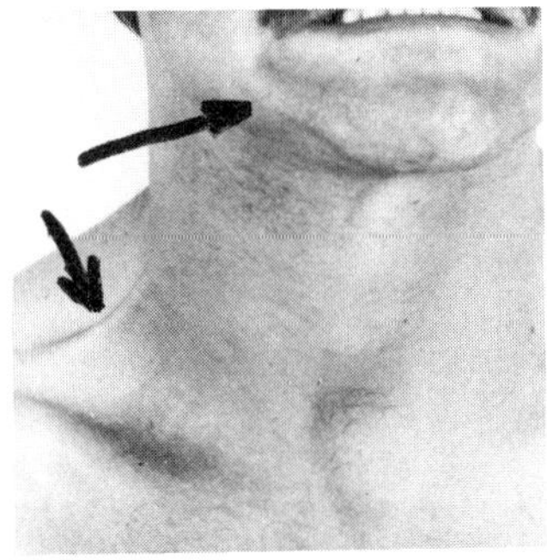

Figure 15-8.

CRANIAL NERVE VII: FACIAL

Motor Portion of Seventh Cranial Nerve

The motor portion of the seventh cranial nerve innervates:

- all facial muscles
- the platysma
- the stylohyoid

Sensory Portion

The sensory portion mediates:

- taste from the anterior two thirds of the tongue
- somatic sensation from a portion of the external ear canal
- autonomic fibers that innervate the lacrimal, submaxillary, and sublingual salivary glands

Observation of Facial Movements

During the initial interview, the patient's facial movements should be observed, and any gross weakness such as the inability to smile or to close the eyelids will be apparent.

Testing Facial Muscles

MUSCLE TO BE TESTED	TEST
frontalis	Patient looks upward and wrinkles the forehead. See Figure 15-4.
orbicularis oculi	Patient closes the eyes tightly and resists attempts to pry them open. See Figure 15-5.
lower facial muscle	Patient shows his or her teeth, purses the lips, blows the cheeks out. See Figures 15-6 and 15-7.
platysma	This muscle will contract when the patient makes a vigorous effort to show the teeth. See Figure 15-8.

Lesions of the Corticobulbar Tract

Lesions of the corticobulbar tracts at any point above the facial nucleus will produce contralateral lower facial weakness with sparing of forehead movement because of bilateral cortical representation of the upper facial muscles. See Figure 15-9.

(Continued)

CRANIAL NERVE VII: FACIAL, Continued

Nuclear or Peripheral Seventh Nerve Lesions

In nuclear or peripheral lesions of the seventh nerve, the entire facial musculature on the same side is weak.

See Figure 15-10.

Sensation of Taste

Taste is not routinely tested unless the patient has peripheral facial weakness. Taste is tested as follows:

- Patient protrudes the tongue, which must be moist.
- Use a wet applicator to apply a substance for identification.
- Patient must not withdraw the tongue until the substance is identified as salty, sweet, bitter, or sour.
- Use these substances:
  - Sodium chloride (salty)
  - Sugar (sweet)
  - Quinine (bitter)
  - Vinegar (sour)

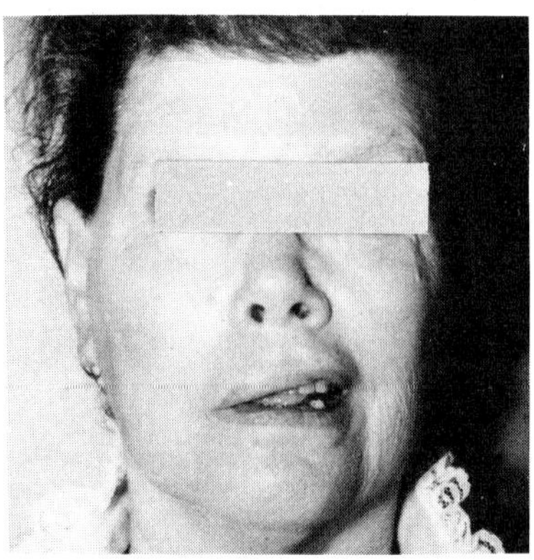

Figure 15-9.

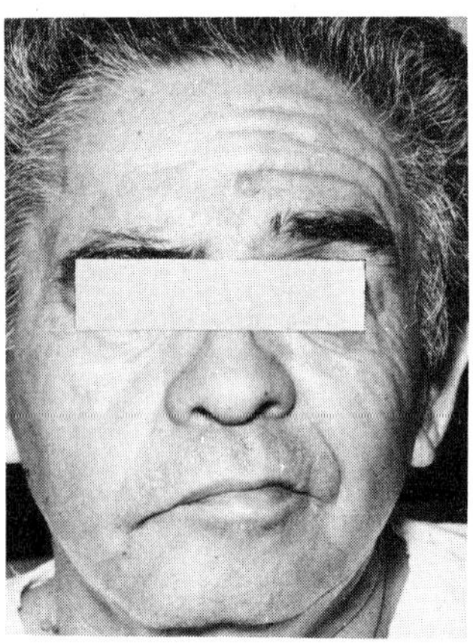

Figure 15-10.

CRANIAL NERVE VIII: ACOUSTIC

Acoustic Nerve	Test for decreased hearing by using voice discrimination or the ticking of a watch. The Weber and Rinne tests, described in Chapter 11, will differentiate neural from conductive hearing loss.

CRANIAL NERVES IX, X: GLOSSOPHARYNGEAL, VAGUS

Screening Procedure

If the patient has no complaints of difficulty with speech or swallowing and neurological disease is not suspected, then observing the palate elevate when the patient says "ah" is all that is required for routine examination.

Glossopharyngeal Nerve

The glossopharyngeal nerve supplies:

tactile and taste fibers	to	posterior third of tongue
tactile fibers	to	nasopharynx and upper pharynx
motor fibers	to	stylopharyngeal muscle

Glossopharyngeal and Vagal Fibers

Due to the intermixing of glossopharyngeal and vagal fibers in the pharyngeal plexus, independent clinical testing of the glossopharyngeal nerve is difficult.

Gag Reflex

- The afferent arm of the gag reflex is mainly mediated by the glossopharyngeal nerve and the motor arm by the vagus. The normal response to a tongue blade touching the posterior wall of the pharynx is contraction of the pharyngeal muscles and elevation of the palate.
- The absence of the gag reflex may be unilateral or bilateral and usually indicates impairment of function of glossopharyngeal as well as vagus nerves. See Figure 15-11.

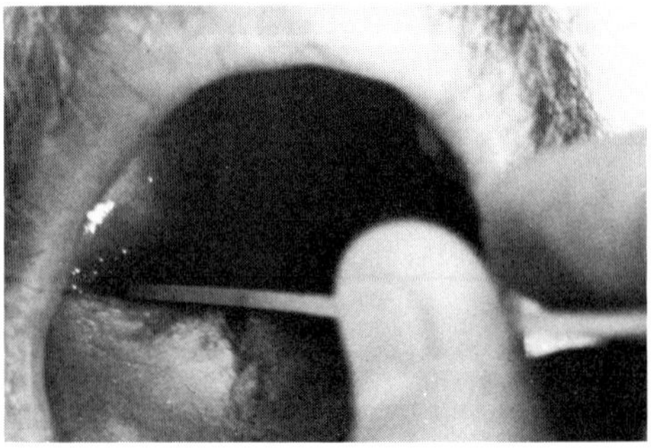

Figure 15-11.

(Continued)

CRANIAL NERVES IX, X: GLOSSOPHARYNGEAL, VAGUS, Continued

Vagus Nerve Impairment

Unilateral impairment of motor function of the vagus leads to ipsilateral palatal and vocal cord weakness or paralysis. When the patient is asked to say "ah," the soft palate will deviate to the normal side.

CONDITION	RESULT
vocal cord paralysis	hoarse voice
weak palate	nasal voice
bilateral vagal lesions	severe dysarthria and dysphagia and regurgitation of liquids through the nose

CRANIAL NERVE XI: ACCESSORY

Screening Procedure

For the screening examination, testing the shoulder shrug against resistance is all that is necessary.

Accessory Nerve

The accessory nerve innervates the:
- sternomastoid
- upper portion of the trapezius

Testing the Muscles

Weakness of the sternomastoid is detected by having the patient rotate the head against resistance to the contralateral side. The patient then elevates the shoulders and the examiner tries to depress them.

NOTE: Since the elevation of the shoulders is principally done by the levators scapulae, the upper trapezius should be observed and palpated in order to detect weakness due to a lesion of the accessory nerve. See Figures 15-12 and 15-13.

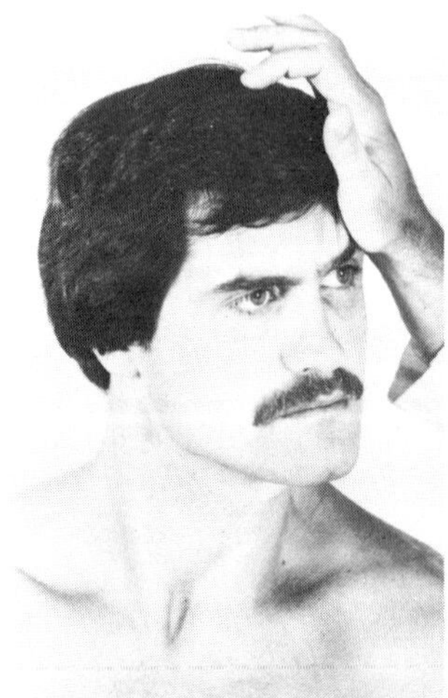

Figure 15-12.

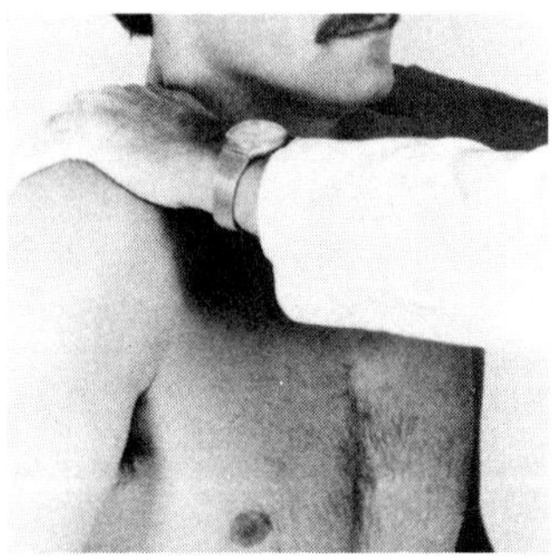

Figure 15-13.

CRANIAL NERVE XII: HYPOGLOSSAL

Hypoglossal	The hypoglossal nerve supplies the: • extrinsic • intrinsic muscles of the tongue.
Disorders of the Hypoglossal	Indications of a lesion of the hypoglossal nucleus or nerve are: • atrophy of one side of the tongue • fasciculations • weakness with deviation of the protruded tongue toward the weak side. See Figure 15-14.

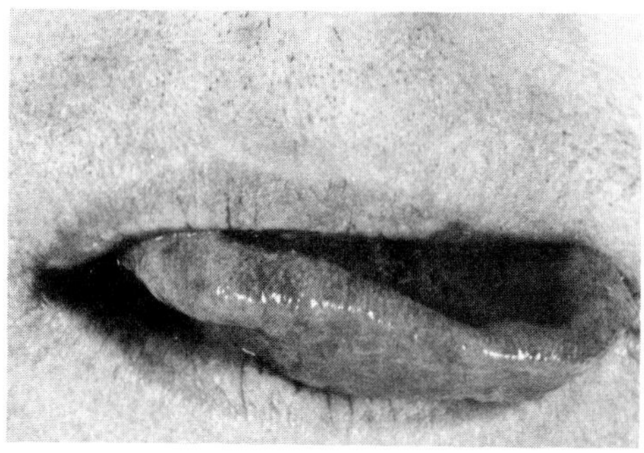

Figure 15-14.

MOTOR FUNCTION: BACKGROUND

Introduction

Motor performance is dependent on:
- intact contractile mechanisms of muscle
- neuromuscular transmission
- cranial and spinal motor nuclei with their respective nerves

These are modified and controlled by the:
- motor cortex
- corticospinal tracts
- extrapyramidal system
- cerebellum

Observation

Initial observations of the patient's posture and spontaneous movements prior to formal examination will frequently yield clues to possible abnormalities in one or more of these systems:

IN DISORDERS OF THE	YOU MAY OBSERVE
upper motor neuron	a pattern of weakness involving the extensor muscles of the arms and the flexor muscles of the leg; the patient is spastic.
extrapyramidal system	the presence of abnormal movements, abnormality of posture, increased tone
cerebellum	incoordination and decomposition of movement

MOTOR FUNCTION: MUSCLE WEAKNESS

Primary Disorders of Muscles

As a general guideline, primary disorders of muscles with clinical weakness result in a pattern of weakness that is mainly proximal.

- Muscular atrophy may be present; however, fasciculations are not seen.
- On occasion, pseudohypertrophy may also be present (e.g., the calves in Duchenne muscular dystrophy).
- Rarely, tenderness of the muscles will be present in polymyositis.
- Deep tendon reflexes, while they may be diminished, are diminished in proportion to the severity of the weakness.

  NOTE: Striking the thenar muscle group with a reflex hammer may produce a contraction lasting several seconds called myotonia. Myotonia is often seen with myotonic dystrophy, but may be present with other disorders.
- Tetany (the involuntary contraction of muscles) may occur spontaneously or may be evoked by compression of the upper arm with a blood pressure cuff that is inflated above systolic pressure (contraction of the muscles of the wrist and finger flexors or Trousseau's sign). The presence of tetanic spasms may also be suggested by percussion on the facial nerve (twitch of the facial muscles or Chvostek's sign). See Figures 15-15 and 15-16.

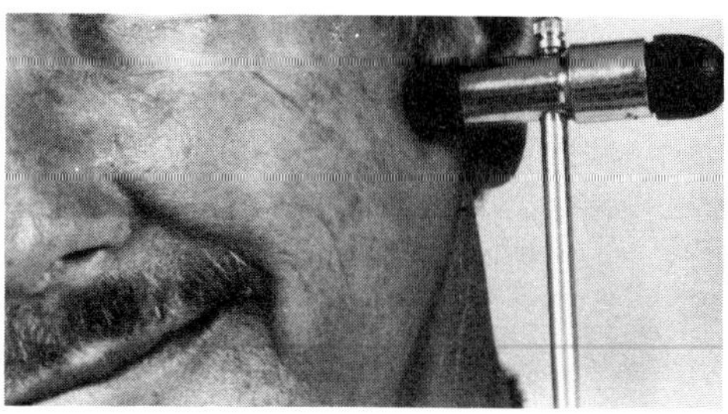

Figure 15-15.

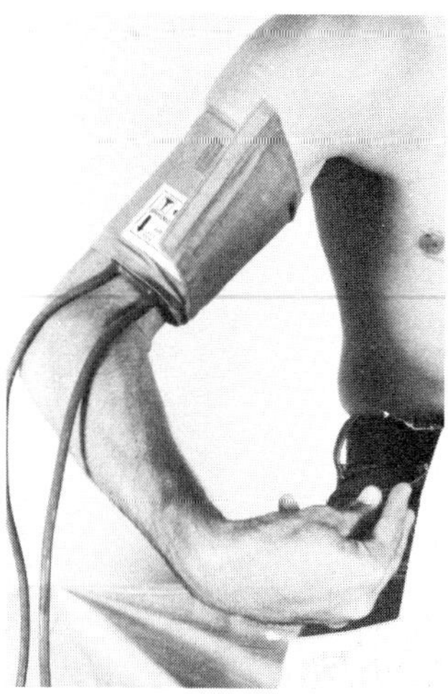

Figure 15-16.

(Continued)

MOTOR FUNCTION: MUSCLE WEAKNESS, Continued

Anterior Horn Cell and Peripheral Nerve Disease

With anterior horn cell and peripheral nerve disease the pattern of muscle weakness depends on whether the pathological process is generalized or is restricted to a peripheral nerve or spinal cord segment.

- Deep tendon reflexes are reduced out of proportion to the amount of weakness present.
- It should be pointed out that while fasciculations are seen in patients with disorders of anterior horn cells and peripheral nerves, they may be present in normal individuals. Benign fasciculations are usually in the calves, the deltoids, or the hand muscles and are accentuated by the patient being anxious or cold.

Neuromuscular Transmission Defects

Disorders of neuromuscular transmission (for example, myasthenia gravis) produce increasing degrees of weakness with repetitive exercise.

- This can usually be demonstrated clinically by repetitively exercising different muscles against resistance (e.g., the deltoid or the iliopsoas).
- On rare occasions, repetitive exercise will result in improved strength (the Eaton-Lambert syndrome, often associated with lung carcinoma).

MOTOR FUNCTION: MUSCLE STRENGTH

Muscle Tone

Muscle tone is tested by the passive movement of a limb through its full range of motion.

- In spasticity there is resistance to passive movement to a point where resistance suddenly decreases (the "clasp-knife phenomenon").
- Steady, plastic resistance throughout the range of motion is typical of extrapyramidal disease.
- The superimposition of tremor on increased tone may produce cogwheel rigidity, as in Parkinson's disease.
- Decreased muscle tone may be seen in cerebellar disease, during spinal shock following acute paraplegia, or immediately following a severe hemiplegic stroke.

Muscle Strength

Muscle strength depends on the age, sex, and occupation of the individual. It is left to the examiner to know what strength to expect for a given individual, and this knowledge comes only with experience. The judgment required is a source of anxiety for a student beginning clinical muscle testing, but there can be no substitute for experience.

NOTE: Evaluating muscle strength in patients with pain or with functional disease can be most difficult. In general, if a muscle contraction, no matter how brief, is normal, then the strength may be judged to be normal (with the exception of patients with myasthenia gravis).

MOTOR FUNCTION: TESTING MUSCLE TONE AND STRENGTH

Testing Procedure

On a routine clinical practice only the following muscle groups need to be tested. If an abnormal weakness is detected, the examiner must consult a reference to determine which nerve provides motor innervation to that muscle.

Value of the Tests

Testing the following muscle groups in the upper extremity allows the examiner to evaluate the function of all major motor nerves, all divisions of the brachial plexus, and all the major cervical nerve roots.

- deltoid muscle
- biceps muscle
- triceps muscle
- finger extensors
- interossei
- abductor pollicis brevis

MUSCLE	TEST	ILLUSTRATION
deltoid	tested by having the patient abduct the arm to 90 degrees; the examiner attempts to depress the arm while the patient resists.	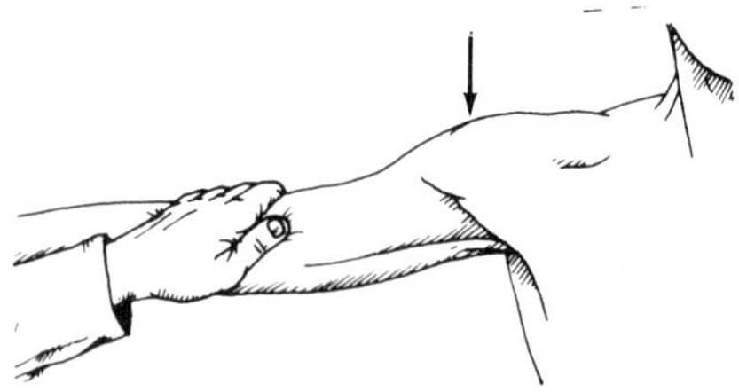
biceps	The patient flexes the forearm, and the examiner attempts to extend it against resistance.	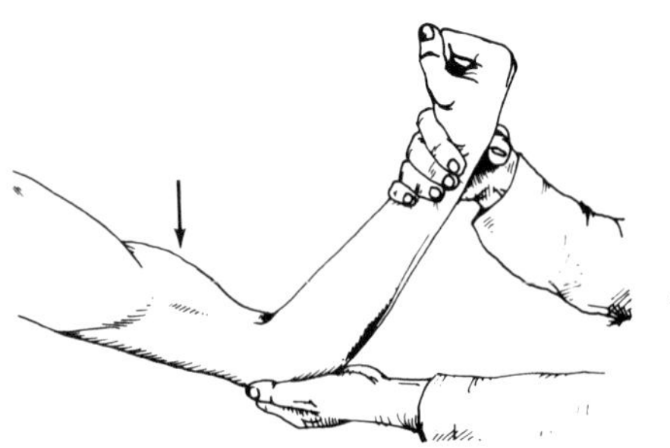

(Continued)

MOTOR FUNCTION: TESTING MUSCLE TONE AND STRENGTH, Continued

MUSCLE	TEST	ILLUSTRATION
triceps	The patient attempts to extend the forearm against resistance.	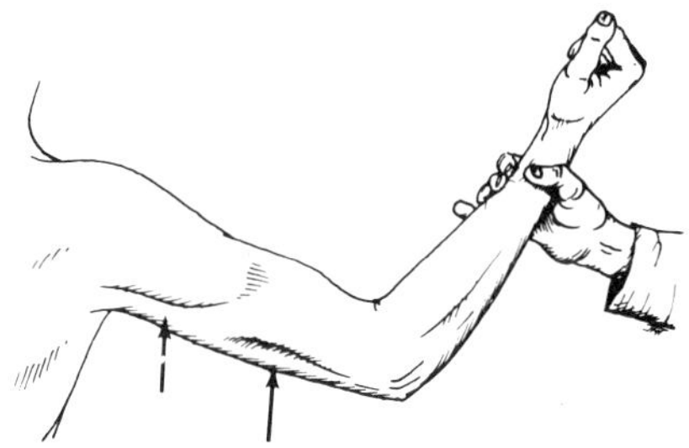
finger extensors	The patient attempts to prevent the examiner from flexing the extended digits at the MP joint. (The patient's hand is firmly supported by the examiner's right hand. Extension is maintained against the resistance of the fingers of the examiner's left hand.)	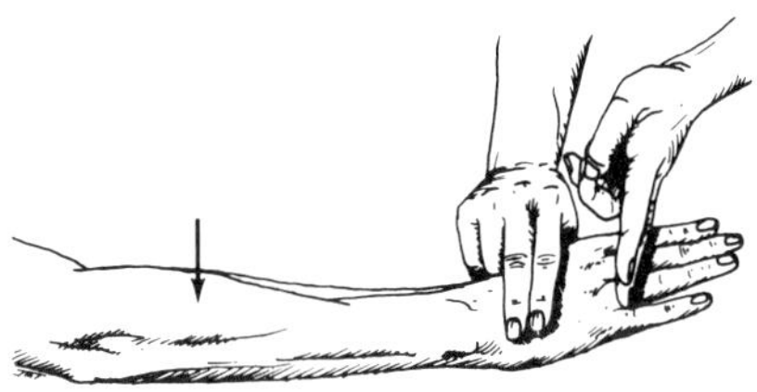
interossei	These should be tested only with the person's wrist and fingers extended, or a false impression of weakness will result. These are tested by asking the patient to spread his fingers while the examiner attempts to resist this movement. (The patient is abducting the index finger against resistance).	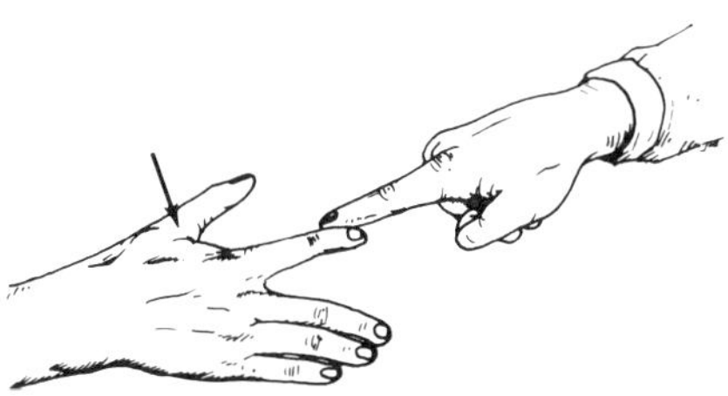

(Continued)

MOTOR FUNCTION: TESTING MUSCLE TONE AND STRENGTH, Continued

MUSCLE	TEST	ILLUSTRATION
abductor pollicis brevis	The patient abducts the thumb in a plane perpendicular to the palm of the hand against resistance.	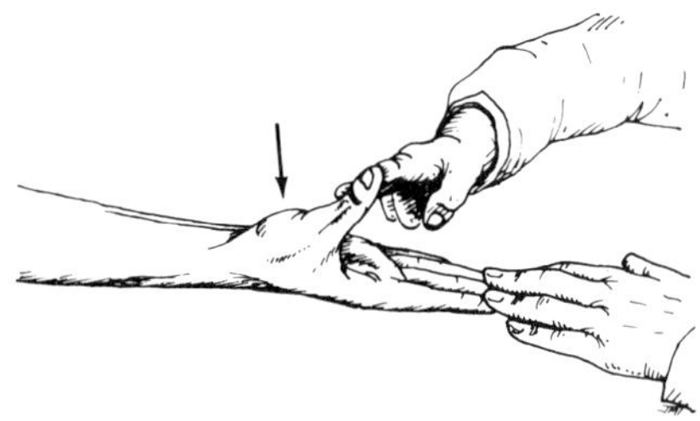

Value of the Tests

The following muscle groups in the <u>lower</u> extremity should be tested:

- iliopsoas
- quadriceps
- hamstrings
- anterior tibial
- gastrocnemius

MUSCLE	TEST	ILLUSTRATION
iliopsoas	The patient maintains the thigh flexed at the hip while the examiner attempts to extend it.	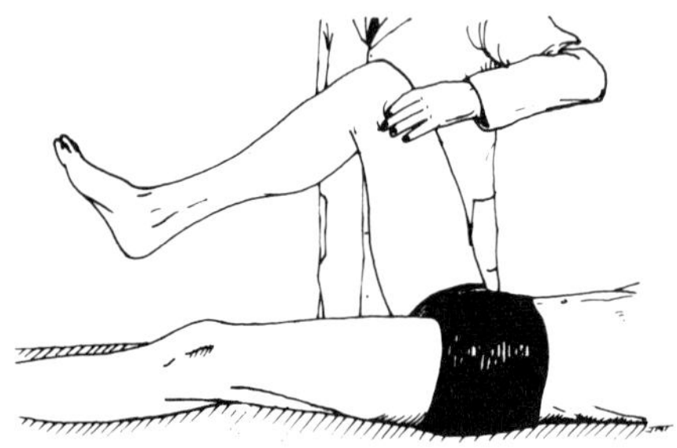

(Continued)

MOTOR FUNCTION: TESTING MUSCLE TONE AND STRENGTH, Continued

MUSCLE	TEST	ILLUSTRATION
quadriceps	With the knee flexed to 90 degrees, the patient attempts to extend the leg while the examiner resists this effort.	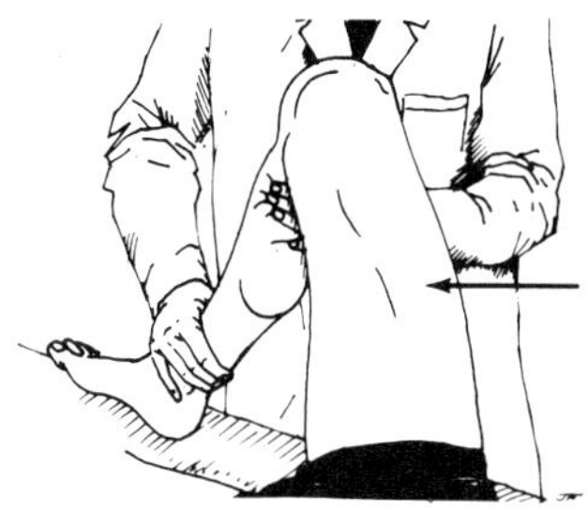
hamstrings	The patient attempts to flex the leg against the examiner's resistance. (The patient lies on his back with the limb flexed at the hip and knee.)	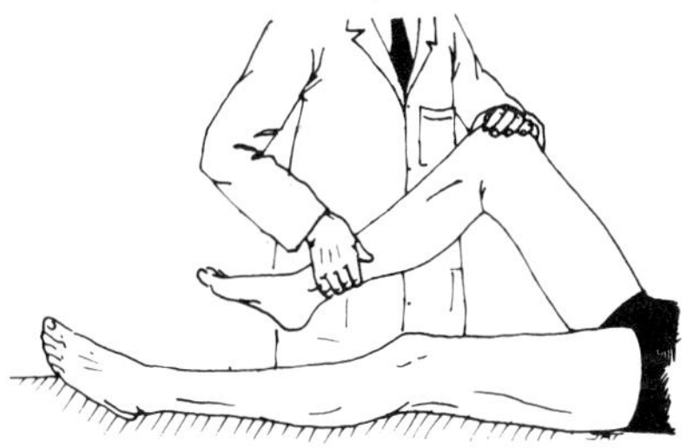
anterior tibial muscles	The patient dorsiflexes his foot; the examiner attempts to plantar flex the foot at the ankle.	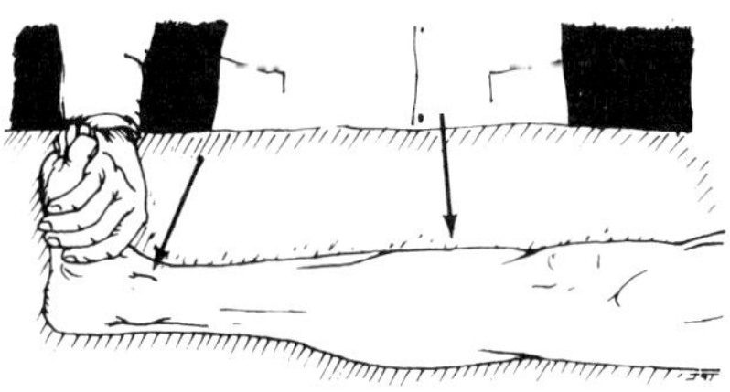

Gastrocnemius	The gastrocnemius is best tested by observing the patient walk on his toes. Significant weakness can be present yet pass undetected by manual testing because the muscle is so strong to begin with.

MOTOR FUNCTION: COORDINATION

Tests of Coordination

- In the finger-nose-finger test the patient moves his index finger quickly and smoothly back and forth between his nose and the examiner's finger. In cerebellar disorders coordination difficulty may be encountered in the hand on the same side as the lesion. See Figures 15-17 and 15-18.
- Rapid alternating movements such as the rapid finger wiggle or patting of the foot may be slowed with disease affecting the cerebellar pathways, extrapyramidal pathways, pyramidal system, and proprioceptive system.
- Cerebellar hemispheric disease will result in an impairment of the movement required in the heel-to-shin test. This test is done by placing the heel on the patella and running it down the tibial surface in a straight line. See Figure 15-19.

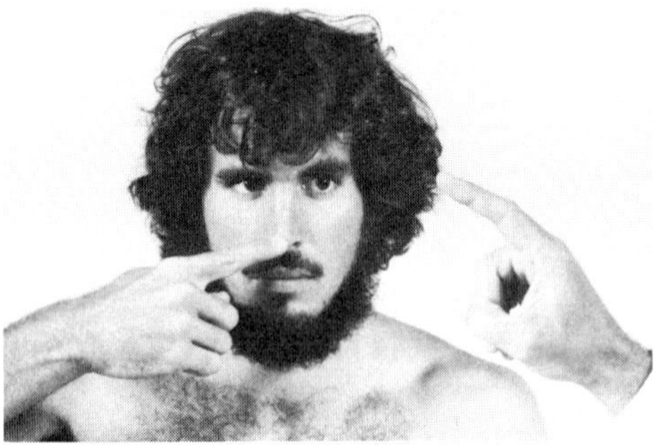

Figure 15-17.

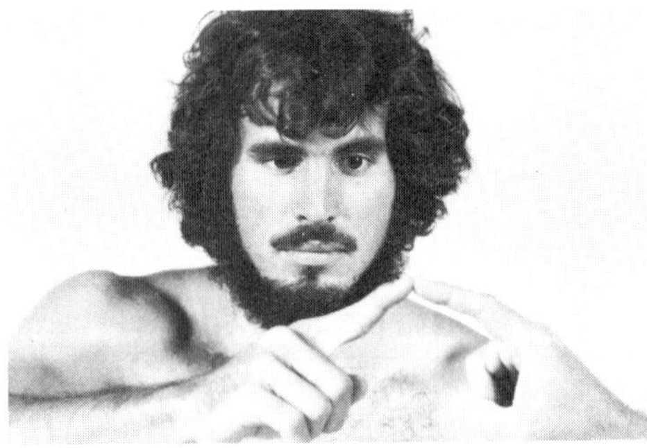

Figure 15-18.

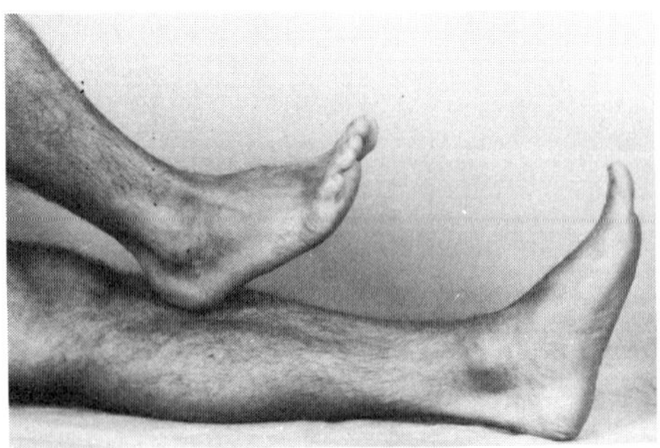

Figure 15-19.

MOTOR FUNCTION: INVOLUNTARY MOVEMENTS

Tremors

Rhythmic involuntary movements are called tremors. For example, Parkinsonian tremor has a regular rhythm of four to six cycles per second and is best seen in moderate relaxation. It often disappears during sleep or complete relaxation, and lessens with voluntary movement. It is often called a "rest" tremor and is distributed in the distal joints of the limbs. The most characteristic feature is the pattern of tremor occurring in the hand in which the thumb beats rhythmically against the flexing fingers.

Familial and Senile Tremors

Familial and senile tremors are characterized by rhythmic oscillation of the head and fingers of the outstretched hand. The tremor is rapid and is accentuated in amplitude by action and emotional stress. They are classified as "action" tremors.

Cerebellar Tremors

Cerebellar tremors are characteristically action tremors with an oscillation perpendicular to the line of movement and increasing in amplitude as the target is approached.

Asterixis

Sporadic loss of tonus in muscles under steady contracture results in brief lapses of posture, with an irregular flapping tremor (known as asterixis). This is best demonstrated with arms outstretched and wrists extended, and occurs in hepatic encephalopathy as well as in many other encephalopathies. See Figure 15-20.

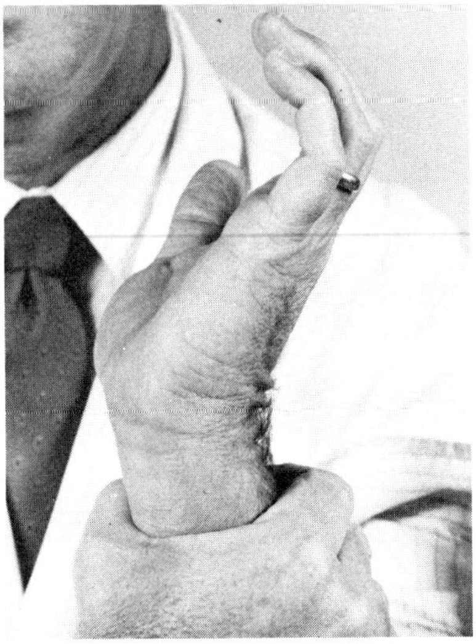

Figure 15-20.

(Continued)

MOTOR FUNCTION: INVOLUNTARY MOVEMENTS, Continued

Athetosis

Athetosis is a rather slow writhing movement of the arms and feet that may be accompanied by a twisting of the neck and retraction of the lips. The hands tend to swing alternately but irregularly between two extremes of posture. One consists of extension at the elbow with supination of the wrist and hyperextension of the fingers. The other consists of elbow flexion with pronation and finger flexion.

Choreic Movements

Choreic movements appear with bilateral disease of the caudate nuclei. These movements are quick and erratic, without an easily discernible pattern. They affect individual digits, wrists, proximal parts of limbs, and the trunk. Twisting or lurching movements of trunk may appear on walking. Smacking and sucking movements of the lips and darting motions of the tongue are common.

Ballistic Movements

Ballistic movements are sudden violent flailing movements of the extremity and are frequently unilateral.

MOTOR FUNCTION: STANCE AND GAIT

Stance and Gait	Standing and walking are largely automatic but are really very complex activities depending on: • adequate muscle strength • coordination • proprioception • vestibular function • vision
Stance	In observing stance, the patient is asked to stand with his feet close together and arms outstretched, first with his eyes open and then with his eyes closed. This is known as the Romberg test. See Figure 15-21.

THIS ROMBERG RESULT	IS FOUND
increased swaying and unsteadiness with eyes closed	in patients with impairment of proprioception as in tabes dorsalis, subacute combined degeneration, and sensory neuropathy
Normal stance is difficult to maintain even with the eyes open, and the patient separates the feet widely in order to stand on a broader, and therefore steadier, base.	in cerebellar disease
tendency to fall to one side	in patients with acute unilateral impairment of vestibular function, the tendency is to fall to the ipsilateral side.

Gait	Gait is usually observed by asking the patient to walk out freely. Many normal patients have a tendency to walk slowly and deliberately when observed by an examiner. An abnormality in gait may be exaggerated and more easily observed by asking the patient to walk a straight line.

(Continued)

MOTOR FUNCTION: STANCE AND GAIT, Continued

Decrease of Associated Movement

Decrease of associated movement, such as arm swing, occurs in hemiplegia or rigidity and is characteristically seen in patients with Parkinson's disease. Further, patients with this disorder walk with slow short steps, stooped forward as if chasing the center of gravity, turn clumsily in one block, and have difficulty in stopping abruptly.

Other Abnormalities

DISEASE/DISORDER	GAIT ABNORMALITY
cerebellar disease	Patient walks with a wide base and staggers or reels laterally. See Figure 15-22.
hemiplegic gait	The leg is circumducted, the knee is held stiffly, and the ankle is plantar flexed.
bilateral spastic paresis of the legs	produces a scissoring of the knees while the legs are moved forward in a jerky manner; often accompanied by extreme compensatory movements of the trunk

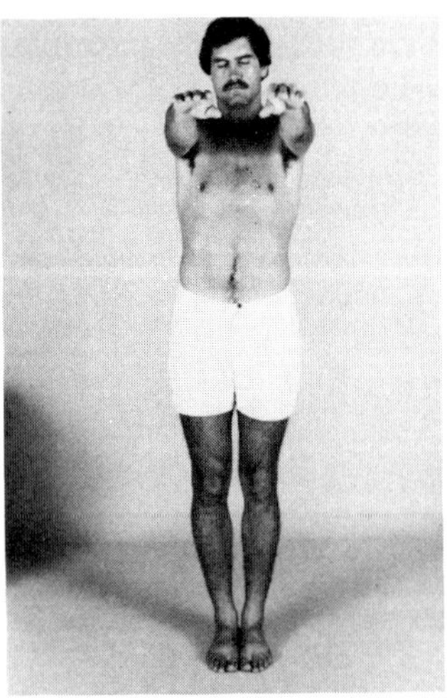

Figure 15-21.

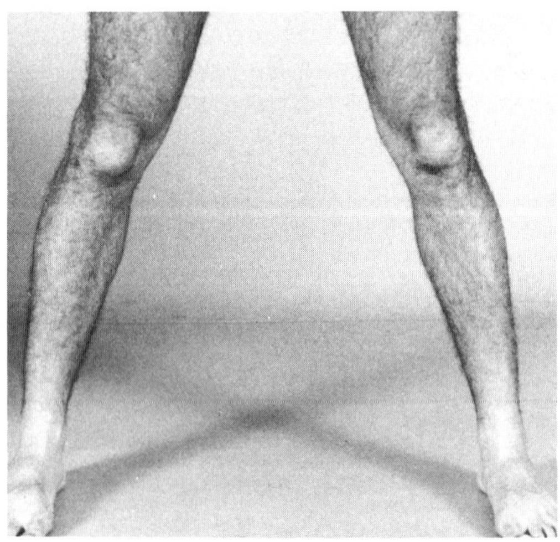

Figure 15-22.

MOTOR FUNCTION: STRETCH REFLEXES

How to Elicit a Muscle Stretch Reflex	Adequate relaxation of the patient is necessary to elicit a muscle stretch reflex. The response is evaluated as to its briskness and ease of elicitation, and is compared with that of the homologous muscle on the other side.
Stretch Reflexes	To test muscle stretch reflexes, (A) the muscle is briefly stretched by a tap on the tendon. (B) Stretch receptors in the muscle (muscle spindles) send impulses via afferent fibers in peripheral nerves and dorsal roots to anterior horn cells. These are excited and (C) send efferent impulses via anterior roots and motor nerves to the same muscle, leading to (D) a brief contraction. This is a simple monosynaptic reflex that may be diminished or lost with interruption of afferent (sensory) fibers. It is also diminished with extensive damage of efferent (motor) fibers or anterior horn cells.
Hyperreflexia	Release of this monosynaptic reflex from the influence of suprasegmental fibers produces <u>hyperreflexia</u> that, when extreme, leads to clonus.
Clonus	Clonus is a rapid repetitive contraction of muscles and is elicited by stretching a muscle briskly and maintaining the stretch. Knee clonus is tested by forcibly pushing patella caudad, and ankle clonus by forcibly dorsiflexing the ankle with the knee supported in the flexed position. In each case, stretch is maintained. See Figures 15-23 and 15-24.
Slow Relaxation After Muscle Contraction	Slow relaxation after muscle contraction is observed in hypothyroidism.
Differences Between Sides	Differences between sides are best detected by eliciting a muscle stretch reflex first on one side and then immediately in the homologous muscle on the other side. If a reflex cannot be elicited or if asymmetries are found, the reflexes should be tested in several different positions to verify its absence, diminution, or hyperactivity.
Reinforcement Maneuver	Reflexes may be brought out by an isometric reinforcement maneuver: pulling against the interlocked fingers or clenching the fist. See Figure 15-25.

(Continued)

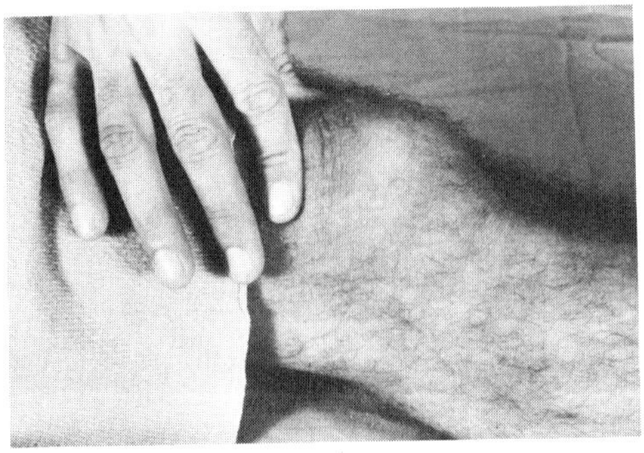

Figure 15-23.

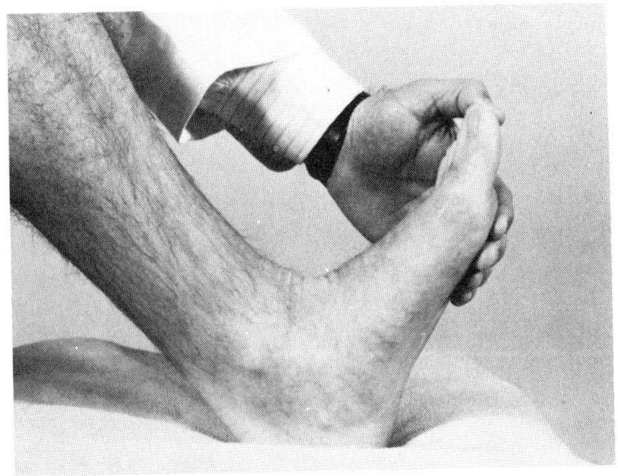

Figure 15-24.

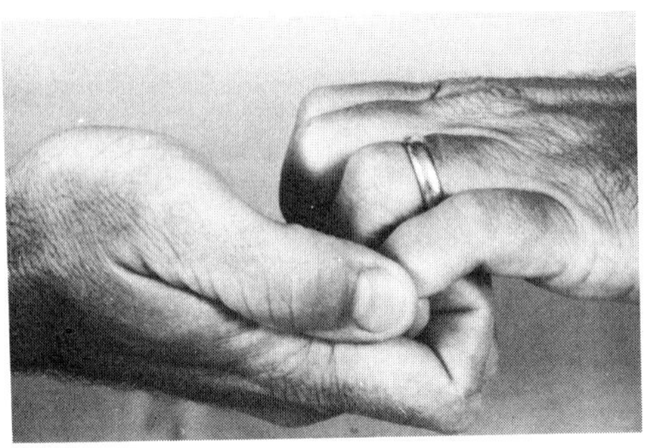

Figure 15-25.

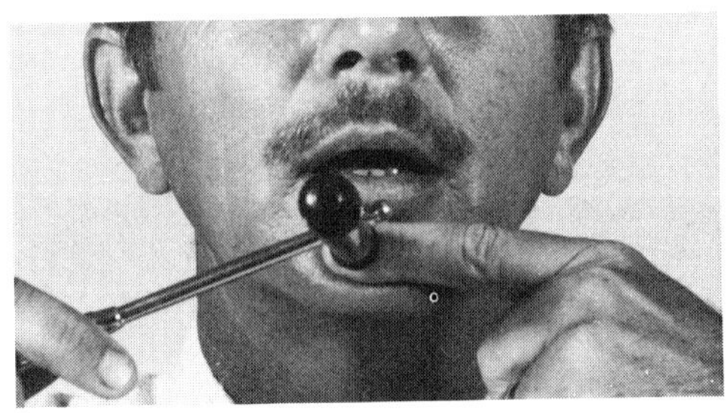

Figure 15-26.

MOTOR FUNCTION: STRETCH REFLEXES, Continued

Testing Stretch Reflexes

All muscles can be made to contract reflexively, but only a few are tested clinically. The following table lists these tests.

REFLEX	ELICIT REFLEX BY	COMMENT
jaw jerk	Having the patient let the jaw sag open, place one finger on the patient's chin and tap with a hammer. See Figure 14-26.	A normal person should have no response or only a faint contraction. The jaw will close briskly in hyperactivity of the reflex in an upper motor neuron lesion.
biceps reflex	Supporting the patient's elbow with your hand, place your thumb over the tendon, and have patient's hand rest on your forearm.	Muscles, if percussed directly, will have a brief contraction; this direct contraction is to be disregarded.
triceps reflex	With the patient's arms folded across the chest or supported by the examiner and the forearm swinging freely, strike the aponeurosis rather than the muscle.	
quadriceps	With the patient's legs dangling when the patient sits at the edge of the bed, strike the tendon just below the patella.	
ankle jerk	With gentle dorsiflexion of the foot, strike the Achilles tendon with the reflex hammer.	This reflex may be decreased or absent in older patients.

(Continued)

MOTOR FUNCTION: PATHOLOGICAL REFLEXES

Hoffmann's Sign	Flicking the patient's third fingernail provides a sudden stretch, which is followed by quick flexion of the fingers. Normally, this contraction is minimal. With hyperreflexia, finger flexion becomes more pronounced and the thumb also flexes (Hoffmann's sign). See Figure 15-27.
Plantar Reflex	Stimulation of the sole of the foot (plantar reflex) produces flexion of the toes (Babinksi reflex). The Babinski sign refers to the pathologic reflex of toe extension. The plantar reflex is tested in a relaxed recumbent patient who has his legs extended. Firm pressure with a blunt instrument is exerted against the sole of the foot on its lateral aspect, and the instrument is moved slowly upward toward the little toe and then across the sole toward the big toe. Dorsiflexion of the big toe and fanning of the other toes constitutes the pathologic reflex (extensor plantar response). At times this response is accompanied by flexion of the thigh at the hip, knee flexion, and dorsiflexion of the foot. This reflex is a normal finding in infants less than 1 year of age. See Figure 15-28.
Other Pathological Reflexes	A group of pathologic reflexes may appear that cannot be ascribed to lesions in any specific location of the brain but are caused by cerebral cortical atrophy and other bilateral diffuse disorders of the cerebral hemispheres: • Snout reflex consists of a quick pursing or pouting expression of the lips. It can be elicited by a light tap beneath the nose. See Figure 15-29. • Palmomental response involves contraction of the mentalis muscle on one side after stroking the palm on the same side with a sharp object. Traces of this are present in about a third of normal individuals, but a brisk response is pathologic. See Figures 15-30 and 15-31.
Sucking and Grasp Reflex	Another group of reflexes is directly attributable to destruction of the medial premotor portions of the frontal lobe. The reflexes are released on the side opposite the lesion. • Sucking reflex is elicited by gently stroking the lips with a tongue blade, moving from the center laterally. In mild form the lips contract reflexively upon the blade. With more severe release, the tongue moves toward the blade and the lips and head follow it as if to take hold of the object. See Figure 15-32.

MOTOR FUNCTION: PATHOLOGICAL REFLEXES, Continued

- Grasp reflex of the hand is elicited by stroking the patient's palm with one's fingers. The patient's fingers are flexed and the thumb opposes, serving to entrap the examiner's fingers in a persistent grasp. The reflex may be released by stroking the dorsum of the hand. See Figure 15-33.

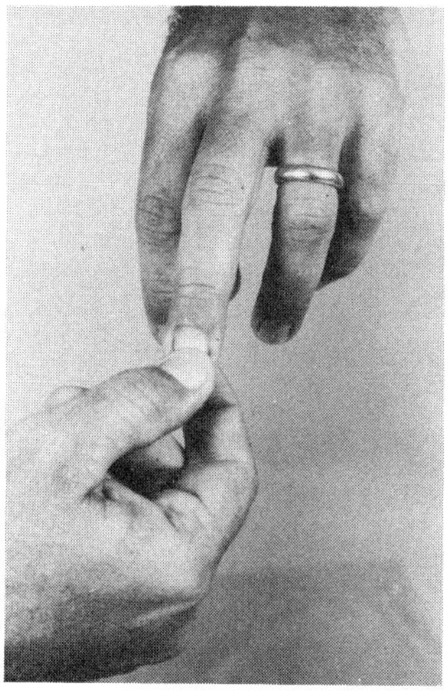

Figure 15-27.

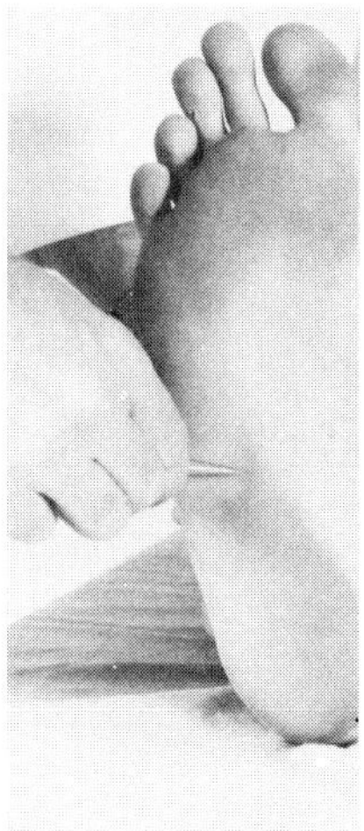

Figure 15-28.

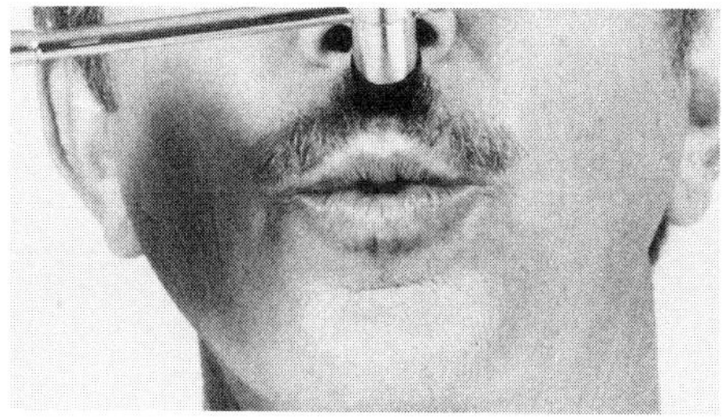

Figure 15-29.

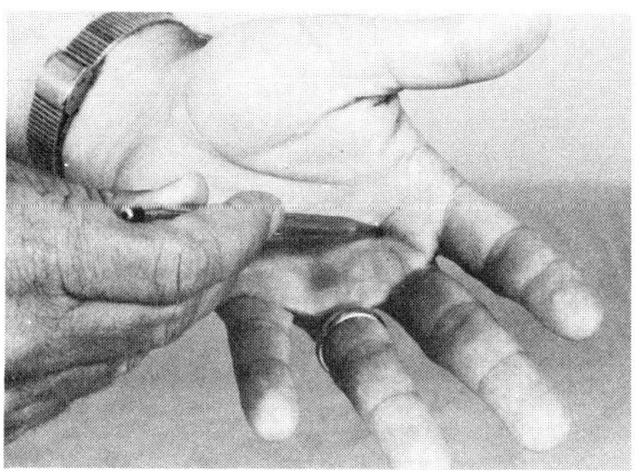

Figure 15-30.

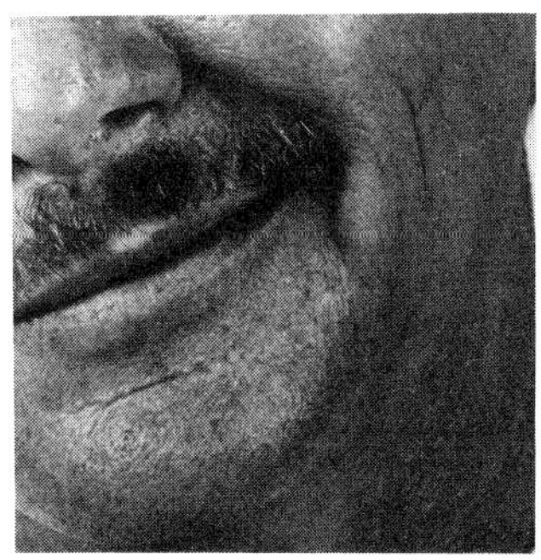

Figure 15-31.

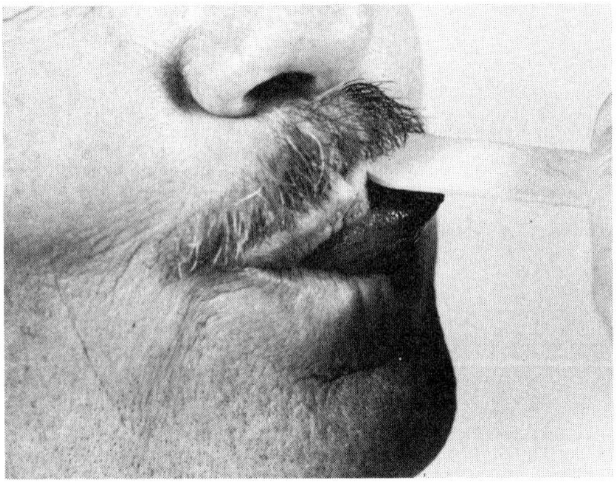

Figure 15-32.

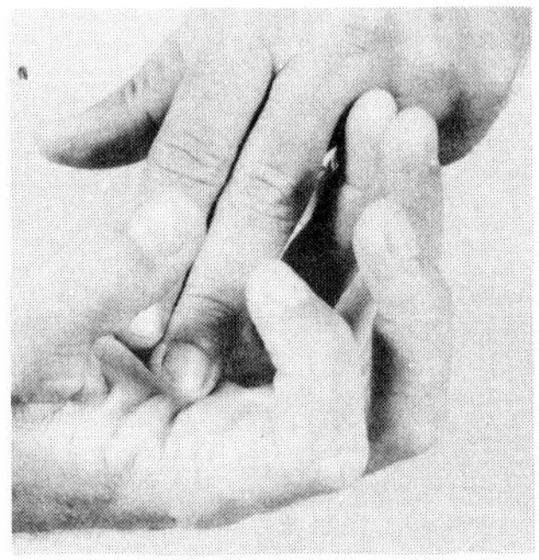

Figure 15-33.

SENSORY EXAMINATION

Sensory Examination	Ideally a patient should be intelligent, alert, cooperative, and not suggestible when undertaking a sensory examination. Only rarely are all of these attributes present in an individual patient at a given time.
Reliable Testing	In order to yield optimal and reliable information, each sensory examination has to be adjusted according to the patient's particular abilities. A fatigued patient may perform poorly and may superficially give the impression of sensory loss, which disappears when the patient is retested after rest.
Painful Stimulus	In a totally uncooperative or obtunded patient, the only sensory modality that can be examined may be pain. The patient's face is observed for grimacing in response to a painful stimulus. Even though this is a very crude sensory examination, it may still provide important information.
Instructions to the Patient	Without the patient's knowing exactly how to respond, the results of a sensory examination will be confusing and the examiner may become frustrated. Therefore, it is essential to explain to the patient what will be done and how he is expected to respond. A brief practice demonstration before the actual testing will quickly clarify any misunderstanding.

(Continued)

SENSORY EXAMINATION, Continued

Note	It is certainly not practical or necessary to examine every square inch of skin surface for every sensory modality in every patient.
Equipment	The equipment needed for a sensory examination is simple and consists of a: • cotton wad • sharp pin • tuning fork (128 Hz is best)
Loss of Sensation	Loss of sensation is usually relative. It is not sufficient to determine whether a patient perceives a painful stimulus as pain.
Intensity of Stimulation	The intensity of the stimulus should be minimal at first and then gradually increased. In areas of sensory impairment a higher threshold is found more frequently than total loss of sensation.
Vibratory Perception	Vibratory perception in the feet and legs may be normally decreased past the age of 60 years. However, a difference between left and right may indicate a significant neurologic deficit.
Peripheral Neuropathies	In peripheral neuropathies involving the legs, the most severe deficits are usually found in the feet and gradually reduced as the stimulus is moved up the leg.
Dermatome	On the other hand, an isolated nerve or root lesion will show a loss corresponding to its dermatome.

EXAMINATION OF INDIVIDUAL SENSORY MODALITIES

Sensory Modalities	Sensory modalities include: • light touch (spinothalamic tract) • pain (spinothalamic tract) • vibratory sense (dorsal columns) • position sense (dorsal columns)
Light Touch	The perception of "light touch" is tested by gently touching the skin with a wisp of cotton. The patient responds with "yes" or "no" whenever he feels the stimulus. The testing should be done at irregular intervals, because the patient may begin to respond repetitively whether or not he feels the stimulus if it is applied at regular intervals. See Figure 15-34.

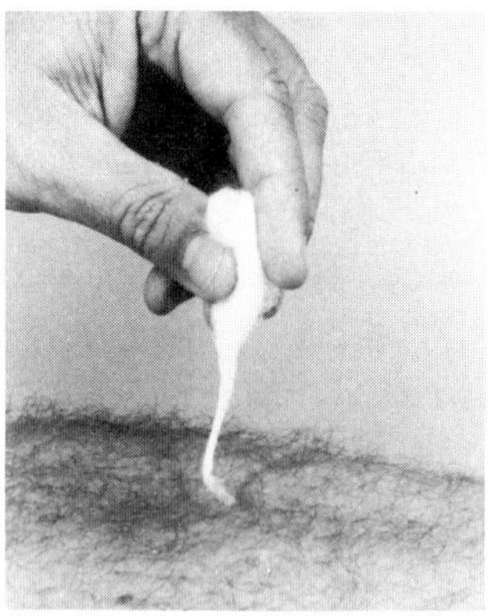

Figure 15-34.

Increased Stimulation	If the patient does not feel the lightest touch, the pressure of the stimulus or the area of stimulation is increased until a response is elicited.
Areas of Decreased Perception	If an area of decreased touch perception is found, the stimulus is then moved from the point of maximal impairment into several normal areas to delineate the exact boundaries of the deficit. It is good to repeat this procedure several times until the same boundaries are determined repeatedly, always testing from the abnormal area into the normal.
Thresholds for Touch	Different areas of the skin normally have different thresholds for touch. The back, buttocks, and thickened parts of the skin require more pressure than do the face or fingertips.

EXAMINATION OF INDIVIDUAL SENSORY MODALITIES, Continued

Pain Perception

Pain perception is usually tested next. Since it is important to apply stimuli of about equal intensity, it has been found helpful to attach a pin to an applicator stick or to use a large safety pin. See Figure 15-35.

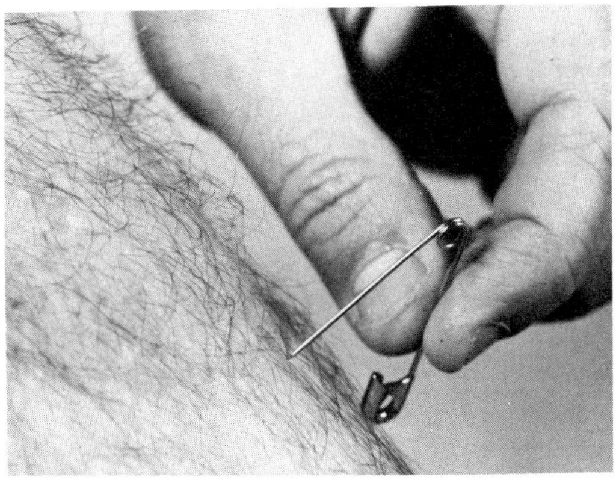

Figure 15-35.

Procedure

The threshold is determined and areas of loss are mapped out in the same manner as was established for "light touch." The skin is usually touched in an irregular fashion either with the sharp end of the pin or the dull head. The patient responds with "sharp" or "dull."

Impairments

In some patients with peripheral neuropathy or tabes dorsalis the initial respose to a painful stimulus may be "dull," only to be corrected within 1 to 3 seconds by the response "sharp." This delayed pain appreciation may be overlooked unless the patient is instructed to watch for this phenomenon.

Other Pain Responses

Poorly localized or deep pain is mediated by a different pathway system from sharp "pinprick" sensation. It is elicited by the application of heavy periosteal or testicular pressure.

Vibratory Sensibility

Vibratory sensibility is not a separate sense, nor is it bone sensibility. Superficial and deep pressure receptors are involved, and a temporal pattern of pressures is perceived as vibration.

(Continued)

EXAMINATION OF INDIVIDUAL SENSORY MODALITIES, Continued

Procedure

Placing a tuning fork over bone mechanically intensifies the stimulus. Usually the vibrating fork is placed over the fingers and toes. Threshold is determined by having the patient respond when he no longer feels the vibration. The tuning fork is then quickly placed on other parts of the body to determine if vibration is still perceived there. The patient's threshold may be compared with that of the examiner. See Figures 15-36 and 15-37.

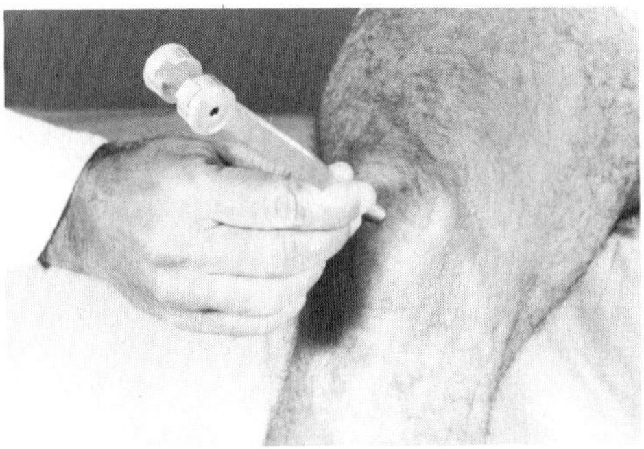

Figure 15-36.

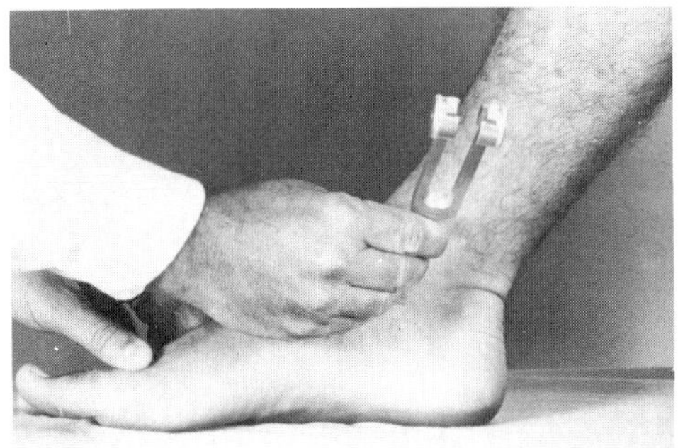

Figure 15-37.

Position Sense

The patient's ability to detect small passive movements is tested by holding a finger or toe between the examiner's fingers. The digit should be held by its lateral surfaces. The patient's muscles should be completely relaxed in order to test joint receptors rather than muscle stretch receptors. See Figures 15-38 and 15-39.

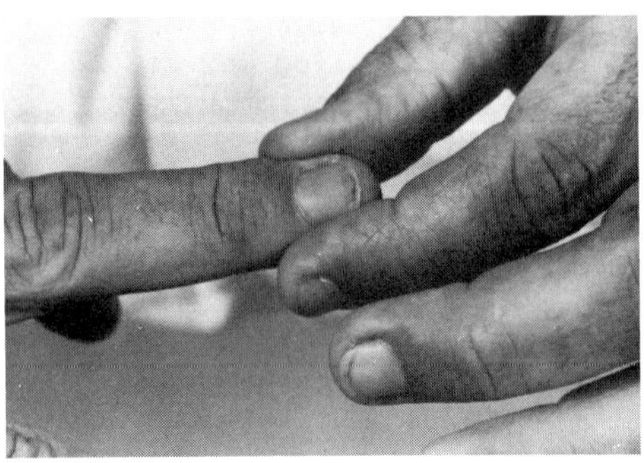

Figure 15-38.

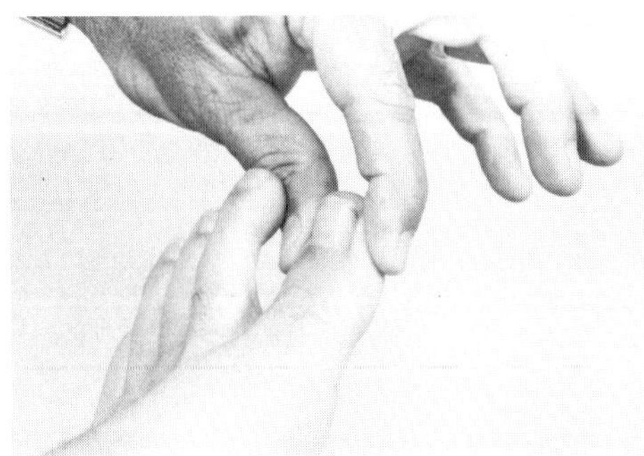

Figure 15-39.

EXAMINATION OF INDIVIDUAL SENSORY MODALITIES, Continued

Procedure	The digit is moved several times up or down 5 to 10 degrees and the patient responds with "up," "down," or "I don't know." The patient should clearly understand that "up" or "down" refers to the last position of the digit and not the midposition. To avoid any misunderstanding, the patient should look at a few movements first, and if he responds properly he is then asked to close his eyes.
Evaluation	A normal person can easily detect movements of a few millimeters. Should the patient be unable to detect finger movements, motion of the hand is then tested.
Hysterical Reaction	A hysterical patient may demonstrate sharp borders to sensation (e.g., the shoulder joint) that do not make neuroanatomic sense. Likewise, the tuning fork may be felt on one side of the forehead (solid bone!) but not the other.
Summary	Once again, if abnormalities in sensation are detected, one must consult a reference to determine the nerve or dermatome involved (see the following diagrams).

(Continued)

EXAMINATION OF INDIVIDUAL SENSORY MODALITIES, Continued

Dermatomes on the Upper Limb

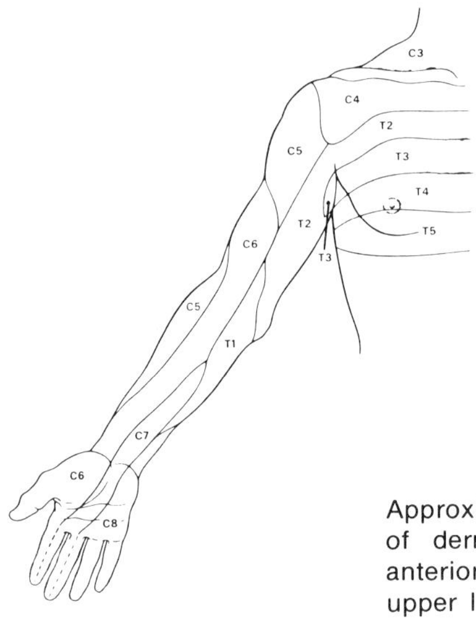

Approximate distribution of dermatomes on the anterior aspect of the upper limb.

Dermatomes on the Lower Limb

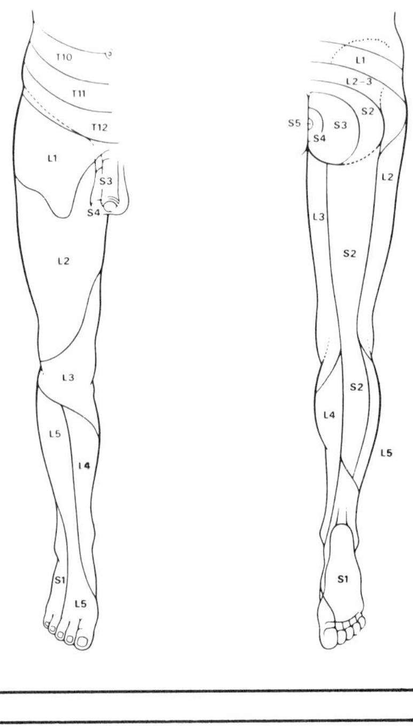

Approximate distribution of dermatomes on the lower limb.

SELF-ASSESSMENT

1. State the characteristics of lower motor neuron weakness.
2. With what types of lesions is fasciculation found?
3. State the characteristics of an upper motor neuron lesion.
4. Describe how to test light touch, pain, position, and vibratory sensations.
5. What kind of nasal disorders are common causes of loss of smell (anosmia)?
6. State the normal diameter of the optic disc.
7. Which nerve is responsible for the afferent limb of the corneal reflex?
8. Which nerve and which division are responsible for innervating the muscles of mastication?
9. Name three things to inspect in muscles.
10. Which nerve innervates the interossei?
11. Which nerve is important in the biceps reflex?
12. Weakness of the flexors in the legs and the extensors of the arms suggests a lesion in the __________________.
13. Rapid alternating movements test which "systems"?
14. Weakness of the lower two thirds of the face is due to ______________.

CHAPTER SIXTEEN

The Female and Male Genitourinary Examination

Alvin L. LeBlanc, M.D., and Donald McDonald, M.D.

The Female Pelvic Examination

INTRODUCTION AND PREPARATION

Overview

The female pelvic examination is composed of four parts:
- preparation for the examination
- the external examination
- the speculum examination
- the digital examination

Preparation of Physician

The physician should wash his/her hands before examining the patient.

Preparation of Patient

Before the examination, a patient must empty her bladder. It is best if the rectum is empty also, but this is not always practical. An attendant positions the patient for the pelvic examination. The presence of an attendant during the examination can:
- comfort and reassure the patient
- help to protect the physician legally
- assist the physician

  NOTE: An attendant must be present during a pelvic examination of a psychotic patient, or when the results of the examination may become legal evidence in criminal proceedings, for example, alleged rape.

Positioning

The nurse helps the patient to assume the dorsal lithotomy position on the examination table.
- The patient is lying on her back.
- The hips are flexed to about 75°.
- The hips are abducted as much as is comfortable.
- The kness are flexed to about 90°.
- The feet are supported in stirrups.
- The knees should be allowed to fall apart as much as is comfortable.
- The knees and abdomen are draped to permit an adequate view of the perineum while avoiding undue exposure.

(Continued)

INTRODUCTION AND PREPARATION, Continued

- The patient has her hands at her sides or folded across the upper abdomen.
  See Figure 16-1.

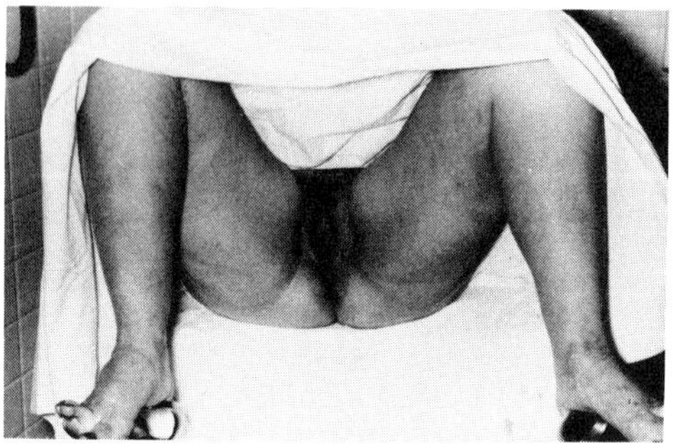

Figure 16-1.

Informing the Patient

The examiner should encourage the patient to breath slowly through her mouth during the examination to relax her abdominal muscles and the hip adductors.

NOTE: The knees are NEVER forcibly separated by the examiner or attendant.

The examiner should inform the patient of each step of the procedure before it is performed.

Position of Hands

The examiner sits or stands before the patient with at least one hand gloved. A right-handed examiner wears a glove on the left hand; a left-handed examiner wears a glove on the right hand.

IF THE LEFT HAND	THE RIGHT HAND
• is gloved	• is ungloved
• is used to separate the labia during inspection of the vulva	• handles instruments
• fingers are used for the vaginal portion of the bimanual examination	• performs the abdominal portion of the bimanual examination

EXTERNAL EXAMINATION

Procedure

After the patient is informed of the procedure to follow, the labia are separated with the thumb and forefinger of the gloved hand, and the vulva and vaginal vestibule are inspected in a regular sequence. See Figure 16-2.

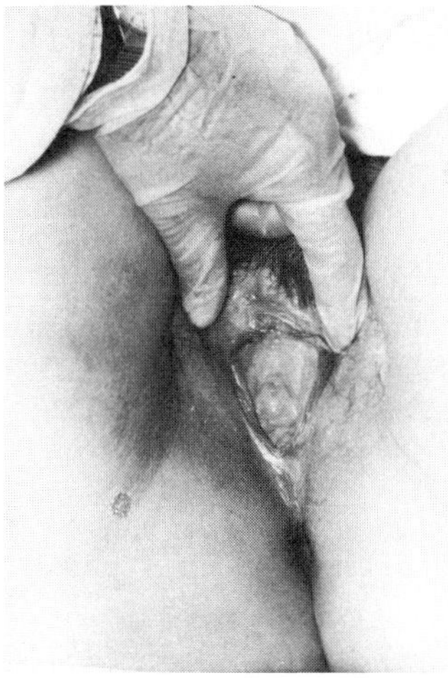

Figure 16-2.

STEP	OBSERVATIONS
inspect perineum	Note any skin lesions and the escutcheon. If the perineum of an adult has a scaphoid appearance (as is seen in children), the genitalia are probably hypoplastic or atrophic.
inspect vulva	Lesions include: • ulcers • abscesses • edema • varicosities • hernias • tumors • abrasions In elderly women the skin of the vulva becomes atrophic and wrinkled. Leukoplakia arises most frequently in such skin.
palpate vulva	Special attention should be devoted to any visible lesion. Neoplasms are usually painless. Abscesses, cellulitis, and some sexually transmitted ulcers are tender.

(Continued)

EXTERNAL EXAMINATION, Continued

STEP	OBSERVATIONS
inspect labia majora	The labia majora of postpubescent, premenopausal women are plump.
inspect labia minora	In nulliparous women, the labia minora are relatively small and lie together. If the perineal muscles are stretched or lacerated during pregnancy and childbirth, the labia minora gape and fall apart.
inspect external urethral meatus	• Prolapsed mucous membrane of the urethra or a urethral caruncle may be infected, red, inflamed, and tender. • A test for acute suppurative urethritis is to "milk" the urethra from the bladder neck downward with the index finger in the vagina by using gentle anterior pressure. This may be a very painful maneuver. Any discharge from the urethra should be cultured and a wet smear and a Gram stain prepared.
inspect clitoris	Abnormal enlargement of the clitoris indicates a masculinizing process.
inspect introitus and hymen	Note the vaginal opening and the hymenal ring. • Bulging of the posterior vaginal wall into or past the introitus is a rectocele. • Bulging of the anterior vaginal wall into or past the introitus is a cystocele or urethrocele. See Figure 16-3. • With uterine prolapse, the cervix may be seen at (or even outside) the introitus. • In virginal women, the hymen varies a great deal in thickness and in flexibility. The structure will generally admit at least one finger. • Some girls may be born with an imperforate hymen. • In nonvirginal patients, remnants of the hymen may become inflammed, red, tender, and swollen in acute vaginitis.

(Continued)

EXTERNAL EXAMINATION, Continued

STEP	OBSERVATIONS
inspect vestibule	The vestibule lies between the labia minora (with the clitoris anteriorly). This area is a common site of vaginitis in younger women and of neoplasms in older women. • The skin within the vestibule is normally softer and more delicate than that of the labia majora and perineum. No hair follicles are located in the vestibule, but it does contain sweat and sebaceous glands that may become infected. • The peri-urethral (Skene's) glands, located at 5 o'clock and 7 o'clock around the urethra, secrete mucus. These glands are often involved in gonococcal infections and sometimes in infections produced by non-sexually transmitted organisms.
inspect greater vestibular gland (Bartholin's gland)	The ducts of the greater vestibular (Bartholin's) glands open into the vaginal vestibule at 5 o'clock and 7 o'clock just outside the hymen. This gland and its duct are frequently the site of gonococcal infections. Additionally, the opening of the duct is easily obstructed in any acute infection and results in a Bartholin abscess. Such an abscess can be seen as a tumor beneath the labia majora that may involve the base of the labia minora, and it is tender with palpation. NOTE: Palpation of the gland or abscess is done by inserting the index finger into the vagina and palpating the mass between that finger and the thumb (see Fig. 16-4). An abscess is tender.

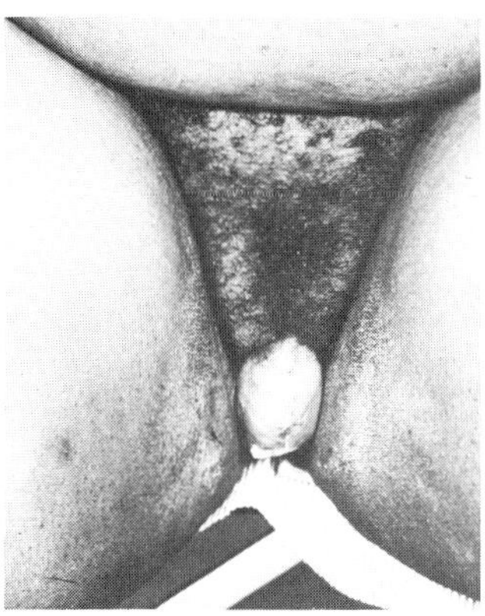

Figure 16-3.

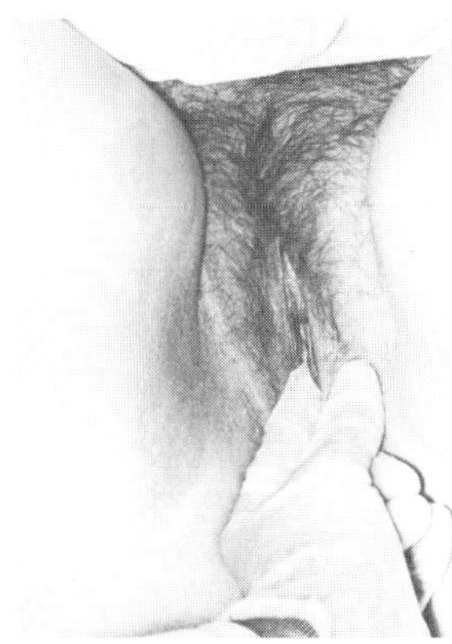

Figure 16-4.

SPECULUM EXAMINATION: PROCEDURE

Introduction

The speculum examination (and cervical smear) is performed after the external examination.

> NOTE: Avoid contamination of the cervical and vaginal smears with lubricant; do not apply the jelly to the speculum at this point. Moisten the speculum with warm tap water.

Speculum Description

The speculum is available in three sizes; the choice of size depends upon the introitus of the patient. The examiner must always check the screws on the speculum before use so that adjustments may be made.

- The set screw that holds the two blades together should be "finger" tight with the blades approximated.
- The set screw on the thumb rest should be loose so the tips of the blades approximate.

Use of the Speculum

Before the examiner begins the speculum examination, he or she should describe the procedure to the patient.

- The speculum is held in the right hand (or left hand of left-handed persons).
- Separate the labia with the thumb and index finger.

OR

- Separate the labia by pulling the skin of the left labium majus laterally (see Fig. 16-5).
- Turn the handle of the speculum 45 to 60 degrees to the side.
- The thumb joint is kept against the underside of the thumb rest to hold the blades of the speculum together.
- The tip of the speculum is inserted into the vagina in the 2 to 8 o'clock or 10 to 4 o'clock plane. Avoid pressure on the external urethral meatus anteriorly (see Fig. 16-6).

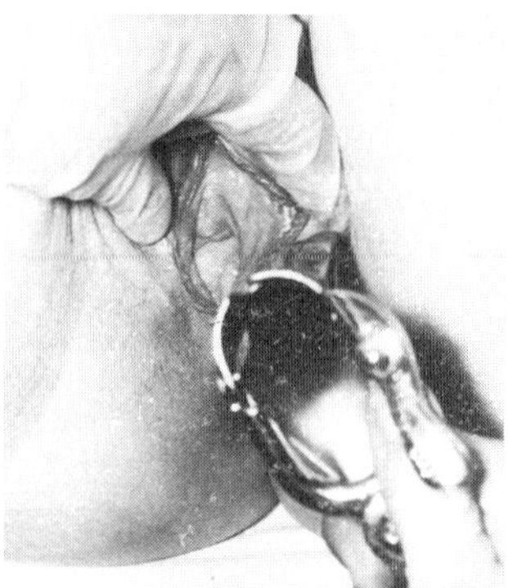

Figure 16-5

Figure 16-6.

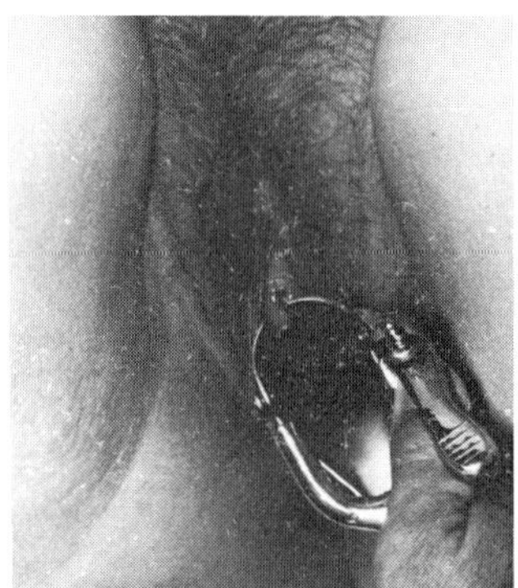

SPECULUM EXAMINATION: PROCEDURE, Continued

<u>NOTE:</u> The speculum may also be inserted by introducing two fingers of the gloved hand through the introitus, and depressing the perineal body backward. The speculum is then put into the vagina over the top of the fingers. This method also avoids pressure on the urethra.

- The speculum is inserted the remainder of the way into vagina, exerting pressure against the posterior vaginal wall.
- Tilt the handle upward and rotate back to the midline (see Fig. 16-7).

  <u>NOTE:</u> During this maneuver, exert posterior pressure to avoid the sensitive urethra.
- With the handle of the speculum depressed, the blades are opened by pressing down on the thumb set (see Fig. 16-8).
- The normal cervix can now be seen at the top of the speculum. If one cannot bring the cervix into view, remove the speculum, palpate the location of the cervix, and reinsert the speculum.

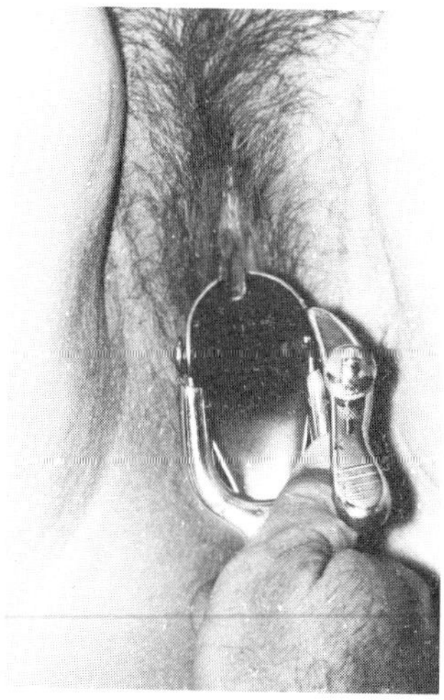

Figure 16-7.

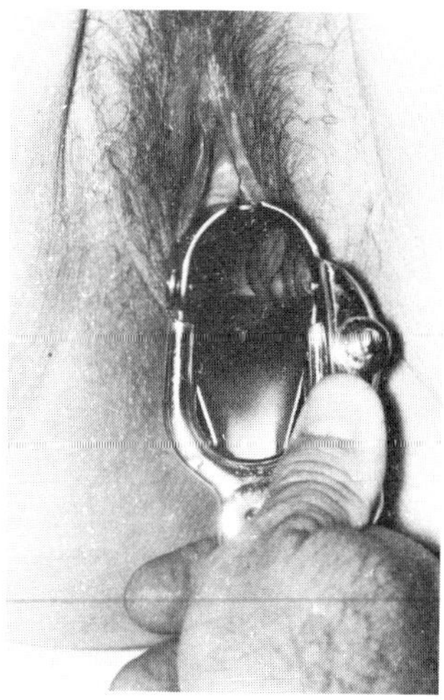

Figure 16-8.

Cervical Smears

Specimens for gonococcal culture and Papanicolaou ("Pap," cytologic) smear should be taken from the cervical os and vaginal vault. The cytologic smear should be taken from the endocervix by scraping the squamocolumnar junction of the cervix.

- A thin wooden spatula that is made expressly for scraping the cervix is used (see Fig. 16-9).

(Continued)

Figure 16-9.

- The spatula is placed against the cervix and is rotated 360 degrees with gentle pressure.

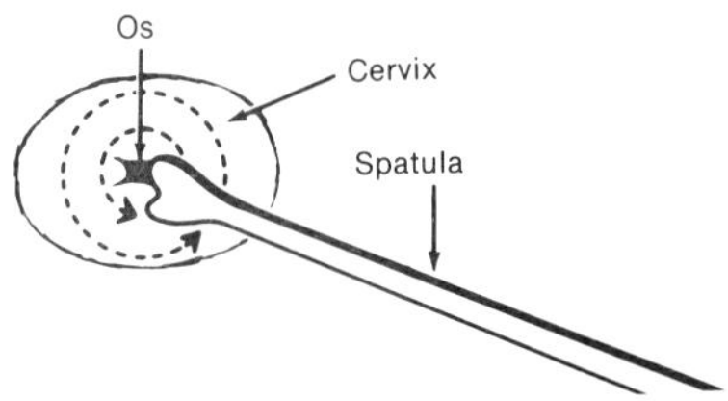

- The material obtained is then transferred to a slide, and the examination of the vagina and cervix begins.

Normal Vaginal Appearance

The appearance and texture of normal (adult) vaginal walls vary somewhat according to age, although, in general, the walls are pink and uniform.

- In a child, the vaginal walls are smooth and delicate.
- In an adult, the epithelium is thicker, heavier, and elastic, with many folds (rugae).
- In a postmenopausal patient, the rugae tend to disappear, and the epithelium is thin and velvety.

Normal Cervical Appearance

The cervix is 2 cm to 3 cm in diameter and protrudes 2 cm to 3 cm into the vagina. The cervix is cylindrical and points posteriorly unless the uterus is retrodisplaced (as in about 20% of women), in which case the cervix points anteriorly. The cervix is normally covered by squamous epithelium and is the same color as the vagina.

SPECULUM EXAMINATION: CERVICAL ABNORMALITIES

CONDITION	DESCRIPTON
early pregnancy	A bluish color is an early indication of pregnancy (Chadwick's sign).
erosion and early carcinoma	A red friable area that extends from the external os may be an extension of the columnar epithelium (which normally lines the endocervix) onto the exterior cervix. A benign erosion cannot reliably be differentiated from a carcinoma by gross inspection. See Figure 16-10 and 16-11.
advanced carcinoma	In advanced carcinoma, the cervix has a friable, rough, granular surface (cauliflower) that bleeds easily. Some cancers, however, particularly if they originate within the endocervix, may not change the appearance of the cervix. See Figure 16-12.
eversion	A "fish-mouth" deformity of the cervix from a prior vaginal delivery will render the endocervical epithelium visible -- an eversion. The exposed columnar epithelium easily becomes infected; this is associated with a thick mucopurulent discharge. The cervix becomes enlarged and edematous. Cysts (nabothian cysts), 1 mm to 3 mm in diameter, often form on its vaginal cervix. See Figure 16-13.
cervical polyps	A dark, red mass (several millimeters to 3 cm in diameter) that extends out of the cervical canal is usually a cervical polyp. Polyps are smooth and uniform and bleed easily. See Figure 16-14.
endometrial polyps and fibroids	Endometrial polyps and prolapsed submucous fibroids may be seen at the cervical os. Fibroids are usually larger than polyps. If a large polyp or fibroid protrudes through the cervix, the cervical canal and its external opening are obviously dilated. Occasionally, the tumor may be so large that the view of the cervix is obstructed.

(Continued)

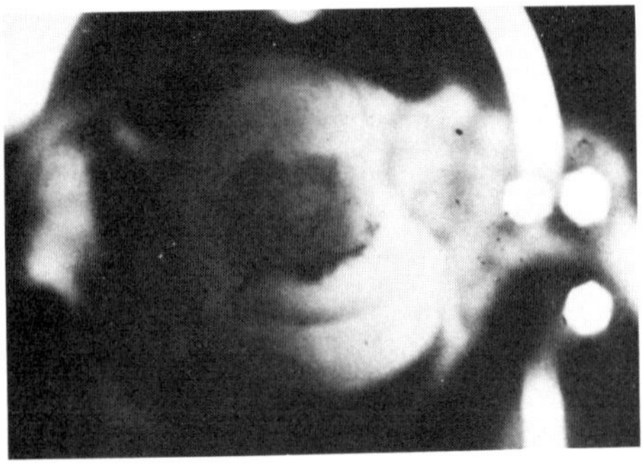

Figure 16-10.

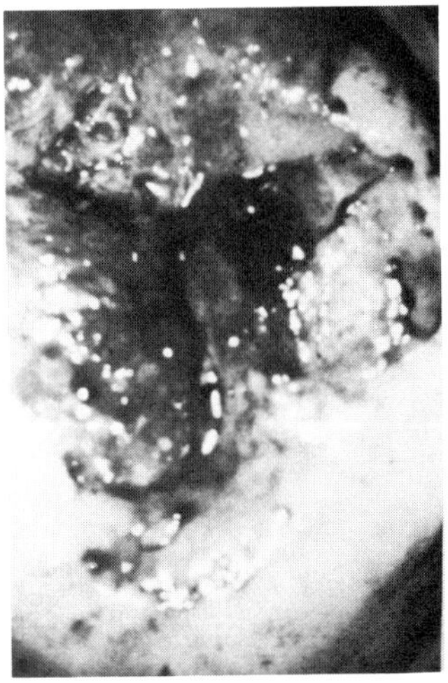

Figure 16-11.

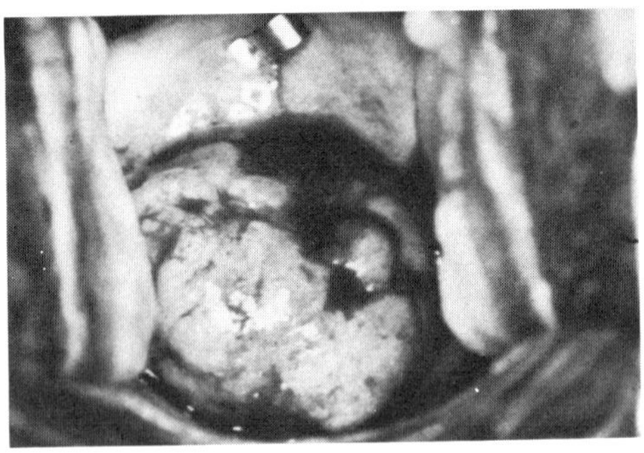

Figure 16-12.

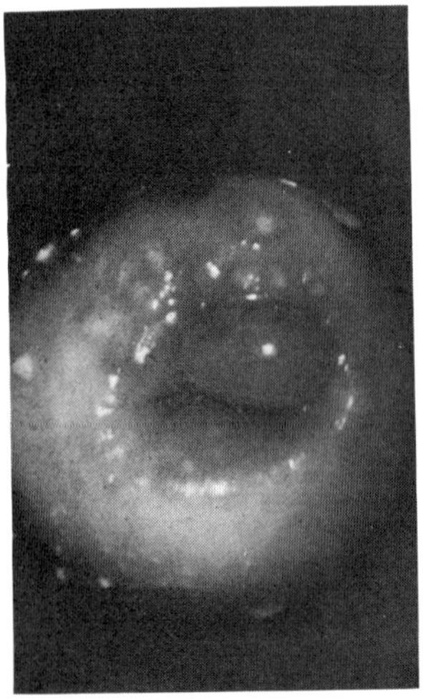

Figure 16-13.

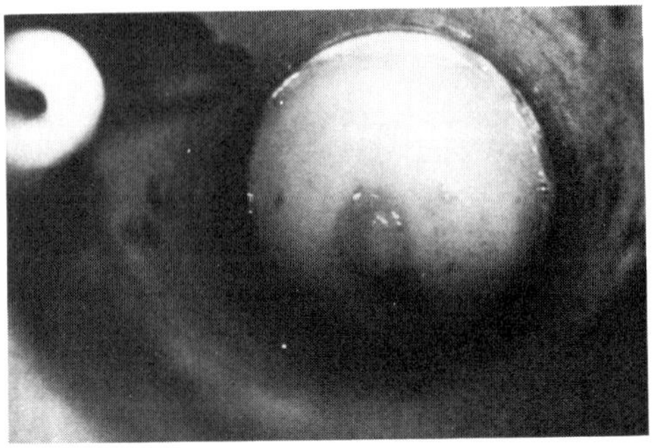

Figure 16-14.

SPECULUM EXAMINATION: CERVICAL ABNORMALITIES, Continued

CONDITION	OBSERVATIONS
vaginal discharge	Any of the aforementioned problems may cause a vaginal discharge. Additionally, sexually transmitted diseases may cause a discharge: • gonorrhea • trichomoniasis • moniliasis • "clue" cell or nonspecific vaginitis (<u>Gardnerella</u> <u>vaginalis</u>) • chlamydial vaginitis and cervicitis • herpes simplex cervicitis A bloody discharge suggests: • erosion • eversion • carcinoma • polyps <u>NOTE</u>: Varying amounts of vaginal secretions are due to changing levels of estrogen and progesterone during the menstrual cycle and are normal.

SPECULUM EXAMINATION: VAGINAL ABNORMALITIES

The following abnormalities may be noted in the vagina.

CONDITION	DESCRIPTION
inflammation	The walls are red and often coated with a discharge.
trichomonas vaginitis	The discharge is thin, yellow, and often frothy, with a musty odor. Small red spots are often seen on the walls, and the cervix has a strawberry appearance. See Figure 16-15.
monilial infection	Monilial (candidal) vaginitis causes a thick, white, curdlike discharge that clings to the vaginal wall (see Fig. 16-16). It is usually associated with perineal pruritis.
nonspecific "clue" cell vaginitis	The discharge tends to be thin and yellow-green and smells "fishy." Squamous cells, containing a large number of adherent gram-negative bacilli, are diagnostic ("clue cells").

(Continued)

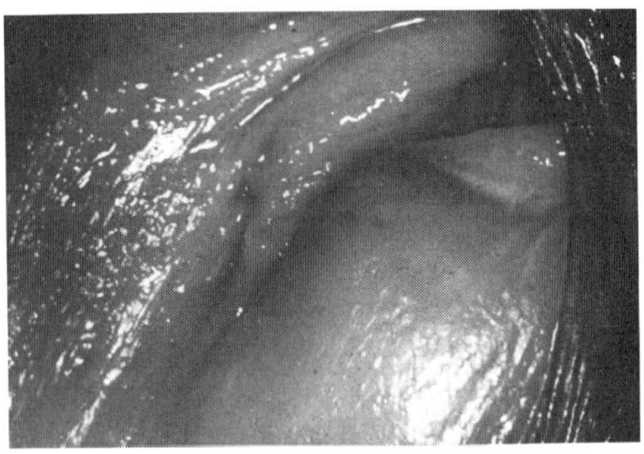

Figure 16-15.

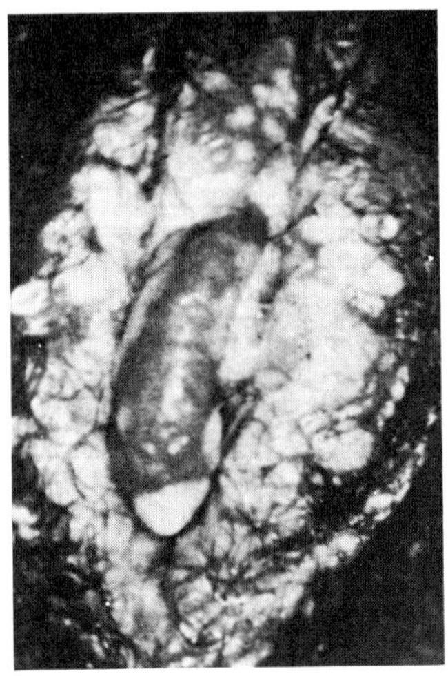

Figure 16-16.

SPECULUM EXAMINATION: VAGINAL ABNORMALITIES, Continued

Diagnosis of Vaginitis

To test vaginal secretions for the specific organisms, several types of smears are used.

STEP	ACTION
1	Gently scrape a small amount of vaginal secretion onto an applicator.
2	Place a drop of the secretion onto three glass slides.
3	• Place a drop of normal saline on the secretion on one slide. • Place a drop of 10% potassium hydroxide on another slide. • Let the third slide dry and prepare a gram stain.
4	Drop a coverslip on the first two slides.
5	Since the strong base on the second slide will destroy the desquamated vaginal cells, the yeast can be seen easily. Motile, flagellated trichomonas can be seen easily on the slide with the saline. "Clue" cells are diagnostic on the third slide.

Completing the Vaginal Exam

Inspect the anterior, posterior, and lateral vaginal walls by rotating the speculum. Keep the blades apart as the speculum is removed and inspect the vaginal walls as the speculum is removed.

Assessing Uterine Supports

When the speculum is withdrawn to near the introitus, instruct the patient to "bear down". If a cystocele or rectocele exists, the vaginal walls, or even the cervix, will protrude into the speculum.

DIGITAL EXAMINATION: BACKGROUND

Introduction

The digital examination consists of palpation of the:

- pelvic muscles
- vagina
- cervix
- bladder
- parametrium
- uterus
- fallopian tubes and ovaries
- rectovaginal septum

Lubrication

Surgical lubricant should be spread lightly over the first and second fingers of the gloved hand and the inner aspect of the labia minora.

Positioning the Hand

Slight posterior pressure should be exerted against the introitus and the posterior vaginal wall with the fingers as they are introduced into the vagina so that pressure on the urethra is avoided. The fingers, hand, and forearm must be held in a straight line, with no extension, abduction, or flexion of the wrist. The third and fourth fingers are flexed completely, and the thumb is hyperextended (see Fig. 16-17). The hand is kept perpendicular to the floor throughout the examination; the palm is never turned up. The flexed third and fourth fingers press against the perineal body.

> NOTE: If the palm of the examining hand is turned upward (a common error), the penetration is stopped as the third and fourth knuckles contact the pubic ramus. The palm of the hand is turned up only when the anterior vaginal wall or the urethra is being palpated.

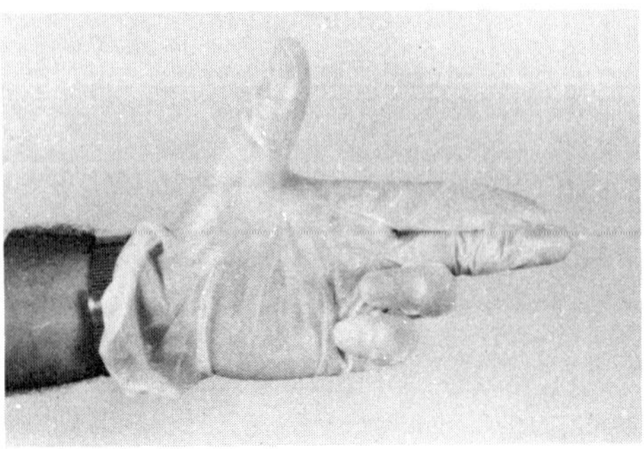

Figure 16-17.

DIGITAL EXAMINATION: VAGINA AND BLADDER

Vaginal Wall

Palpate the vaginal walls as the fingers are introduced; various characteristics may be observed.

- Scars from previous surgery or childbirth are indurated.
- Tumors or cysts may be palpated.
- The relaxation or redundancy of the vaginal walls may be assessed.
- An imperforate hymen may prevent digital access to the vagina; a partially perforate hymen may allow penetration only with the fifth finger.

  NOTE: If an imperforate hymen or a tight hymenal ring restricts the entrance, the internal genitalia may be evaluated by a rectoabdominal bimanual examination, described later.
- A partial or complete vertical, longitudinal septum attached to the anterior and posterior walls of the vagina is often associated with a double cervix or bicornuate uterus. See Figure 16-18.

Evaluation of Vaginal Musculature

The patient must be able to cooperate for an examiner to evaluate pelvic muscles.

PROCEDURE	POSSIBLE FINDINGS
Insert the first and second fingers into the vagina. Ask the patient to tighten her perineal muscles or vagina about the fingers.	Normally, the examiner will feel pressure as the fingers are elevated against the pubic arch.
Turn the fingers palm down, separate the fingers, and depress the perineal muscles posteriorly. Palpate the thickness of the perineal body. Ask the patient to strain or "bear down" as with a bowel movement.	A rectocele will be felt as a bulge between the fingers. Weakness of the anterior vaginal wall will also be evident as bulging of the urethra or bladder floor downward when the patient strains (urethrocystocele). If the uterine supports are weak, the cervix may fall into view.

(Continued)

DIGITAL EXAMINATION: VAGINA AND BLADDER, Continued

Examining the Bladder

The bladder is palpated for tenderness, tumor, or induration by compressing it between the hand on the abdomen and the fingers in the vagina.

- The normal empty bladder is neither tender nor palpable.
- Inflammation of the bladder or bladder neck will cause tenderness.

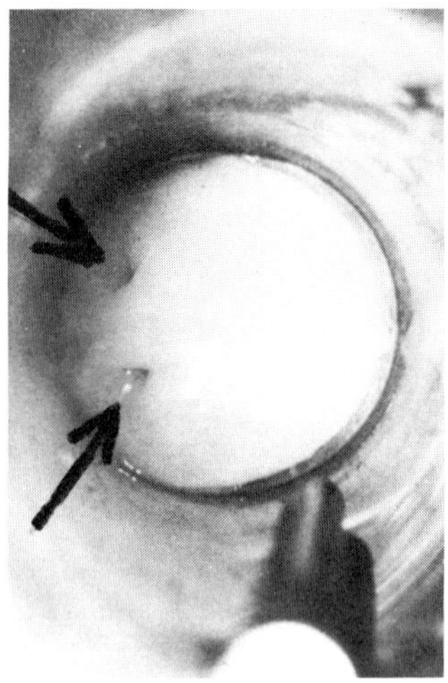

Figure 16-18.

DIGITAL EXAMINATION: CERVIX AND PARAMETRIUM

Examining the Cervix

The cervix should be evaluated for:
- size
- shape
- position
- mobility
- regularity
- consistency
- lesions

Size of Cervix

The examiner should determine the length of the cervix and compare it with the size of the uterus. In normal adults, the length ratio is 1:2. The ratio is 2:1 in children or in women with hypoplasia of the uterus. The external opening (os) of the cervix is normally 3 mm to 5 mm in diameter.

Consistency of the Cervix

The normal adult cervix is firm, round, and smooth. Advanced cervical cancer is hard. Cancer also causes a granular, cauliflowerlike (in both feel and appearance) tumor. Pregnancy will make the cervix soft. Smooth, small, tense cysts on the cervix are nabothian cysts.

Position of the Cervix

The cervix and os normally point downward and posteriorly in the midline from the apex of the anterior vaginal wall. The normal position of the cervix and the direction in which it points, however, may vary.

Conditions of the Cervix

CONDITION	POSSIBLE CAUSES
change in the direction of the cervix so that it points upward	retrodisplacement of the entire uterus
change in position and axis	A tumor of the uterus or other pelvic organ that displaces or pushes the body of the uterus, as well as the cervix, to the side (e.g., inflammation and fibrosis or cancer in the parametrium) may retract the cervix to the side.
immobility (fixation) of the cervix	• carcinoma • endometriosis • pelvic inflammatory disease NOTE: The cervix normally moves freely about 2 cm to 3 cm in any direction.

DIGITAL EXAMINATION: CERVIX AND PARAMETRIUM, Continued

CONDITION	POSSIBLE CAUSES
Tenderness on movement of the cervix	• pelvic inflammatory disease • ruptured ectopic (tubal) pregnancy • endometriosis • pelvic peritonitis (ruptured viscus) NOTE: Because movement of the cervix, especially from side to side, stretches the pelvic peritoneum and broad ligament, movement of any irritated pelvic peritoneum will produce tenderness.
descent of the cervix into the vagina	uterine prolapse
deformed cervix	lacerations suffered during childbirth
protrusion of a spongy mass through the cervical os	cervical polyp, which is soft and varies in size from a few millimeters to 2 cm in diameter
cervical os wide enough to admit the tip of the index finger	• products of conception • endometrial polyp

Parametrium

The pelvic soft tissue adjacent to the cervix and the lower segment of the uterine corpus is the parametrium, which extends laterally and posteriorly. The parametrium contains the vascular supply and the lymphatics that drain the cervix.

- The parametrium becomes indurated and tender with pelvic infections.
- The parametrium will be both indurated and immobile with advanced carcinoma.
- The posterior portion of the parametrium, containing the uterosacral ligaments, may be nodular and cyclically tender with endometriosis.

DIGITAL EXAMINATION: UTERINE CORPUS

Examining the Uterine Corpus

Palpate the uterus, noting:

- position
- mobility
- size
- shape
- consistency

The uterus is palpated bimanually, using an ungloved hand on the lower abdomen and the gloved, intravaginal hand.

Positioning the "Vaginal" Hand

The intravaginal hand is positioned as noted earlier--extended fingers with the hand and forearm held in a straight line.

Positioning the "Abdominal" Hand

The fingers of the ungloved hand are placed just below the umbilicus. During the examination, the abdomen is palpated as the hand is brought slowly downward toward the pubis.

NOTE: Do not press too close to the pubis because the abdominal wall will move downward, making the uterus difficult to feel.

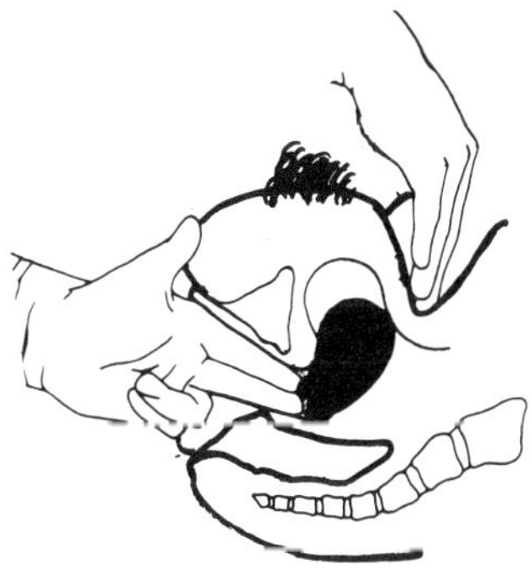

Procedure

When the uterus (or a pelvic tumor) is pressed with the "abdominal" hand, movement will be perceived by the hand in the vagina. The fingers in the vagina should then palpate in the anterior vaginal fornix. The uterus (in its normal anteflexed position) is palpable here and its width, size, and regularity can be evaluated by both hands. Depressing the anterior abdominal wall further will usually bring pressure on the posterior part of the lower part of the uterus, which is normally firm and identical in consistency to the uterine fundus.

(Continued)

DIGITAL EXAMINATION: UTERINE CORPUS, Continued

Uterine Corpus Examination

The lower uterine segment and the corpus are evaluated by spreading the fingers in the vagina as shown. The fingers press into the lateral vaginal fornices and are moved along the lateral walls of the uterus. While the fingers in the vagina steady the uterus, the hand on the abdomen palpates for enlargement and other abnormalities of the fundus.

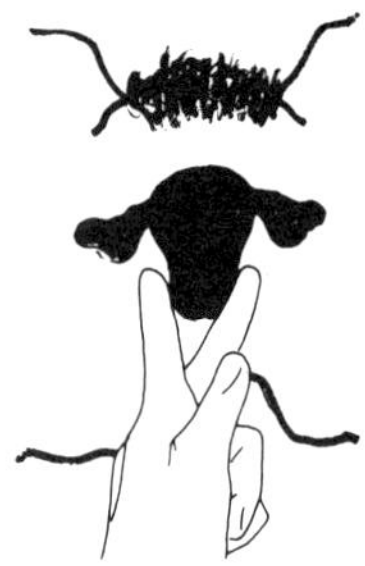

Anteroposterior View

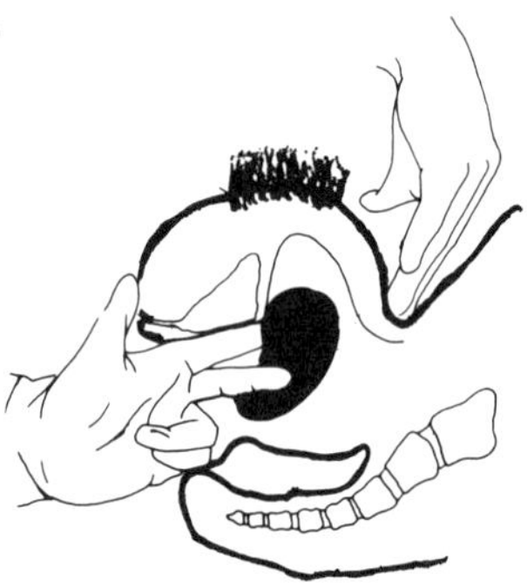

Lateral View

(Continued)

DIGITAL EXAMINATION: UTERINE CORPUS, Continued

Pregnancy	In early pregnancy, the uterine corpus softens so that it can be compressed easily (Hegar's sign). This sign of pregnancy can often be observed before much enlargment of the uterus has occurred.
Fibroids (Leiomyomata)	The uterine body may be enlarged by fibroid tumors that are firm, smooth, and rounded and usually appear as nodules within the uterus. They vary in size from 2 cm to 20 cm. Cystic degeneration of uterine fibroids will produce easily compressed, irregular uterine masses. Uncomplicated fibroids are not tender; areas of tenderness will occur in tumors only if infarction or hemorrhage is present.
Retro-displacement and Fixation	In about 20% of normal women, the uterus is retrodisplaced: the fundus lies in the cul-de-sac and is palpable behind the cervix. Normally, the body of the uterus can freely be moved anteriorly if gentle, steady pressure is applied by the fingers in the vagina. Occasionally, this must be done using a rectal bimanual technique if the fundus cannot be lifted otherwise. Fixation of the uterus in a retroflexed position may be due to: • peritoneal adhesions caused by inflammatory disease • scarring and infiltration with endometriosis • cancer All three can cause fixation and immobility of the uterus in any position.

DIGITAL EXAMINATION: ADNEXA

Examining the Tube and Ovary (Adnexa)

The ability to palpate the tube and ovary (the uterine adnexa) takes experience to develop and requires that the examiner know that:

- the normal tube is not palpable
- the normal ovary is about 2 cm by 3 cm, is sensitive to pressure, and should be palpated between fingers in the vagina and fingers on the abdomen
- the ovaries lie just above the lateral vaginal fornices

Bimanual Examination

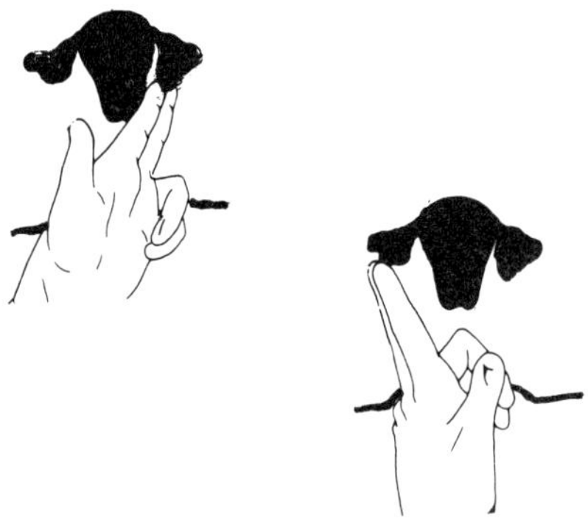

The fingers on the patient's left lower abdomen should exert deep pressure (directed slightly toward the midline) at the level of the anterior superior iliac spine. At the same time, the fingers in the lateral fornix should be directed slightly laterally and anteriorly to feel the ovary being pressed toward them. The process is reversed on the right side. Pressure should be relatively gentle; the ovaries are sensitive, and excessive pressure will cause discomfort and tightening of the patient's abdominal muscles.

Findings

FINDING	COMMENTS
ovarian tumors	When the ovaries enlarge, they occupy the posterior half of the pelvis. Thus, ovarian and tubo-ovarian masses lie posterior to the uterine corpus and displace it forward. Such masses may become so large that they fill the pelvis or stretch the ovarian pedicle such that they escape the pelvis and enter the lower abdomen. Ovarian tumors may be: • cystic • solid • cystic and solid Cystic tumors can be compressed between the examining fingers; they are usually smooth, and range from very tense to very soft. Solid tumors are firm and cannot be compressed; they may be either smooth or nodular. Nodules on the suface of either a cystic or a solid mass indicate a malignant neoplasm.

(Continued)

DIGITAL EXAMINATION: ADNEXA, Continued

FINDING	COMMENTS
tenderness	Tenderness of a mass in the adnexa indicates an acute inflammatory disease that may be: • tubo-ovarian abscess • bleeding or necrosis within a tumor • ectopic tubo-ovarian pregnancy • infarction of the ovary or ovarian tumor caused by torsion of the pedicle that contains its blood supply. NOTE: Any acute tubal infection almost always involves the ovary. With such an infection, the tube and ovary usually cannot be distinguished from each other: instead they feel like a single, tender, indurated mass.
fixation	Chronic or repeated pelvic inflammatory disease (salpingo-oophoritis) usually causes fixation of the adnexa and, at times, cystic enlargement of the tubes. Movement of the enlarged tube and ovary produces pain.
colon masses	Masses that originate in the sigmoid colon may be confused with adnexal tumors. Such masses (often carcinoma or diverticulitis of the colon) tend to be in the left side of the pelvis. Carcinoma of the cecum and appendiceal abscess may be felt in the right side of the pelvis. NOTE: Fecal material in the sigmoid colon or rectum may be mistaken for pelvic masses. Gentle pressure on the feces will usually change its shape, whereas such pressure will not affect the shape of other masses.

DIGITAL EXAMINATION: TWO RECTAL PROCEDURES

Vaginorecto-abdominal Method

The rectovaginal or vaginorectoabdominal examination is performed by:
- inserting the index finger into the vagina
- inserting the third finger into the rectum

The rectal septum and the cul-de-sac then can be palpated. The examination must be employed if the introitus will admit only one finger. Some of the other uses of the technique are to:
- assess the relationship of the upper vagina to the rectum
- evaluate weakness, integrity, and induration of the rectovaginal septum
- palpate abnormalities in the cul-de-sac

The remainder of the bimanual examination is done as described for the vaginal bimanual examination. Additionally, this examination must explore the rectum as described in Chapter 14, Abdomen and Lower Extremities.

Rectoabdominal Examination

The rectoabdominal examination may be performed:
- as a part of the routine evaluation of virginal women
- when a finger cannot be introduced because of a tight hymenal ring or vaginal atresia
- when the vagina is malformed after radiation therapy for cancer of the cervix or after vaginal surgery

The Male Genitalia Examination

PENIS

Inspect and Palpate Prepuce and Penile Shaft	The prepuce should be retracted and the skin, mucosa, and glans penis examined for cleanliness and lesions, including adhesions, ulcers, or tumors. If any skin or mucosal lesions are present, wear gloves because some lesions are infectious. The normal prepurce is soft and pliable. The corpus cavernosum is normally soft and regular; note any areas of tenderness or induration.
Phimosis	If the prepuce cannot be retracted over the glans, the condition is called phimosis. This may require surgical incision to enable exposure of the glans penis. Phimosis may cause adhesions of the prepuce to the underlying glans penis. The prepuce must not be forcibly retracted over the prepuce, which may cause splitting of the foreskin, causing infection, scarring, and contracture and leading to worsening phimosis.
Paraphimosis	The prepuce can sometimes be partially retracted over an edematous, inflamed glans. Reduction of the skin forward to cover the glans may then become impossible; this is paraphimosis. See Figure 16-19.
Examine Meatus	The urethral meatus should be inspected for size and position. The meatus is very small in boys with meatal stenosis due to a thin membrane at the meatal opening.
Hypospadias	Hypospadias is a congenital anomaly in which the urethral meatus lies on the ventral aspect of the penis, and may be on the glans, penile shaft, scrotum, or perineum. Also, the prepuce is incompletely fused on the ventral surface and forms excessive foreskin on the dorsal side. The scrotum must be thoroughly examined for gonads, since chromosomal or endocrinologic abnormalities may cause hypospadias. Ventral curvature of the penis, called chordee, is due to a restricting band of tissue between the glans and the meatus, and is frequently associated with hypospadias. A chordee may be present in the absence of the hypospadias.

(Continued)

PENIS, Continued

Epispadias

A related defect of different embryologic origin is epispadias. This condition also involves the meatus; the opening is located on the glans or the dorsal shaft. The defect may involve the puboprostatic urethra, the bladder neck, or, in extreme epispadias, failure of closure of the symphysis pubis.

Other Conditions

NAME	DESCRIPTION/CAUSE	ACTION
exstrophy	developmental anomaly in which the anterior walls of the bladder and of the lower abdomen fail to fuse and the bladder mucosa is exposed	
urethral discharge	gonorrheal, chlamydial, or ureaplasmal in origin (see Fig. 16-20)	Obtain cultures and Gram stain.
primary syphilis	firm, painless ulcer on the prepuce, along the coronal sulcus, or on the glans penis (see Fig. 16-21)	Examine scrapings by dark-field microscopy.
epidermoid carcinoma	indurated, raised, firm, sometimes ulcerated lesion; advanced lesions are cauliflower-like.	Confirm the diagnosis with a biopsy.
condyloma latum	infectious lesions of secondary syphilis; moist, wartlike lesions on the glans penis, prepuce, or scrotum	Dark-field and serologic tests establish the diagnosis.
condyloma acuminatum	venereal viral warts (see Fig. 16-22)	
priapism	sustained painful erection, often associated with sickle cell anemia or spinal cord lesions	

(Continued)

PENIS, Continued

NAME	DESCRIPTION/CAUSE	ACTION
Peyronie's disease	localized fibrotic thickening of the corpora cavernosa causing angulation of the shaft; plaques may be palpated along the penile shaft or corpora cavernosa (see Fig. 16-23).	Dupuytren's contracture of the palmar fascia may also be present.
urethral stricture	results from periurethral fibrosis	

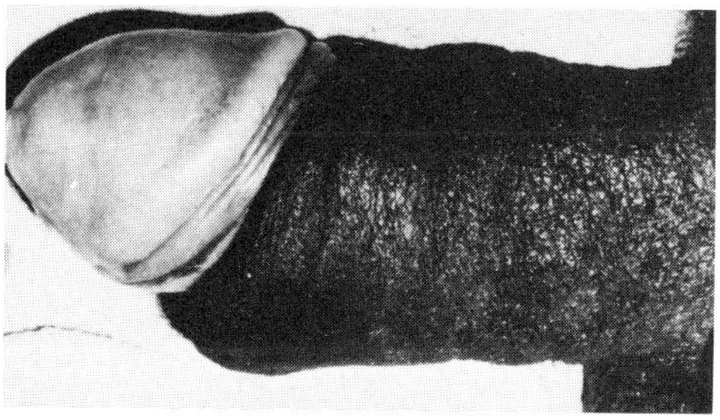

Figure 16-19.

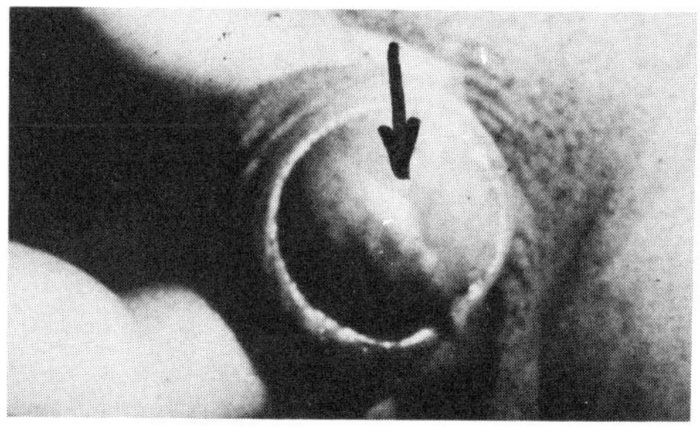

Figure 16-20.

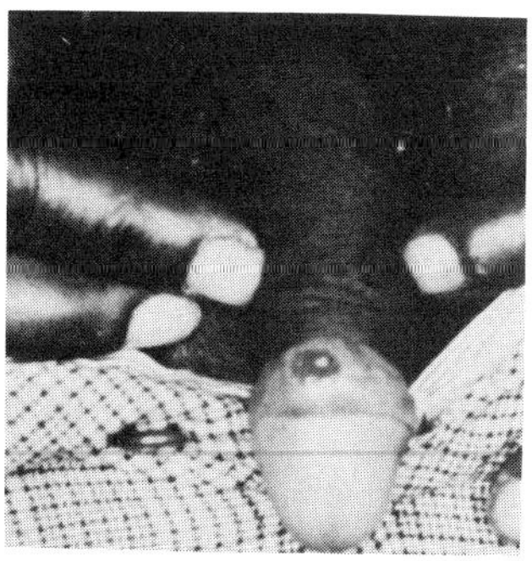

Figure 16-21.

Figure 16-22.

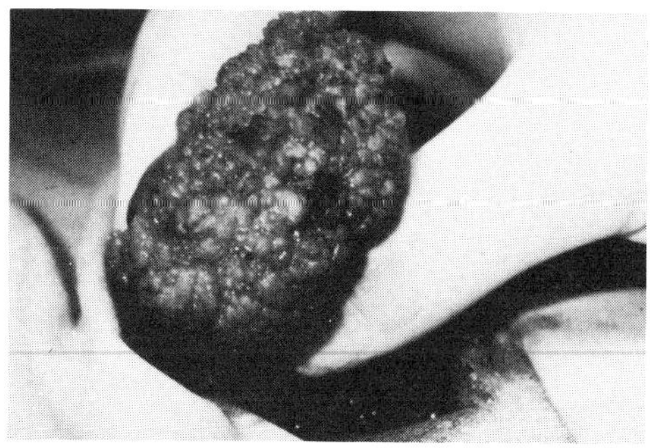

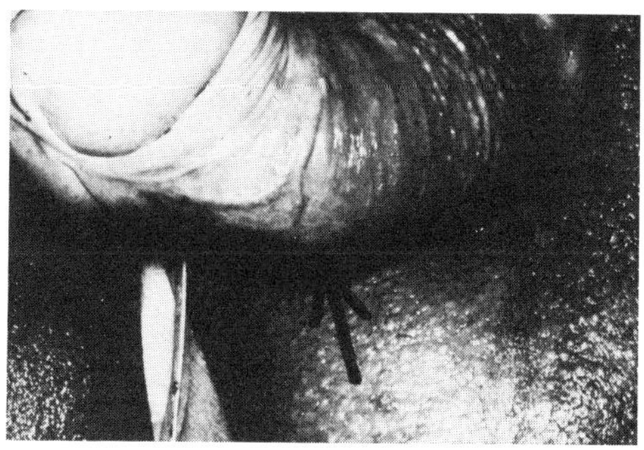

Figure 16-23.

SCROTUM

Description

The scrotum is a musculocutaneous pouch that contains the:
- testes
- epididymes
- spermatic cords

It functions as a thermal regulator, keeping the testes cooler than normal body temperature. The left scrotal sac usually hangs lower than the right due to the greater length of the left spermatic cord. Normally, both testes are in the scrotum at or shortly after birth.

WHEN THE INDIVIDUAL IS	OR THE SCROTUM IS	THE SCROTUM
old and debilitated	warm	• is elongated • is flaccid
young	cold	• is wrinkled • is short • firmly hugs the testes

Palpation

The scrotum and its contents can be palpated with the patient in a standing or recumbent position. However, examination must be gentle. Furthermore, stimulation of the scrotum or inner thigh may elicit the cremasteric reflex (cephalic retraction of the scrotum) and cause a "migratory testis" to be retracted into the inguinal canal.

Congenital Defects

Congenital defects of the scrotum may occur alone or in association with ambiguous external genitalia.

DEFECT	DESCRIPTION
bifid scrotum	often associated with hypospadias and other developmental anomalies of the penis (see Fig. 16-24)
undescended testes	abscence of the scrotal pouch or unilateral failure of development of the scrotum

(Continued)

SCROTUM, Continued

Edema	Edema of the scrotum may be the result of: • systemic disease, such as: • congestive heart failure • cirrhosis of the liver • renal disease OR • localized disease, such as: • carcinoma of the prostate • torsion of the testes in young men • debilitation associated with hypoproteinemia or malignancies Unilateral scrotal edema in an older man that cannot be otherwise explained should arouse suspicion of carcinoma of the prostate. Massive scrotal swelling (elephantiasis) caused by lymphatic blockage with microfilaria occurs in tropical climates. Nonfilarial lymphatic fibrosis also can produce scrotal edema.
Hydrocele	Intrascrotal tumors are frequently encountered. The most frequent tumor is a hydrocele, which is an accumulation of fluid in the tunica vaginalis (see Fig. 16-25). The cystic character of the hydrocele is easily appreciated on palpation. Light readily transilluminates a hydrocele. A hydrocele may occur anywhere along the cord into the inguinal canal. A hydrocele may mask epididymal and testicular tumors and obscure normal testes. Aspiration of fluid from a hydrocele is a definitive diagnostic procedure. Differentiation of a hydrocele from a hernia may be difficult, especially if the hernia cannot be reduced. Bowel sounds may be audible in a hernia.
Spermatocele	Another fluid-filled scrotal mass is a spermatocele or cyst of the epididymis. These cystic structures can also be transilluminated. Fluid in these cysts usually contains sperm because the spermatocele originates from a lobule of the testis that does not communicate properly with the epididymis. The obstructed ductule fills with fluid, forming a cystic structure. The spermatocele is discrete from the testis, and one can feel two masses; the upper mass is the spermatocele, and the lower one is the testis.

(Continued)

SCROTUM, Continued

Varicocele

A varicocele is an abnormal, tortuous collection of spermatic veins. The scrotal contents feel like a bag of worms when the patient is standing. The outline of the veins can sometimes be seen through the scrotal wall, to which they add a bluish tint when transilluminated (see Fig. 16-26). When the patient is supine, the veins disappear.

Varicoceles rarely occur before puberty, and are nearly always on the left due to higher insertion of the spermatic vein into the left renal vein. If the right scrotum is involved, spermatic vein obstruction due to extrinsic pressure from a retroperitoneal tumor (lymphoma or hypernephroma) must be suspected.

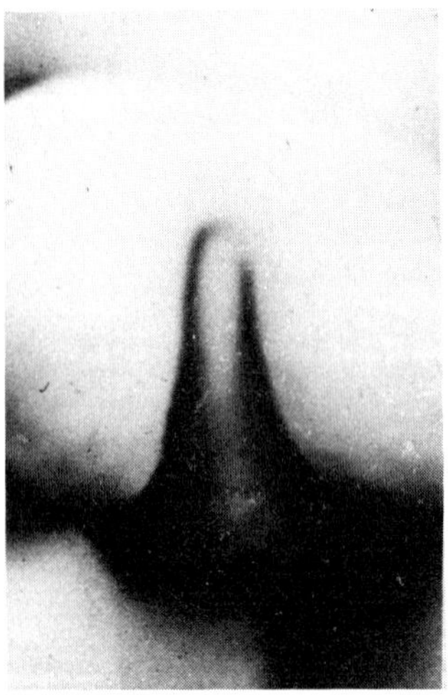

Figure 16-24.

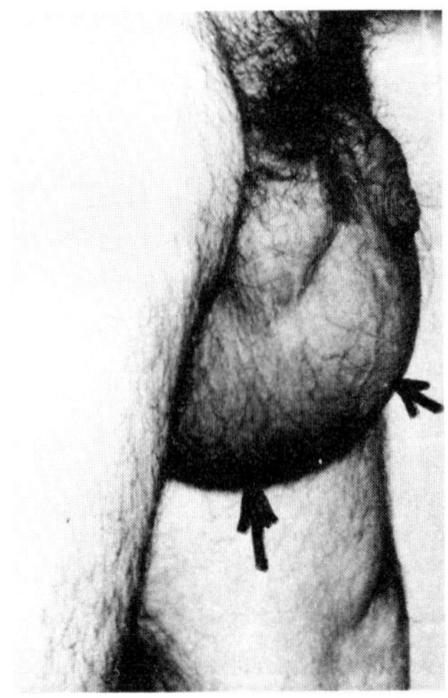

Figure 16-25.

TESTIS

Description

The normal testis lies with its long axis in a vertical position, but it may lie in a transverse position, in which case intrascrotal torsion is more likely to occur. The normal adult testis is firm and smooth; atrophic testes are small, soft, and almost mushy. Firm atrophic testes may follow mumps orchitis.

Neoplasm

A neoplasm of the testis is:

- painless
- asymmetric
- firm
- heavy
- sometimes nodular

The overlying skin is rarely attached to the underlying tumor. The mass never transilluminates unless an accompanying hydrocele masks the tumor.

Torsion of the Spermatic Cord

Torsion of the spermatic cord with infarction of the testis is frequently confused with acute epididymitis. The scrotum is swollen and red, and the testis is exquisitely tender and elevated. The mass cannot be transilluminated, making precise examination almost impossible. The patient is reluctant to stand and will grab the examiner's hand to prevent manipulation of the cord and testis. The spermatic cord above the twist is also tender. If recognized in the first 4 hours, the twisted testis may be rotated surgically to prevent necrosis.

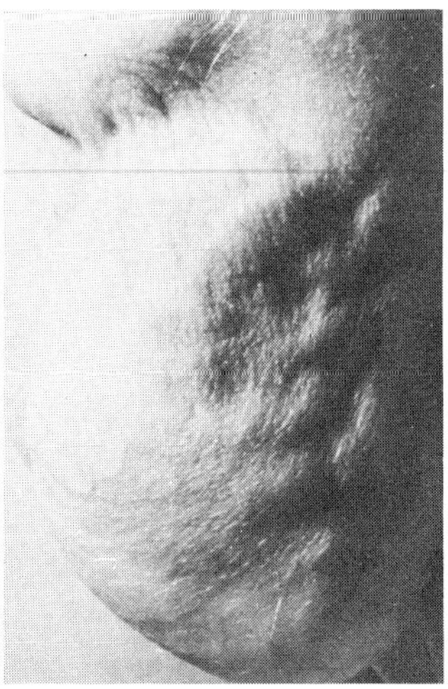

Figure 16-26.

EPIDIDYMIS

Epididymis	The epididymis lies along the posterior border of the testis. It is palpable as a ridge of about the same consistency as the testis. Nodularity indicates chronic infection or fibrosis.
Acute Epididymitis	Acute epididymitis is a common intrascrotal inflammatory lesion. Acute infection of the epididymis produces a firm, exquisitely tender enlargement of the entire epididymal body, occasionally with extension along the spermatic cord. The scrotal wall is usually swollen and reddened. Acute epididymitis may be encountered at all ages, but occurs most often in young adult men.
Chronic Epididymitis	In chronic epididymitis, abscesses may result in suppuration of the testis and scrotal wall. Enteric bacilli or mycobacteria can usually be cultured from the urine or pus.
Tuberculous Epididymitis	A "cold abscess" that has been present for months is usually tuberculous. In tuberculous epididymitis, the prostate, seminal vesicles, and vas deferens are usually beaded or nodular.

PROSTATE

Positions for Examination

Several positions for examining the prostate offer different advantages.

POSITION FOR PATIENT	ADVANTAGE
• standing beside the bed or examining table, leaning forward with the chest on the bed or table • lying on a bed in a knee-chest position	allows for satisfactory digital examination of the prostate
lying on a bed on his back with his knees drawn up	provides for less satisfactory digital exam than above, but permits bimanual examination of the bladder region

Contraindications

Digital rectal exams should <u>not</u> be done in these cases:

CONDITION	REASON
acute myocardial infarction	These patients tend to have an exaggerated vagal reflex from the sphincter ani, and rectal examination may precipitate an arrhythmia or heart block.
active suppurative urethritis	Massage of the prostate can cause infection to disseminate down the vas deferens and into the epididymis, causing epididymitis.
severe neutropenia or agranulocytosis	Bacteremia may result from manipulation.

(Continued)

PROSTATE, Continued

Procedure

The gloved examining finger should be well lubricated and introduced gently into the anal orifice. If this is carried out too rapidly or vigorously, the procedure may be painful and result in sphincter spasm, in which case the examiner will have to allow the patient to relax before continuing the examination. The examiner should first examine the lower rectum, and then the prostate, which can be palpated on the anterior rectal wall.

Anatomy

The lateral lobes in the normal adult are about 3 cm by 4 cm. A median groove extends along the posterior surface between the two lateral lobes. A slightly enlarged lobe is about 5 cm by 5 cm. A markedly enlarged gland might occupy most of the anterior pelvic outlet.

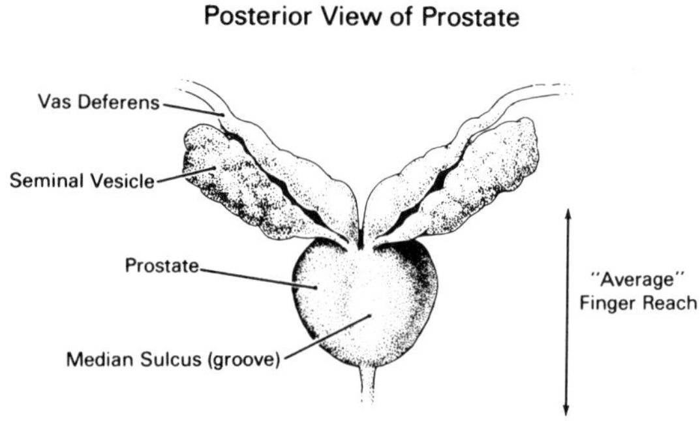

The anatomy of the prostatic region.

Enlargement

Enlargement of the prostate gland and resulting interference with urination occurs in about two thirds of men over age 60. The palpable enlargement may not be proportional to the degree of obstruction, since a small gland may produce complete obstruction because of hypertrophy or neoplasia of the median urethral prostate.

Palpation

The normal prostate is smooth and firm. The median groove is obliterated when the lobes of the prostate are hypertrophied or involved with carcinoma. The seminal vesicles extend laterally from the upper prostatic edge beneath the bladder and are usually not palpable unless they are diseased. If secretions are produced by prostatic palpation or massage, a specimen should be placed on a glass slide for microscopic examination.

(Continued)

PROSTATE, Continued

Abnormalities	Soft, even fluctuant, texture suggests prostatic abscess. A stony hard nodularity may involve small areas or the entire gland; these areas suggest granulomatous prostatitis, prostatic calculi, prostatic tuberculosis, or carcinoma. Carcinoma of the prostate tends to extend beneath the base of the bladder and the region of the seminal vesicles to form a shelf or plateau. Usually this periprostatic invasion is limited by fascia, but once this barrier has been broken, circumferential extension about the rectum occurs.
Spinal Cord Lesions	A detailed examination of the function of the sacral spinal cord must be done if the man has: • impotence • inability to ejaculate • urinary incontinence • loss of voluntary bowel control Inability to perceive touch, pain, and temperature in the perineal and scrotal areas suggest the presence of cord lesions. A patulous anal sphincter reflects a defect at S3, S4, and S5, the same segments that supply the urinary sphincter.

THE ABDOMEN IN RELATION TO THE GENITOURINARY SYSTEM

Masses Asymmetry of the abdomen caused by masses or distended bladder should attract the examiner's attention. One can often see a renal mass because it causes a prominence below the costal margin anteriorly and in the flank.

Palpation Right renal masses are best palpated by placing the right hand with the fingers parallel to the ribs about 4 cm below the costal margin or below an obvious mass. The left hand is placed in the costovertebral angle below the twelfth rib. As the two hands are brought together, the patient is asked to take a deep breath, which causes the mass to brush against the upper hand. Pressure applied to the mass anteriorly may be transmitted to the posterior hand. Often a retroperitoneal mass can be ballotted between the two hands.

Bladder The bladder is not palpable or percussible unless it is abnormally distended. When the bladder is abnormally full, a midline suprapubic mass may be palpated and percussed, but a thick or tense abdominal wall may obscure these findings.

Hernias The best way to examine the inguinal region and scrotum is with the patient standing. This will allow any mass to fall away from the surrounding tissue so that it is easier to palpate. It also clarifies the position of masses with respect to the testes, for as the patient stands, the structures will fall into their normal anatomic orientation. The most common scrotal mass is an inguinal hernia. This usually presents as a mass in the upper scrotum, but it may be very large, involving the entire scrotum. In the indirect hernia, the sac will describe a course similar to the processus vaginalis of the testis, which forms the lining membrane (tunica vaginalis) surrounding the testis. The indirect inguinal hernia is a part of the patent processus vaginalis. A hernia does not transilluminate in an adult, but in children the thinness of the bowel may allow transillumination.

SELF-ASSESSMENT

1. Diagram the normal external female genitalia as viewed in the lithotomy position.

2. Diagram the normal internal female genitalia as viewed sagittally.

3. Describe the appropriate method for inserting a vaginal speculum.

4. At which point in the examination does one apply lubricant to the speculum or examining fingers?

5. Describe structures and abnormalities to be noted in:
   a. perineum and vulva
   b. vagina
   c. cervix
   d. uterus
   e. adnexa

6. A backward tilting of the uterine corpus is normal.
   a. true
   b. false

7. Early cervical carcinoma cannot be readily distinguished from a cervical erosion by inspection.
   a. true
   b. false

8. Profuse thin yellowish or green discharge that is bubbly is suggestive of:
   a. monilia vaginitis
   b. trichomonas vaginitis
   c. "clue" cell vaginitis
   d. none of the above

9. Which of the following scrotal abnormalities usually presents <u>without</u> pain?
   a. hydrocele
   b. testicular tumor
   c. spermatocele
   d. all of the above
   e. a and c

(Continued)

SELF-ASSESSMENT, Continued

10. A hernia located within the scrotum is usually:
    a. an indirect hernia
    b. a direct hernia

11. Seminal vesicles are not normally palpable on rectal examination.
    a. true
    b. false

12. The cervix is usually palpable through the anterior rectal wall.
    a. true
    b. false

13. The anorectal junction is palpable on rectal examination.
    a. true
    b. false

14. A have irregular nodule, producing asymmetry of the prostate and a variation in its consistency, is suggestive of:
    a. prostatitis
    b. prostatic stones
    c. carcinoma of the prostate
    d. all of the above
    e. a and c only

15. On rectal exam, how much of the prostate is palpable?
    a. all of the gland
    b. posterior surface
    c. anterior surface

ANSWERS TO THE SELF-ASSESSMENT

6. b
7. a
8. b
9. d
10. a
11. a
12. a
13. b
14. c
15. b

CHAPTER SEVENTEEN

The Pediatric Patient

Joan R. Hebeler, M.D.

INTRODUCTION

Goals

In evaluating children, each student should be able to:

- obtain an appropriate history from the parent, guardian, or older child
- perform a physical examination on a newborn, an older infant or toddler, and a preschool child
- record the resulting data on appropriate forms and charts
- identify normal and abnormal physical characteristics

Objectives

After mastering this chapter the student should be able to:

1. obtain and record an appropriate history
2. modify and adapt the general physical examination for adults to:
   - newborns (birth to 4 weeks)
   - infants (1 month to 2 years)
   - preschool children (2-5 years)
3. perform the general physical examination on a newborn
4. perform the examination on an infant:
   a. establish rapport on an age-appropriate level
   b. identify gross motor and fine motor skills and personal-social skills for age
   c. use a parent's or an assistant's help to examine the infant's chest, heart, lungs, and abdomen
   d. examine head, eyes, ears, nose, and throat, using appropriate restraint techniques (e.g., parent, assistant, mummy wrap, or papoose board).
   e. examine the hips, feet, and legs
   f. examine the external genitalia
   g. perform a neurologic examination
   h. obtain a blood pressure
5. perform the examination on a preschool child:
   a. establish and maintain rapport and control of the examination
   b. identify sinus arrhythmia and normal heart sounds; identify increased splitting of pulmonary second sound with inspiration, physiologic third sound, and functional murmurs; identify a venous hum (a continuous murmur, louder in diastole, heard best at the base of the neck, and increased in intensity by the upright position and by inspiration); and a carotid bruit

(Continued)

INTRODUCTION, Continued

c. identify gross motor and fine motor skills, language, and personal-social skills appropriate for age
d. perform a screening orthopaedic examination, examine the back for scoliosis or lordosis; evaluate the lower extremities for everted or inverted feet, pes planus, genu valgum, or genu varum

6. determine and record on age- and sex-appropriate grids:
   - height
   - weight
   - head circumference

THE INTERVIEW

Introduction

Two types of skills are necessary to obtain an adequate pediatric history. These involve:

- conducting a good interview
- being thorough in completing the basic components of the history

The most important part of patient evaluation is a clear and reliable account of the patient's or informant's reasons for seeing the physician and of the expectations with regard to medical assistance. The ultimate effectiveness of recommendations and therapy is in part dependent upon the patient's or informant's attitude toward the physician. The length and depth of the interview will vary with circumstance, and in acutely ill patients the interview may consist of an initial brief session to get enough information to initiate rational treatment.

Overall Goals

In conducting the interview the physician and the informant should be as comfortable and undisturbed as possible. For all ages, an unhurried, friendly, and genuinely interested attitude is a prerequisite. Pencil and paper tend to inhibit free communication, so don't start writing--just listen. While the ultimate goal is to discover facts, one must also uncover associated feelings and less obvious problems, some of which may be difficult for the informant to relate. The initial part of the interview should be an unstructured, getting-acquainted period, and the physician should not be disappointed if relatively little factual material is obtained. In fact, some of the informant's observed attitudes may prove more useful than specific answers to direct questions.

Reactions to the Physician

Families and patients react to the physician in many different ways:

- Some will express hostility, which is most often only a mask for the intense fears and anxieties generated by illness and should be met with understanding and patience on the part of the physician.
- Some are overly cooperative and eagerly provide an essentially positive response to all questions.
- Others downgrade all symptoms.
- Others may edit by addition or subtraction of findings "to help you," the physician.
- Occasionally an anxious parent exhibits the desire to believe that the physician dealing with their child's life is omniscient, and is thereby easily steered by the unwary physician into grossly inaccurate responses.

(Continued)

THE INTERVIEW, Continued

Basic Guidelines

The pitfalls listed above can be avoided by following these guidelines:

- Use open-ended statements and questions.
- Be careful not to imply guilt or criticism by the way the questions are phrased.
- In the initial part of the interview, do very little steering except when it becomes apparent that the informant has need for encouragement or guidance.
- The interview should be communication from the informant to the physician, and the physician should be a good listener.
- Avoid submitting premature diagnostic explanations and criticisms.

Interviewing the Parent

Interviewing may well begin with the family so that the physician may see the interaction of patient and family and sense areas to be explored. However, in many instances individual sessions are desirable. It is good to let the family know almost from the beginning that this is the plan so that they will not feel compelled to bring out inappropriate material in the presence of the spouse or child.

Interviewing the Child

Much of what has been said above applies to the interview with the child. It is essential that the physician and the patient establish rapport, and the technique for doing this will vary with the age and the subject.

The Very Small Child

In the very small child (0–2 years), obtaining relevent information through direct interview is not practical, since speech is generally limited to labeling and making requests. The 3-year-old child, however, can answer most questions appropriately, participate in conversations using short, adult-like sentences, and express a variety of feelings.

(Continued)

THE INTERVIEW, Continued

The Preschool Child

In the preschool child (4-5 years) speech provides a simple, often frank medium of communication once a dialogue is established. For the latter purpose, a number of word games or ideas may be useful. The child's responses are effective "ice breakers" and can provide the basis for additional open-ended conversation.

- Example 1: Ask the young child what his response would be if a good fairy gave him three wishes. Two answers may be very traditional, the third often relates a real concern.
- Example 2: Draw on a sheet of plain white paper single-lined faces: one with a happy expression, one appearing angry, and one worried or sad. Just the act of drawing for the child often pleases him, and he is then willing to tell you what the faces are doing, sometimes name them, and tell why they are reacting as they appear to be reacting.

The School-Age Child

In the school-age child, the above technique may be useful, but as the child gets older, one may wish to use more mature questions, which develop along the lines of open-ended opportunities for expressing what they like to do or don't like to do. This may involve exploring the child's:

- normal age-related interests
- peer relationships
- long-term plans for education or career

A reasonable knowledge of current events of interest to the age group is essential. If the child seems intellectually retarded, questioning at the performance age is more suitable.

INTERVIEW CONTENT

Format	The pediatric history contains six basic components: • heading • chief complaint • present problems • patient profile • past medical history • family history • review of systems
Heading	In the heading, be sure to include all of the following: • name • date • unit history number • date of birth • referring physician or agency • address • telephone
Chief Complaint	Record the reasons the family has consulted a physician. These may be single, as in the case of an acute episode, or multiple. It is often helpful to list these problems and review them with the parent as a basis for subsequent recording of the present illness.
Present Problems	The story of the problems elicited in the interview should be developed in chronologic and orderly form. This may require retracing some steps, re-asking some questions, and in-depth exploration of specific areas. The chronology of symptoms is a foundation for assembling a meaningful history. Whenever possible, begin the history with the first relevant departure from a state of good health. In developing the present illness, resist the temptation to make an early diagnosis and thereby shape the story to fit the "textbook" history.

(Continued)

INTERVIEW CONTENT, Continued

Interpreting vs. Recording	It is permissible and often highly desirable to indicate in the present illness an interpretation of a certain series of events, but if done, this material should be set off in brackets to indicate that this is an editorial addition and may, in fact, be misleading. This is most useful when recording medication received or diagnostic studies done for which the parents' understanding is rather vague. When a symptom or complaint is mentioned, do not abandon it, but indicate later if it became worse, stayed the same, or resolved. While dates are useful, a more meaningful story may be assembled if events are related as days prior to admission. Avoid vague time markers such as "Monday" or "last week." If the history just doesn't seem to "make sense," don't edit it into a logical state--one of the best clues to the common problem of accidental poisoning is a history that just doesn't fit!
Patient Profile	Two factors must be remembered while caring for children: • The child does not exist alone; he or she is a dependent member of a family subject to the stresses, weaknesses, and strengths of at least one other person. • The infant and child are ever-changing entities throughout the developmental years. Whereas this is also true of adults, the changes are far more dramatic in children.
Health, Development, and Social Factors	Health, development, and social factors are always closely interrelated, and consideration must be given to each of these areas for both diagnosis and management of medical conditions. Social stresses may cause illness, may prevent recovery from illnesses with other causes, and may delay development. Developmental delays may be due to biological causes and may cause severe social stresses. Illness of any type may cause developmental delays on a biological or social basis. Therefore, the patient profile is of utmost importance. Because the layperson is often unaware of the above associations, the informant does not always offer this information and at times may be resistant to giving some of these details. Skillful interviewing reduces the resistance and obtains useful data.

(Continued)

INTERVIEW CONTENT, Continued

Data Collection in the Patient Profile

The information sought may be divided into two categories:

- factual
- an interpretation of attitudes and feelings of the family members

Both direct and indirect methods can be used to ascertain the data and usually a combination of these two methods is necessary. History of past development and what the child can do is obtained with direct questions. What the child actually does at present may be obtained indirectly. Growth grids and forms are helpful aids to follow the developmental patterns of a given child.

Types of Development

Development may be divided into:

- physical growth -- heights, weights, head circumferences, osseous changes, and tooth eruption
- physical development -- gross motor, fine motor, vocalization, and speech
- mental or intellectual development
- psychosocial development

Physical Development

History-taking for physical growth is often inaccurate, and charts and grids should be obtained. If these are not available, measurements at specific dates should be sought. Baby books kept by parents are most useful for this information. If dates are not known, comparisons to the growth of other siblings or peers have to suffice.

Gross Motor Development

Specific gross motor developmental steps should include the age at which the child:

- held head up
- turned over
- sat alone
- crawled
- stood alone
- walked
- rode a tricycle
- skipped
- rode a bicycle

(Continued)

INTERVIEW CONTENT, Continued

Fine Motor Development

History of fine motor steps is more difficult to obtain unless it has been recorded on a scale. Examples include such items as:

- grasping a rattle
- picking up a pellet
- stacking blocks
- using a pencil
- coloring
- cutting with scissors

These skills can be demonstrated on physical examination.

Language Development

Language is of such importance to families that parents usually remember the age of first words, sentences, and intelligible speech. These should be recorded. In infants, the approximate number of words used by the child is significant.

Psychosocial Development

The history of psychosocial development is as reliable and important as neuromuscular development. It manifests itself as behavior of the child. Under 1 year of age, two types of social interactions should develop:

- discriminative smiling
- distress at separation from the mother-figure.

BETWEEN THE AGES OF	THE INFANT
3 weeks and 3 months	occasionally smiles at various nonspecific stimuli
3 months and 6 months	smiles at the human face or similar objects
6 months and 7 months	shows discriminative smiling, limited to familiar or well-liked faces only
7 months and 9 months	becomes upset by the approach of a stranger
12 months and 20 months	shows distress caused by separation from the mother

(Continued)

INTERVIEW CONTENT, Continued

Additional Psychosocial Patterns	The child continues to have behavior characteristic of specific ages. This is related to the physical growth and development for that age. Psychosocial developmental patterns include: • bedwetting • temper tantrums • soiling • jealousy • curiosity • impulsivity • restlessness • nightmares • fears • enuresis • encopresis • anxiety • bizarre behavior • destructiveness • sex knowledge and activity If present, details of precipitating events, reactions of parents, siblings and peers to the behavior, and management of the child should be obtained.
Collecting Data	One method of obtaining much of the developmental information indirectly is to have the parent describe in detail a typical day of the child. It should include exactly what the child does on his own, the parental reactions, instructions to the child, and feelings, conflicts, and attitudes of individuals involved. This method provides a means of evaluating overprotectiveness, rejections, overindulgence, coerciveness, consistency of patterns, and discipline. As one obtains the facts of development, one should also inquire as to how each person felt about certain steps, behavior, and management by himself or the other parent.
Review of Systems	The review of systems is a systematic inventory of potential problems largely done in a question-answer format. The emphasis will vary with the age of the subject and the complaint. It is usually appropriate to indicate to the parent beforehand that this is an inventory and not specifically related to the complaints under consideration. Such an explanation will allay anxiety.

PAST MEDICAL HISTORY

Content	The past medical history contains a variety of information. The pertinent content will differ depending upon the age of the subject and nature of the problem to be considered. The suggestions to follow should be used selectively and as a guide.
Pregnancy	The following information concerning the pregnancy may be pertinent: • length • health of mother • infections • bleeding • falls • accidents • surgery • drug therapy • diagnostic x-rays • planned? • parents' perception

Birth and Neonatal Period	The following information concerning the labor and delivery may be pertinent:
	• labor
	  • spontaneous?
	  • induced?
	  • complications?
	  • length?
	• type of presentation
	• use of forceps
	• anesthesia
	• birth weight and length
	• presence of:
	  • cyanosis, bleeding, convulsions, jaundice
	  • cry (shrill, high-pitched, weak)

Feeding	Method of feeding and problems with feeding should be identified. • breast or bottle? • sucking reflex • feeding satisfactory for both mother and child? • formula and feeding schedule • appetite • diarrhea • vomiting • solid foods started when? • time of weaning and difficulties encountered

(Continued)

PAST MEDICAL HISTORY, Continued

Diseases and Hospitalizations	The interviewer should inquire about: • general health • allergies to drugs • accidents, injuries, poisoning • hospitalization and dates • specific treatments • operations--type, date, place, complications
Immunizations and Childhood Illnesses	The status of immunizations or whether the child has had the illness, with dates, should be obtained for: • typhoid • pertussis • diphtheria • tetanus • polio • rubella • rubeola • mumps • varicella • *Hemophilus influenzae*, type B • pneumococcal vaccine • MMR vaccine (measles, mumps, rubella) • influenza vaccine

FAMILY HISTORY

Mother and Father	The following information should be obtained about the parents. • age, health, education, and occupation • if mother works outside the home, information concerning provisions for child's care and stability of arrangements. • appraisal of personality (anxiety, affect, hostility, distortions, reliability, general tone of relationship with the child, overprotection, rejection, ambivalence)
Siblings	Obtain information concerning siblings about: • abortions, stillbirths, neonatal deaths, and erythroblastosis fetalis • ages and state of health
General	Inquire about any family history of: • tuberculosis, syphilis, convulsive disorders, or congenital malformations • chronic disease in the parents and how this has affected the child • the presence of similar illness in the household or community

EXAMINATION OF THE NORMAL NEWBORN (BIRTH-4 WEEKS)

Observation

Refer to Guidelines for the Newborn Examination. Observe the infant for 3 to 5 minutes before disrupting the behavior to remove his or her clothes. Look for:

- activity level
- cry
- color
- general state of alertness

Remove all of the baby's clothing, leaving only a loosely attached diaper to keep from getting wet. Observe again. This time look for:

- activity level: lethargy, irritability
- color: cyanosis (peripheral or central), jaundice, redness
- respiration: rate, depth, symmetry of motion, retraction, utilization of accessory muscles
- movement of extremities: symmetry
- character of cry (if present): high-pitched, low, mewing

Supine Examination

While the infant is supine and quiet, evaluate the anterior chest, lungs, heart, abdomen, genitalia, and extremities.

NOTE: The order of the examination is different from that of the adult so that disruption of normal behavior, causing restlessness and crying, are postponed until later in the examination.

1. By observing the chest, identify the point of maximal intensity (PMI) of the heart, which is usually noted in the fourth intercostal space (ICS), 1 cm to 2 cm lateral to the left sternal border.
2. After having identified the PMI, palpate along the left side of the sternum and note any lift or heave that indicates excessive right ventricular activity.
3. Palpate the clavicles for crepitation. Fractures may occur during an uncomplicated delivery.
4. Palpate the breasts. A firm, round breast bud is present in boys and girls. A drop of clear fluid is often noted draining from the nipples. Both the swelling and discharge result from maternal hormones and are normal.
5. Gentle, direct percussion with the finger on the chest may show gross differences in aeration between left and right sides. For example, one side will be hyperresonant if a pneumothorax is present, which may occur spontaneously during or after birth. Little information is gained about heart size, and time should not be spent percussing for heart borders.

(Continued)

EXAMINATION OF THE NORMAL NEWBORN (BIRTH-4 WEEKS), Continued

6. Listen to the heart sounds at the PMI, along the left sternal border, and below the clavicles. The heart valve areas described for adults are decreased in size in the newborn. The heart is more centrally located; the right ventricle is relatively larger and presents anteriorly, making it difficult to identify valve areas. It is better to measure the distance of a sound from the sternal border and record the interspace in which it is found than to state that the sound is in the "pulmonary area" or "mitral area."

   Count the apical heart rate and try to distinguish between the first and second sounds. Splitting of the second sound is difficult to assess at a heart rate of 140, which is normal for a newborn. Learn to identify variations in splitting of the second sound in an older child.

   Frequently, a systolic ejection murmur is audible in the second intercostal space 1 cm to 2 cm lateral to the sternum. It is caused by a ductus arteriosus that is still patent. A patent ductus at this age does not produce the continuous machinery murmur characteristic of a patent ductus after age 6 years.
7. Listen over the chest for crackles. Breath sounds seem much louder on auscultation of the newborn than in the adult. Compare breath sounds on each side of the chest: pneumothorax or atelectasis will produce a marked difference between the left and right sides. If the infant is crying, sounds will have increased transmission through consolidated lung. The identification of variations in transmission of sound during crying is comparable to asking an adult to repeat "99."
8. Observe the abdomen. Contour is important. Abdominal contour should be rounded. A scaphoid or empty abdomen indicates that the usual contents are somewhere else--usually in the chest. A sunken abdomen is one of the clinical signs of congenital absence of the diaphragm with herniation of the stomach and intestines into the left side of the chest. A distended abdomen may be associated with infection or a perforated viscus.

(Continued)

EXAMINATION OF THE NORMAL NEWBORN (BIRTH-4 WEEKS), Continued

9. Look at the umbilical cord. Identify one vein and two arteries on a fresh cord. Finding a single umbilical artery suggests the presence of intra-abdominal congenital anomalies. Palpate the umbilical vessels that course posteriorly from the umbilicus deep to the abdominal muscle toward the pubis. Gentle pinching of the vessels produces a sensation similar to plucking a violin string if the vessles are normal. If the vessels are soft and indistinct and there is associated redness of the skin, infection of the vessels may be present.
10. Auscultation of the abdomen is the same for older individuals.
11. Palpate the abdomen. Gentleness is crucial to a satisfactory examination. Holding the infant's thighs in a flexed posture with the left hand while palpating with the right will relax the anterior abdominal muscles. While this technique may assist palpation of the abdomen, it is not always necessary. The liver edge is sharp and palpable 2 cm to 3 cm below the right costal margin and extends to the midline, sometimes beyond. The spleen is not palpable. Gentle palpation to the paravertebral area will reveal the kidneys. Abdominal masses such as ovarian or omental ones, polycystic kidneys, and neuroblastoma can be identified by palpation. A persistently palpable bladder may mean congenital obstruction of the urethra.
12. Palpate the femoral area for the artery and masses. A reliable method for finding the femoral artery is to place the thumb on the anterior iliac spine and the index finger at a point halfway between the two. The femoral artery usually lies immediately below the index finger. Apply light pressure to avoid overcoming the systolic pressure and obliterating the pulse. Femoral hernias may occur. Because a femoral hernia in a female may contain an ovary, it is essential to identify the abnormality and plan for surgical treatment.

(Continued)

EXAMINATION OF THE NORMAL NEWBORN (BIRTH-4 WEEKS), Continued

13. Examine the genitalia.
    - Male: Identify the location of the urethra. In the infant with hypospadias, it will be situated somewhere between the tip and base of the penis. The finding of hypospadias in a newborn is an absolute contraindication to circumcision because the prepuce is utilized in surgical repair. The prepuce usually fits tightly over the glans and is not easily retracted. Do not force the prepuce back during the examination; it will be easy to retract when the infant is older. Palpate both testes. The infant has a vigorous cremasteric reflex, which is easily activated to retract the testicles out of the scrotum. Often this finding is misinterpreted as "undescended testes." To prevent this misinterpretation, place one or two fingers of one hand over the inguinal area before palpating the testicle with the other hand. Testes should be firm and smooth and measure about 1.5 cm in the longest diameter. If the scrotum is large, place a small light source behind or to the side of it and transilluminate the mass. Hernias may also be noted.
    - Female: Separate the labia majora: identify the clitoris and urethral and vaginal openings and observe for posterior labial fusion. The clitoris often appears large, but is actually less than 1.5 cm in length. Mucous vaginal discharge is usually present. There is usually increased pigmentation of the genital area in both males and females.
14. Examine the anus. Separate the buttocks and observe the anal opening for patency. Note any small fissures or tears. Though a common source for "blood in the stools" in infants, such fissures are best observed with a pediatric anoscope.

(Continued)

EXAMINATION OF THE NORMAL NEWBORN (BIRTH-4 WEEKS), Continued

15. Examine the infant for dislocated hips.
    a. Observe for the normal flexion contracture of the hips. Extend one of the infant's legs while the other is flexed at the hip and internally rotated (see figure). Observe for an angle formed by the extended leg. A dislocated hip will permit complete straightening of the leg. Repeat this process with the other leg.

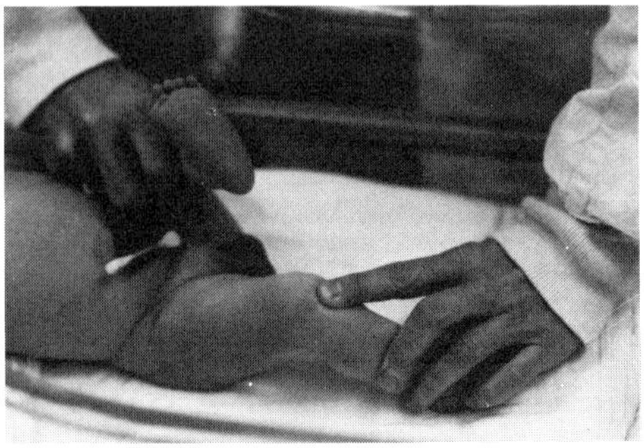

    b. Flex both legs at the hips. Place the tips of the fingers over the heads of the femora and the thumbs around the knees; abduct the legs. If there is resistance to abduction beyond 45°, consider dislocated hips or another reason for adduction tightening. If the hips are dislocated, one may also feel a sensation like one ice cube gliding over another, as the femur slides into the acetabulum.
16. Examine the extremities. Extend both legs and note length discrepancy or asymmetry of the inguinolabial fold in females. Observe for clubbed feet. If feet or ankles turn in or out but can be easily moved through a full range, they demonstrate retention of intrauterine posture. Look at the bottoms of the feet. There should be one axis from heel to forefoot. If two axes are noted, the infant may have an adducted forefoot. If the foot can be moved easily to proper alignment, observe several times before referral because the axis may be positional. Toe grasp is usually elicted during this segment of the examination. Hands and feet should also be observed for extranumerary digits or unusual appearance of creases or other abnormalities; for example, rocker-bottom feet or simian creases.
17. Observe the skin. Look for petechiae, nevi, pustules, and erythema. Superficial hemangiomata are often seen on the eyelids, the nape of the neck, and the back of the head. Bluish-black discoloration, monogolian spots (no relationship to Down syndrome or mongolism) are often seen. Superficial hemangiomata and mongolian spots are innocuous and usually fade during the first year.

(Continued)

EXAMINATION OF THE NORMAL NEWBORN (BIRTH-4 WEEKS), Continued

18. Observe the head. Measure the fontanelle size and note any depressions or bulgings. Observe for edema of the scalp, molding, and cephalohematoma (subperiosteal hemorrhage). Measure head circumference and record the largest of three measurements.
19. Examine the ears for abnormalities in position, deformity, and patency of the external auditory canal. (Otoscopic examination is precluded by the presence of vernix caseosa in the canal.) Hearing can be checked by clapping or other noise. The expected response is a blink or decreased activity.
20. Observe the nares for patency and listen with the stethoscope over each one to make sure the air passes through the nostril.
21. Observe and palpate the lids. Note the conjunctivae. Observe for the presence or absence of discharge and abnormalities. Note the pupil and blink response to bright light. Ophthalmoscopic examination is limited to eliciting the "red reflex." It is used to identify the presence of opacities in the lens or retinal masses. The usual round yellowish-red reflection of light from the retina will be distorted by a lens opacity or an intraocular mass.
22. Examine the mouth for cleft lip. Observe and palpate the palate for evidence of cleft. Many newborns have Epstein's pearls, which are 2-mm pearl-like lumps on the hard palate. These are normal. The uvula can usually be observed, and the gingivae should be inspected for malformations, including the presence of teeth or mucous inclusion cysts.
23. The neck should be inspected for small remnants of the branchial arch system. The entire course of the sternocleidomastoid as well as the thyroid areas should be explored, noting pits, swellings, or masses.

Prone Examination

Turn the baby over and continue the examination.

1. Observe and palpate the skull for edema or cephalohematoma.
2. Observe and palpate the spinous processes from the base of the skull to the coccyx, looking for pits, hair tufts, hemangioma, mongolian spots, or nevi.
3. The gluteal folds should be symmetrical. Asymmetry suggests dislocation of the hips.
4. Listen to the lung fields, noting crackles or differences in aeration between sides.

(Continued)

EXAMINATION OF THE NORMAL NEWBORN (BIRTH-4 WEEKS), Continued

Neurologic Examination

Careful observation of the infant throughout the examination often precludes the need for a "special" neurologic examination. Reflex responses have resulted from examination procedures used to elicit other data.

EXAMPLE: Examination of the mouth usually produces a suck-and-root reflex, and examination of the feet and hands elicits grasp reflexes.

All of the following should be evaluated:

a. Moro startle or embrace reflex. If there is a brisk change in position or a sudden noise, the infant will respond by adducting the arms and legs and subsequently abducting the extremities (figure a). This should be quick and symmetric. Asymmetry of response suggests central nervous damage on the opposite side or peripheral nerve or musculoskeletal damage on the same side. The reflex is present at birth and disappears after 1 to 3 months.

b. The tonic neck reflex is elicited by gently turning the infant's head. The infant will assume a fencing position with the face toward the extended arm (figure b). Observe for symmetry. The reflex is present at birth and disappears after 5 to 6 months.

a

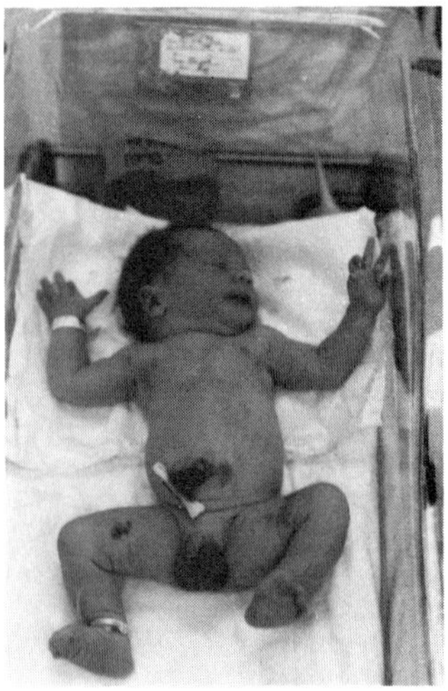

b

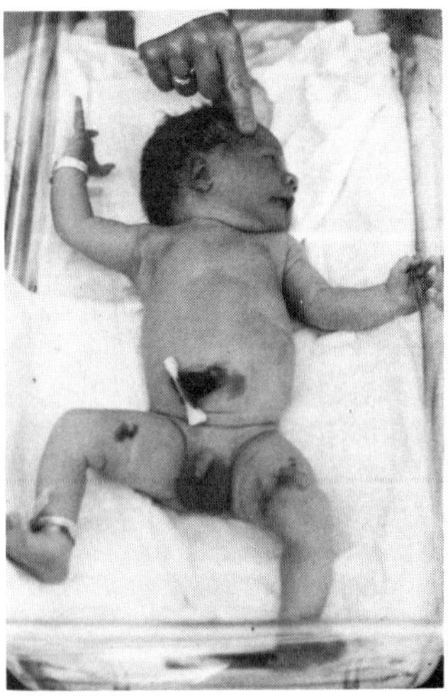

(Continued)

EXAMINATION OF THE NORMAL NEWBORN (BIRTH-4 WEEKS), Continued

c. The rooting reflex is elicited by touching the side of the infant's cheek (figure c). person touching the cheek and begin to suck. It is present at birth and disappears after 3 to 4 months.

c

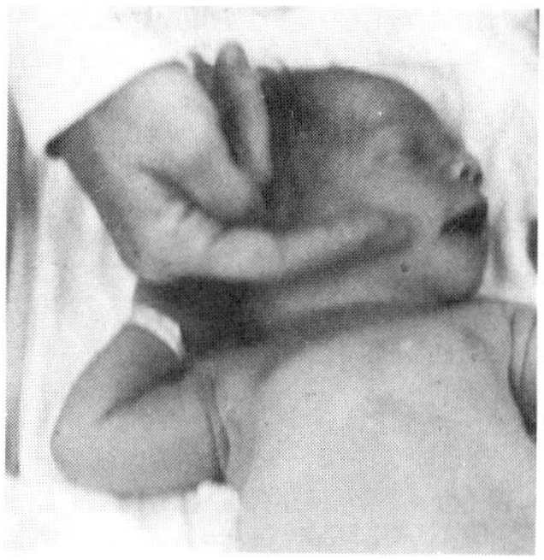

d. Suck response is elicited by stimulation of the mouth or lips (figure d). It should be vigorous and sustained. It is present at birth and disappears after 12 months.

d

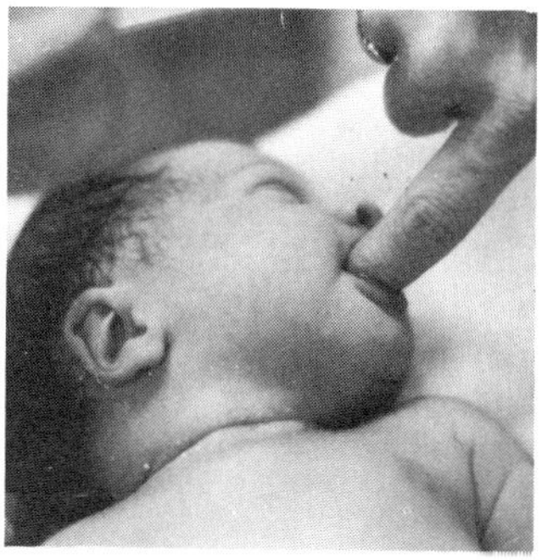

e. Palmar and plantar grasp reflexes are elicited by placing your finger in the palm or on the sole of the infant's foot near the toes. Flexing of the fingers or toes into a grasp is elictied (figure e). It should be symmetrical and brisk. Slow or inordinately sustained grasp is abnormal. Palmar grasp is present at birth and disappears after 4 months. Plantar grasp is present at birth and disappears between 8 and 15 montho.

e

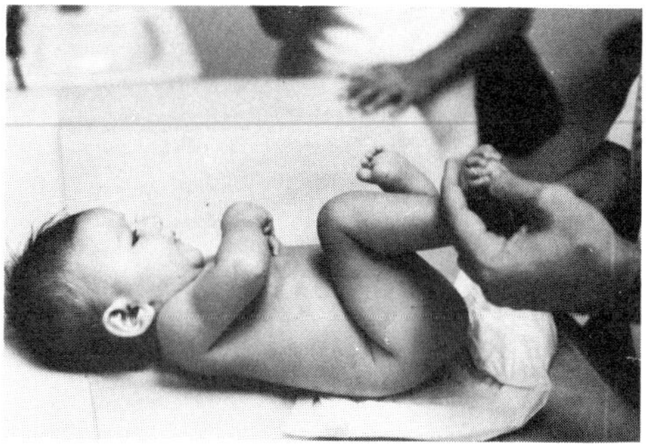

f. A Babinski response is usually present at birth and is elicited by stroking the bottom of the foot (figure f). It disappears after 1 to 2 years.

f

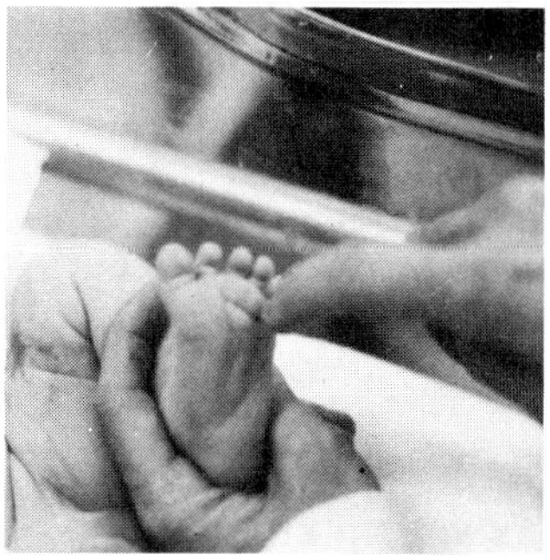

(Continued)

EXAMINATION OF THE NORMAL NEWBORN (BIRTH-4 WEEKS), Continued

g. Reflex response to sound stimulation produces blinking.

h. Reflex response to light produces eyelid closure.

i. Cranial nerves are examined best by careful observation of the baby's face during crying, noting the symmetry of movement of both sides of the face and flattening of a nasolabial fold. Gross response to sound can be elicited by clapping or slamming a door (also produces Moro reflex).

j. Deep tendon reflexes are elicited by direct tapping with the examining finger. Those reflexes in the newborn are usually brisk and "hyperactive" by adult standards.

k. Three beats of ankle clonus can often be found in normal newborns.

Comment

Most of the special reflexes observed in the newborn are called "primitive" and will disappear as the infant's central nervous system myelinates. The retention of these reflexes beyond the expected age of disappearance indicates abnormalities, including cerebral palsy or other central nervous system defects. Become familiar with the normal reflexes in this age group and be alert to their retention.

EXAMPLE: An active tonic neck reflex in a 14 month old is abnormal.

GUIDELINES FOR THE NEWBORN EXAMINATION

- general
  - Wash your hands.
  - Observe before touching.
  - Handle the infant with ease.
  - MODIFY the sequence in response to the infant:
    - Quiet infant: observe, palpate, and listen; defer disturbing examinations.
    - Crying infant: quiet the infant; then begin the examination.
    - Infant who does not stop crying: perform the examination and note the infant's behavior.
  - length and weight
- head
  - Observe molding.
  - Palpate the sutures and fontanelles.
  - Measure head circumference.
- ears
  - Check hearing by holding the child, having the mother speak, and observing whether the child turns his or her head toward the sound.
  - Observe the external ear and canal.
- nose
  - Palpate.
  - Look in.
- eyes
  - Observe whether the child's eyes follow you during the examination.
  - Observe and palpate the lid.
  - Check the conjunctivae.
  - Check the pupil and blink to bright light.
  - red reflex (for cataracts)
- mouth
  - Get a good look at the palate and oral cavity.
  - Palpate the oral cavity.
- neck
  - Check mobility.
  - Check for masses.
- chest
  - respiratory rate
  - Check the clavicle.
  - Check the breasts.
  - palpation
  - percussion
  - breath sounds (front and back, side to side, superior right and left)
- heart
  - Palpate (lower left sternal border and epigastrium).
  - blood pressure
  - Listen over the valve areas.
  - Palpate the brachial and femoral pulses.
  - apical rate
- abdomen
  - general observation
  - Examine the cord.
  - liver
  - spleen
  - kidneys
  - masses
  - bladder
- genitalia
  - male--meatus and testes
  - female--separate the labia.
- rectum
  - Look by separating the buttocks.
- back and extremities
  - Observe the sacral area.
  - Palpate the spinous processes.
  - range of motion, all extremities
  - Check for dislocated hips.
- neurological
  - muscle strength and tone, upper and lower
  - grasp
  - rooting
  - sucking
  - Moro
  - head control
  - stepping and placing
  - deep tendon reflexes
  - Babinski
  - tonic neck reflex
  - facial nerve palsy

NOTE: It is preferable to examine the newborn in the presence of one or both parents.

EXAMINATION OF THE INFANT AND TODDLER (1 MONTH - 2 YEARS)

Introduction

Refer to Guidelines for the Infant-Toddler Examination. The usual order of examination of the child in this age group is to begin with the interview of the parents and proceed to those items of the examination that are not threatening or intrusive. The initial period of observation can provide a great deal of information about the respiratory rate, activity, mood, and vocalization, thereby predicting how the child will react to the examiner.

Chest Exam

Examination of the chest can be done with the infant at rest in the mother's lap. Note the location of the PMI by observation and palpation. The PMI is usually in the 4th intercostal space 1 cm lateral to the sternal border. Listen along the left sternal border and below the clavicles. If a murmur is present, note its location and listen over the back and axillary areas. Count the heart rate and note the presence of sinus arrhythmia. Listen over the lung fields for crackles and other abnormalities; auscultate both sides, back, and front. Remember that breath sounds are much louder in the young child than in the adult. Look at the child's chest and back for any abnormalities.

Abdominal Exam

Observe the abdomen for shape, listen to bowel sounds, and palpate the abdomen gently for the liver, spleen, kidneys, and abnormal masses. This can often be done with the child on the mother's lap. If the infant does not object, place him on the examining table. In general, the younger infant will not object as strongly as the infant approaching 1 year of age (figure a). If the infant is examined on a table, diversion by the parent will permit the physician to examine the abdomen with ease. Palpate the femoral pulses and examine the external genitalia (figure b).

a

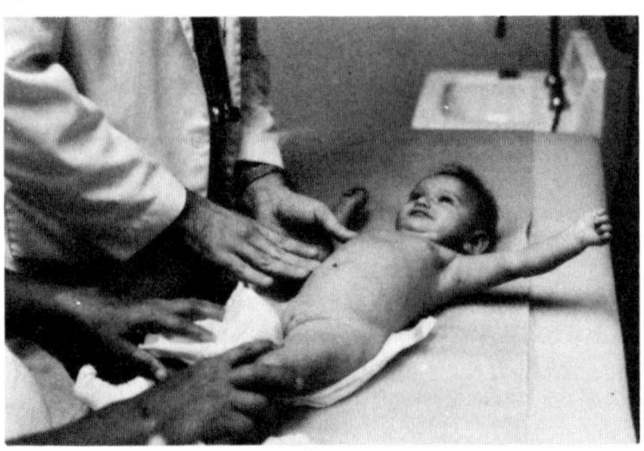

b

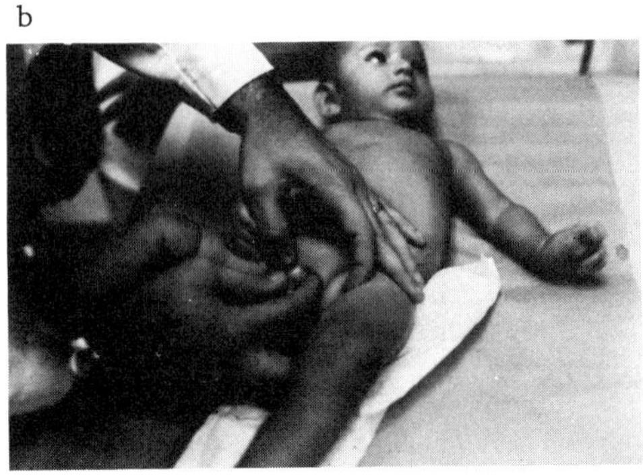

(Continued)

EXAMINATION OF THE INFANT AND TODDLER (1 MONTH - 2 YEARS), Continued

Neurological Examination	Neurologic examination can be started at this point by gently tapping the knee and the Achilles tendons with your finger. Note the presence of the plantar reflex (Babinski). The biceps and triceps reflexes should be elicited. The child's cranial nerves are also checked.
Neuromuscular Maturation	Neuromuscular development progresses from head to foot and from central to peripheral portions of the body. That is, infants can raise their heads before they walk and can look at objects before they can handle them.
Progression of Gross Motor Development	Babies raise their heads from a lying position at about 4 weeks; crawl, pull up, stand, and walk by about 1 year.
Language	Language development progresses from undifferentiated noises that require little tongue coordination to well-articulated words and sentences by the age of 2 years.
Fine Motor Coordination	Fine motor coordination of the hand begins with its use as a rudimentary paddle with inaccurate banging, waving motions. It is then used as a bat to swat at objects within reach. Hand coordination proceeds to opposition of the thumb and forefinger as an accurate tool to pick up objects.
Emotional Development	Emotional development and its progress can be observed during the examination by noting the response of the infant to the parent and examiner. Look for and document smile, attachment, recognition of parent, irritability, or lack of response. At approximately 8 to 9 months of age, infants may become difficult to examine because they are beginning to experience "stranger anxiety." This demonstrates that infants prefer their parent or caretaker. One may or may not be able to decrease this reaction. The examination should be completed as quickly and efficiently as possible. Parents will often say that this is what the child does when he is around anybody, but some parents will say "he is afraid of white coats." Between 18 months and 2 years, children may be at the peak of their normal negative stage. Ignore the noise and complete the examination as efficiently as possible.

(Continued)

EXAMINATION OF THE INFANT AND TODDLER (1 MONTH - 2 YEARS), Continued

Examination of the Head and Neck

Examination of the head and neck can be started at this point. Many infants and young children dislike these procedures, and assistance from the parent is helpful. Measure head circumference. Palpate the fontanelle, and if it is palpable, note whether it is bulging or depressed. Generally, fontanelles are not palpable after 2 years of age. Examine the neck for masses and other abnormalities and around the ears for any evidence of branchial arch remnants.

Examine the external auditory canal with the otoscope. In general, infants do not cooperate with this examination; however, it is worth trying unrestrained. Look first into each ear and evaluate the canal and tympanic membranes. Conclude with the examination of the mouth.

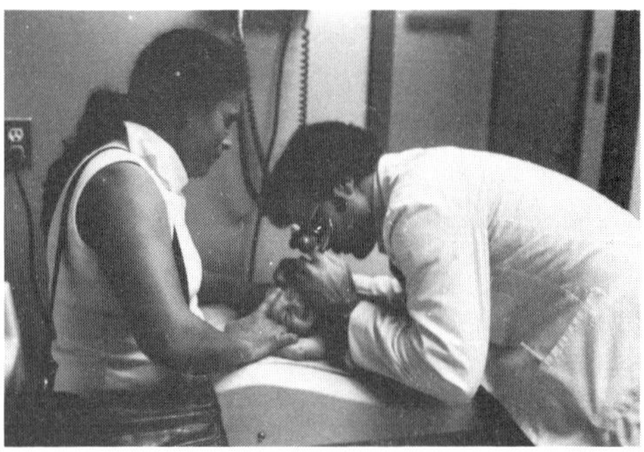

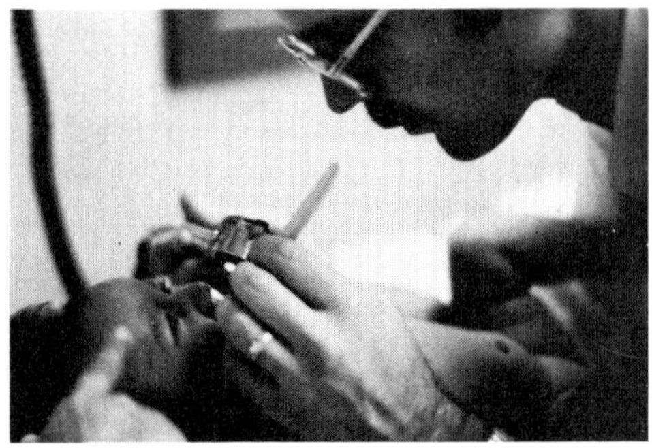

Restraining Techniques

If the child resists examination, appropriate restraining techniques should be utilized. This will ensure that the examination is concluded as quickly as possible for the child and also provide the opportunity for a reliable examination. Several ways of restraining the infant are available. Most people who examine children develop a preferred method. It is essential that the child be as comfortable as possible and that the examination be as efficient and accurate as possible. Some of the following restraining methods are commonly used. An assistant, a parent, or another adult will permit a better examination.

(Continued)

EXAMINATION OF THE INFANT AND TODDLER (1 MONTH - 2 YEARS), Continued

Examination of Ears (on Lap)	The examiner is free to place the palm of the hand against the child and use the fingers to manipulate the ear if necessary. The heel of the hand holding the otoscope should be rested against the child's head so that if the child jumps, the hand holding the otoscope will move and the child will not injure the external canal with the speculum. The use of a fisted grip on the otoscope, as if employed for hammering, is too rigid and can result in jamming the otoscope into the child's ear canal if he jumps unexpectedly. As a less desirable alternative, the parent or assistant holds the child on the lap with the child in a sitting position. The child's back is toward the examiner. The child's arms are around the parent and his head rotated to the right (or left) with the chin over the shoulder. The parent or assistant restrains the child in this position.
Examination of Nose and Mouth (on Lap)	The child's position is shifted so that the child sits facing the examiner. The parent uses one arm to encompass the child's arms and trunk. The other arm is placed around the child's forehead so that the child's mouth is forward. The examiner can then examine the nares with a light. The mouth is examined using a tongue blade in one hand and a light in the other hand. Insert the tongue blade between clenched jaws and gently push posteriorly over the tongue. The child generally cries or gags and opens the mouth at some point. The examiner then quickly and gently eases the tongue blade to the back of the tongue. The light is focused on the posterior pharynx. Observe the anterior pillars, uvula, tonsils, and lymphoid tissue on the posterior pharynx.
Examination of the Ears (Child face up on the Table)	The child is face up on the table with the head turned to the right or left. The parent places his elbows next to the child's hips and holds the child's arms extended along his chest and abdomen, preferably at the elbow so that the child cannot bend his arms. The parent leans his body across the child's legs, if necessary, to control the child's kicking and to let the child know that he is very close. The examiner can then use one hand to control the child's head and ear, and the other hand to hold a light.

(Continued)

EXAMINATION OF THE INFANT AND TODDLER (1 MONTH - 2 YEARS), Continued

Otoscopy and Pneumatoscopy	Pneumatoscopy is necessary for adequate examination of infants' and childrens' tympanic membranes and middle ears. Pneumatoscopy is best accomplished by first adequately restraining the child, either with the parent or a papoose board, then straightening the external auditory canal with the left hand or right hand (in the case of the left-handed person). While the other hand that holds the otoscope rests upon the skull (or upon the hand of the person restraining the child's head), the landmarks and light reflex of the tympanic membrane are adequately visualized. If cerumen obstructs adequate visualization of the tympanic membranes, it must be removed by suction or irrigation. After adequate cleansing of the external auditory canal, the otoscope is gently slipped in so that the tympanic membrane is visualized; then with the left hand a seal is obtained so that the speculum is airtight by pressure exerted anterior to the external auditory canal. Following this, gentle blowing should cause the tympanic membrane to move like a "flag in a breeze."
Cloth Restraints	Cloth restraints are usually reserved for diagnostic or therapeutic procedures rather than an examination. Occasionally, cloth restraints may be needed, particularly to examine the ears of a vigorous 2 year old. The methods require a sheet or a commercially available cloth wrapper with Velcro strips to keep the wrap closed.
Sheet Restraint	The child is placed face up on the center of a sheet that has been folded in half. The fold is placed at the level of the child's shoulder. One side of the sheet is folded over the child's shoulder and passed under his trunk so that the arm is secured to the side. The same is done on the other side. The bottom portion of the sheet is then wrapped around the child's lower trunk and legs for immobilization. If one arm is required for drawing blood, it is left free.
Measurements	Head circumference, length, and weight should be obtained before or after the general examination and plotted on a growth grid. Variation from "average" measurements should be noted.
Blood Pressure	The correct cuff width is one half the circumference of the extremity. Blood pressure readings are obtained by palpation or auscultation as for the adult. A Doppler probe is often used for newborn and ill infants.

GUIDELINES FOR THE INFANT-TODDLER EXAMINATION

- general
  - Introduce yourself and/or establish and maintain a rapport.
  - length and weight (may be done after the examination)
  - Observe without touching.
  - MODIFY the examination sequence in response to the child:
    - Do all observation without disturbing. Palpate and listen before doing disrupting examinations such as the ENT segment.
    - If the child is upset, attempt to quiet him, then do the examination.
    - If the child cannot be calmed, perform the examination with appropriate assistance from a parent.

- head
  - Observe, measure and plot.
  - Palpate the sutures and fontanelles
  - Examine the hair and scalp.

- ears
  - Check the hearing (by some means).
  - Observe the external ear and canal.
  - Look in with an otoscope.

- nose
  - Look in.

- eyes
  - Observe and palpate the lid.
  - extraocular movements
  - cover test
  - Observe the pupil.
  - pupillary reaction to light and accommodation
  - Check the vision (by some means).
  - Observe the conjunctivae.
  - Use the ophthalmoscope.

- mouth
  - Get a good look at the oral mucosa and palpate.
  - Observe and count the teeth.
  - Use the tongue blade.

(Continued)

- neck
  - Palpate the anterior and posterior cervical nodes.
  - Palpate the thyroid and trachea.
  - range of motion
  - Check the clavicles.
  - Palpate the supraclavicular nodes.

- chest
  - Observe (retractions, etc.).
  - respiratory rate
  - palpation (fremitus)
  - percussion
  - breath sounds (side to side, front <u>and</u> back)
  - Palpate the axillary nodes.

- heart
  - Palpate (thrill and PMI).
  - Listen over the valve areas.
  - Palpate the brachial and femoral pulses simultaneously.
  - Palpate the other pulses.
  - Determine the blood pressure.
  - Determine the pulse rate.

- abdomen
  - Auscultate for bowel sounds.
  - Palpate and measure the liver.
  - spleen
  - costovertebral angle
  - deep masses
  - percussion
  - Palpate the inguinal nodes.

- genitalia
  - male--meatus <u>and</u> testes
  - female--separate the labia.

- rectum
  - Look by separating the buttocks.

GUIDELINES FOR THE INFANT-TODDLER EXAMINATION, Continued

- back and extremities
  - Observe the sacral area.
  - straightness of the back
  - Observe the legs, knees, and ankles.
  - Observe the feet.
  - leg length
  - hips
  - range of motion of joints (upper <u>and</u> lower)

- neurological (in addition to above)
  - mental status
    - response to stimuli
    - developmental level--gait (when applicable), crawling, sitting, pulling up, language
  - cranial nerves
    - Observe the facial movements.
    - open mouth, smile, show teeth, close eyes, wrinkle brow
    - gag and uvula
  - motor
    - muscle mass and tone
    - strength--proximal, distal, upper and lower
    - coordination--handling toys, spontaneous play, sitting, walking, crawling
  - reflexes
    - infantile (Moro, suck, tonic neck)
    - deep tendon (four areas)
    - Babinski
    - clonus
  - sensory

EXAMINATION OF THE PRESCHOOL CHILD (2-5 YEARS)

Introduction

Refer to Guidelines for the Preschooler Examination.

The techniques used to examine the preschool child are the same as those used for adults. The most frequent change made to facilitate the examination on such children is to modify the sequence of the examination. For example, nonintrusive procedures are done first; the examination of the ears and throat is done last. Many preschoolers can be examined using the same sequence as that used for adults. Use the initial observation portion of the examination to select a sequence to use.

Modified Sequence

a

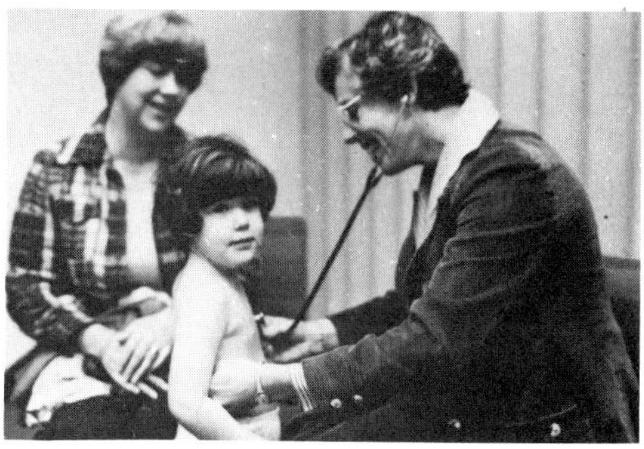

The most important part of the examination is the time spent establishing a rapport with the child. This can be accomplished by spending a few minutes talking to the child. Ask about the patient's pet or toys, and allow the child to handle the examining equipment. The examination of the chest, heart, and lungs can be imitated with the child standing nearby (see figure a).

b

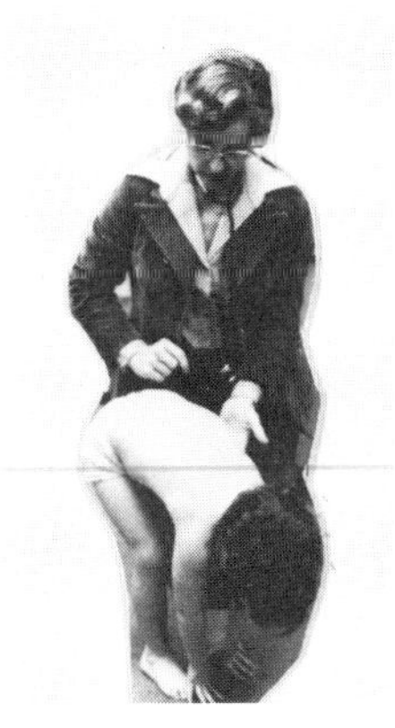

c

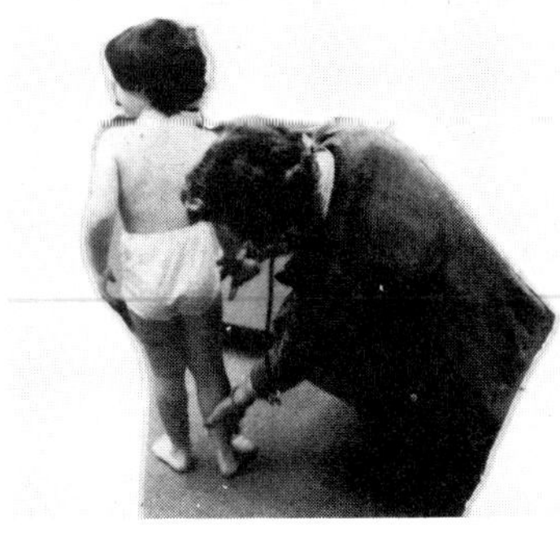

The screening orthopaedic examination (figure b), described later in this section, and the neurologic examination (figure c) may be done next because these are often interpreted by the child to be games. This can serve to increase trust in the examination procedure.

EXAMINATION OF THE PRESCHOOL CHILD (2-5 YEARS), Continued

d

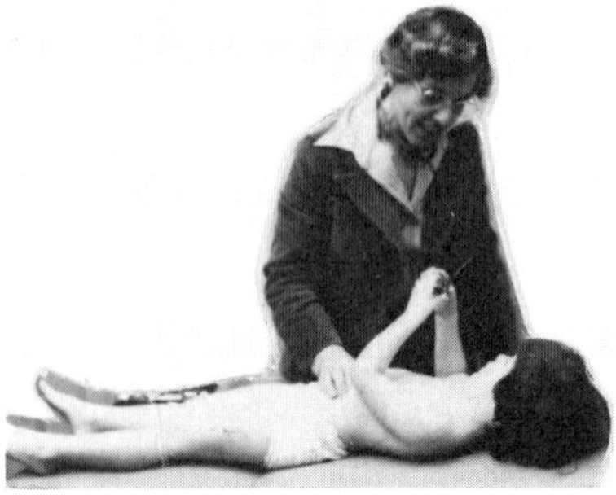

The child is then placed on the examining table. Evaluation of the chest (figure d), heart, lungs, and blood pressure is completed. The abdomen (figure e), the genitalia, and anus are inspected. The neurologic, back, and extremity examinations are completed.

e

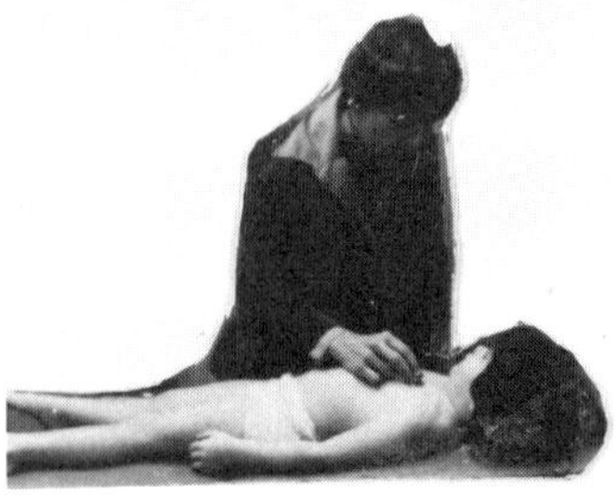

The examination of the child on the table is ended by evaluation of the eyes, ears, and throat.

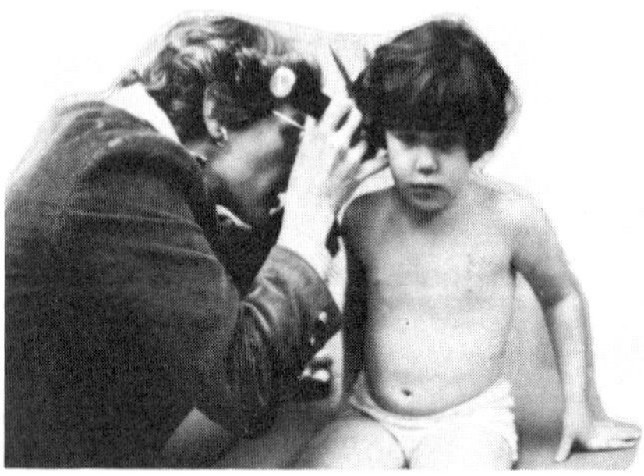

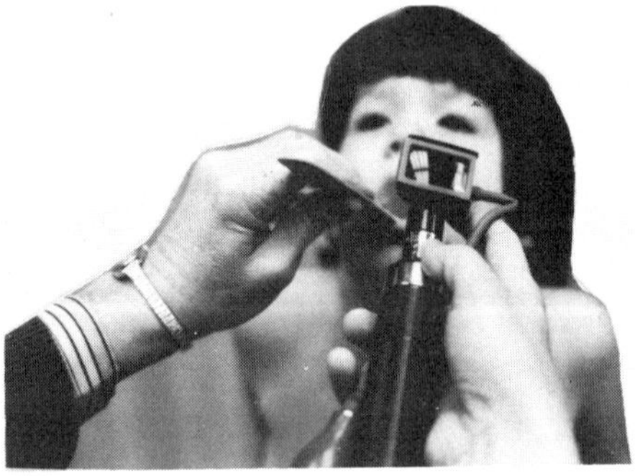

Orthopaedic Examination	The orthopaedic examination screens for scoliosis, knock-knees, bowlegs, and inverted feet.

(Continued)

EXAMINATION OF THE PRESCHOOL CHILD (2-5 YEARS), Continued

Examination of the Back	Facing the child's back, look at the scapulae and hips. These should be level and symmetric. If one shoulder or hip is lower than the other, consider that a discrepancy between the lengths of the legs or scoliosis of the back may be present. Ask the child to bend forward and touch the floor. The back should make a smooth curve. If the curve formed by the back is flattened or the paravertebral muscle mass is prominent on one side, consider the possibility of scoliosis. Screening for excessive lumbar lordosis is difficult. Ask the child to stand sideways and as straight as possible. Some lordosis is expected. Ask the child to pull in the stomach and buttocks. If no change in lordosis is noted and the child also has difficulty performing a forward bend to touch the floor, consider referring the child for orthopaedic evaluation.
Examination of the Legs	Examine the child for knock-knees or bowlegs. Some degree of "normal" bowing can be expected until 1½ years of age, and "normal" knock-knees are expected from 2½ to 5 years. To examine for alignment of the legs, ask the child to stand facing away and to put his legs together. • The presence of bowlegs is suggested when the distance between the knees is greater than 2 cm. This impression is further confirmed if the child's ankles overlap when the child is asked to bring the knees together. • The presence of knock-knees is suggested when the distance between the ankles is greater than 2 cm. It is further confirmed if the child's knees overlap when the child is asked to approximate the ankles.
Examination of the Feet	Examine the child for everted (pronated, flat) or inverted feet by looking at the Achilles tendons with the child facing away. Normally the Achilles tendons are perpendicular to the floor. When feet are pronated or everted, the Achilles tendons will angulate out from perpendicular to the floor. When the feet are inverted, the Achilles tendons will angulate in from a line perpendicular to the floor.

GUIDELINES FOR THE PRESCHOOLER EXAMINATION

- general
  - Introduce yourself.
  - Establish and maintain a rapport with child and parent.
  - height and weight
  - Observe the child.
  - MODIFY the order of the examination for age and response.

- head
  - Observe, measure, and plot.
  - Palpate abnormalities.
  - Examine the head and scalp.

- ears
  - Check the hearing (by some means).
  - Observe the external ear and canal.
  - Look in with an otoscope.

- nose
  - Palpate the maxillary sinus.
  - Look in.

- eyes
  - Observe and palpate the lid.
  - extraocular movements
  - cover test
  - Observe the pupil.
  - pupillary reaction to light and accommodation
  - Check the vision (by some means).
  - Observe the conjunctivae.
  - Use an ophthalmoscope.

- mouth
  - Get a good look at the oral mucosa and palate.
  - Observe and count the teeth.
  - Use a tongue blade.

- neck
  - Palpate the anterior and posterior cervical nodes.
  - Palpate the thyroid and trachea.
  - range of motion
  - Check the clavicles.
  - Palpate the supraclavicular nodes.

- chest
  - Observe.
  - respiratory rate
  - palpation
  - percussion
  - breath sounds (side to side, front <u>and</u> back, right middle lobe)
  - Palpate the axillary nodes.
  - Palpate the epitrochlear nodes.

- heart
  - Palpate (thrill and PMI).
  - Listen over the valve areas.
  - Palpate the branchial and femoral pulses simultaneously.
  - Palpate the other pulses.
  - Determine the blood pressure.
  - Determine the pulse rate.

- abdomen
  - Auscultate for bowel sounds.
  - Palpate and measure the liver and spleen.
  - costovertebral angle
  - deep masses
  - percussion
  - Palpate the inguinal nodes.

- genitalia
  - male--meatus and testes
  - female--separate the labia.

- rectum
  - Look by separating the buttocks.

- back and extremities
  - Observe the sacral area.
  - straightness of back
  - Observe the approximation of the knees and ankles for knock-knees, bowlegs.
  - Observe the heel cord (everted or inverted feet).
  - Observe the feet (metatarsus varus).
  - leg length equality
  - hip
  - range of motion of joints--upper and lower

(Continued)

GUIDELINES FOR THE PRESCHOOLER EXAMINATION, Continued

- neurological (in additon to above)
  - mental status (appropriate for age)
    - response to stimuli
    - developmental level
  - gait
    - tandem walk
    - heel-and-toe walk
  - cranial nerves
    - bite; open mouth
    - smile, show teeth, close eyes, wrinkle brow
    - gag and uvula
    - stick out and wiggle tongue
  - motor
    - muscle mass and tone
    - strength--sample proximal and distal, upper and lower
    - coordination--finger-nose; finger-finger; rapid alternating movements
  - reflexes
    - deep tendon reflexes
    - clonus
    - Babinski
  - sensory

PHYSICAL MEASUREMENTS

Introduction

Accurate assessment of a child's growth is an essential ingredient of the medical evaluation. Measurements are obtained using standardized methods and plotted on an appropriate growth grid. The usual measurements obtained include:

- reclining length for infants and toddlers (birth to 3 years) OR standing height for children over 3 years of age
- head circumference of children under the age of 3 years and in older children if clinically indicated
- weight

There are other measurements that can be obtained; height, weight, and head circumference are the minimum parameters required to assess growth. These measurements provide essential data for health supervision of children. Further changes in weight accurately reflect the status of hydration in infants who have diarrhea or vomiting.

Growth Grids

Measurement data are plotted on one of many standardized growth grids available for use. Grids are developed from measurements made on groups of children. Some are based on the collection of longitudinal data from a single group of children (Boston grids); others use cross-sectional data from several groups of children (UTMB Department of Pediatrics from Faulkner data). Grids exist based on measurements of special groups; for example, norms have been derived from a group of black children. It is therefore important to remember that a single grid does not represent the normal, but rather provides a standard against which a given child can be compared. Examples of the growth grids are included in this chapter.

(Continued)

PHYSICAL MEASUREMENTS, Continued

Weight	Balance the infant on a scale without clothes (a). Older children may retain underwear (b). Record weight and any variations in clothes left on the patient (c).

a

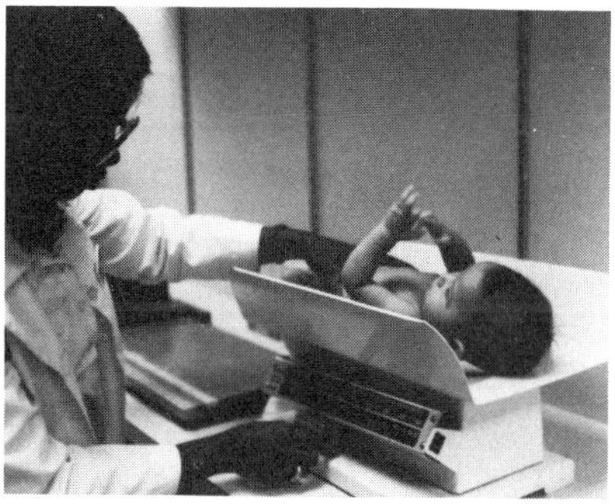

b

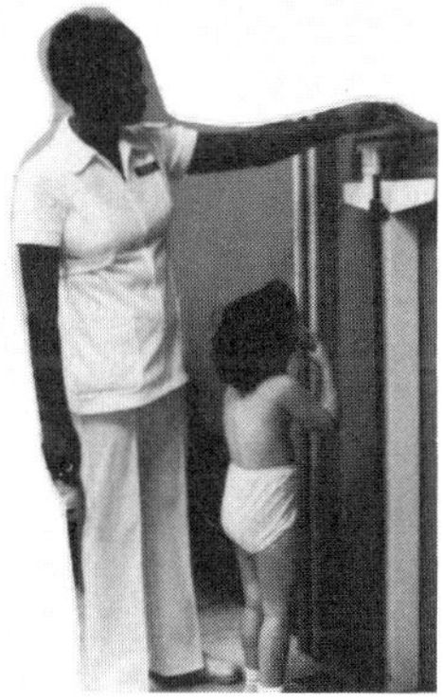

c

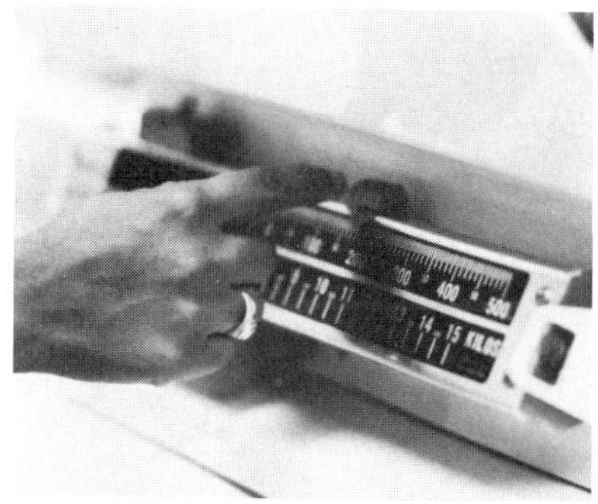

Length or Height	To obtain a reclining length, place the infant on a measuring board with his head firmly against the fixed end of the board. Slide the moveable end of the board against the sole of the foot flexed to 90° (a). To obtain a standing height, place the child against a measuring tape fixed to the wall. Make sure that the heels are on the floor and firmly against the wall (b). Make sure that the child is standing straight. Use a right angle between the wall and the top of the child's head (c).

a

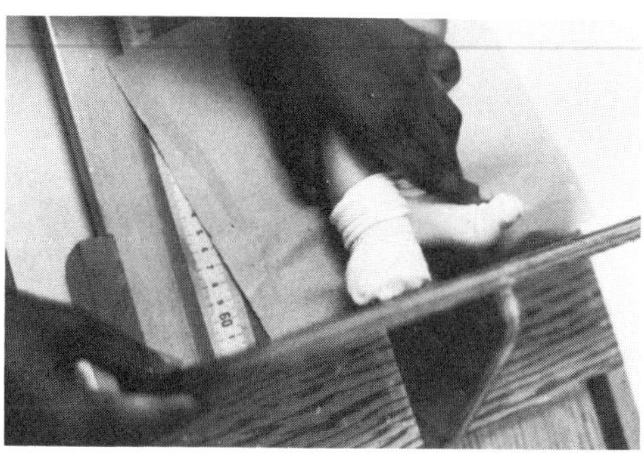

b

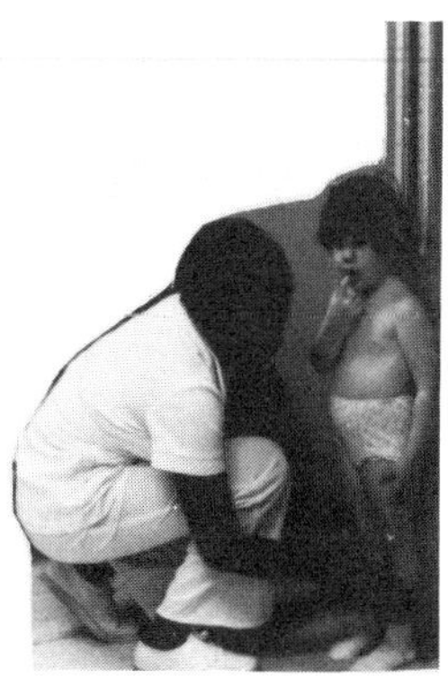

c

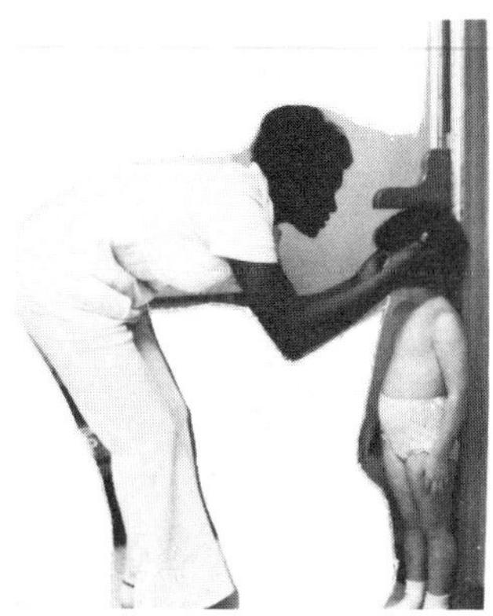

(Continued)

PHYSICAL MEASUREMENTS, Continued

Head Circumference	Wrap a metal or paper tape around the largest circumference of the head (a). Obtain three measurements and record the largest number. Take care to exclude the ears, braids, and barrettes (b).

a

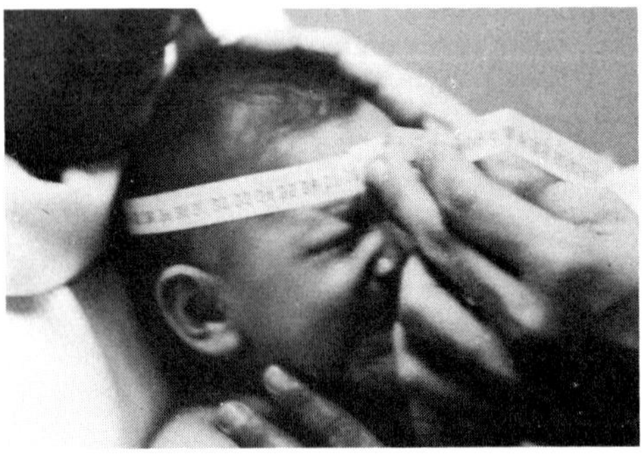

b

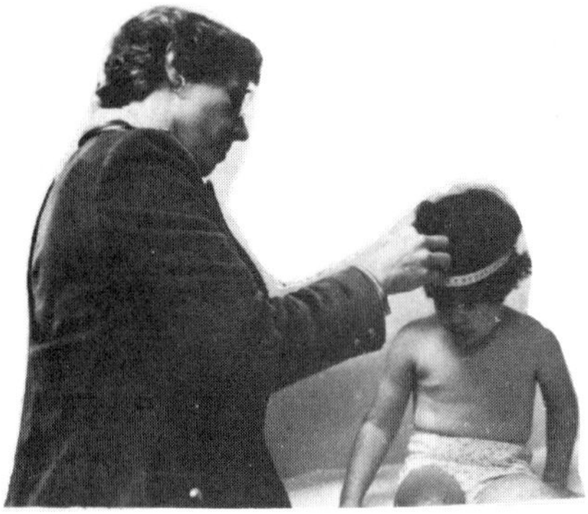

GROWTH GRIDS

Growth Grids

Height, weight, and head circumference are plotted on growth grids. A child's measurements can be compared to those of a number of children of the same age to note if the measurements fall within the expected limits for age. The patient whose measurements are above the 95th percentile or below the 5th percentile on appropriate grids is likely to have a growth problem. A single set of measurements provides less reliable information about growth than multiple sets collected over time. Deviations from standard growth curves for height, weight, or head circumference require further evaluation. Any persistent deviation requires evaluation for organic and/or environmental causes for the abnormality.

Examples

The growth grids that follow illustrate growth patterns. Several examples of deviant patterns are provided on the following pages.

- Patient A: Normal pattern
- Patient B: Decelerated weight and height growth. This may be the result of a number of problems including underfeeding, chronic renal disease, or malabsorption.
- Patient C: Normal growth pattern
- Patient D: Accelerated weight and height growth. This may be the result of a variety of problems including obesity, gigantism, or adrenal tumor.
- Patient E: Accelerated head-circumference growth (macrocephaly). This may be the result of hydrocephalus.
- Patient F: Decelerated head-circumference growth (microcephaly), probably resulting from abnormal brain growth or craniosynostosis.

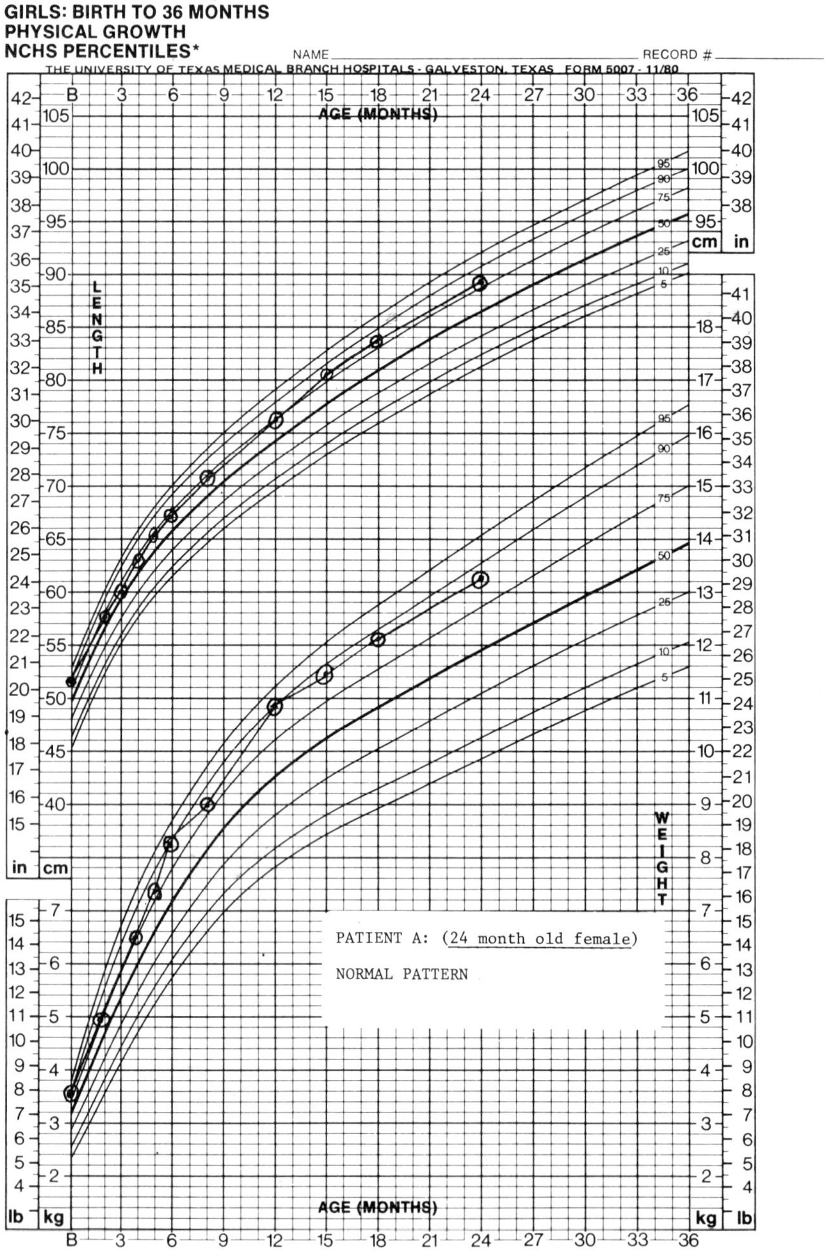
GIRLS: BIRTH TO 36 MONTHS
PHYSICAL GROWTH
NCHS PERCENTILES*
NAME
RECORD #
THE UNIVERSITY OF TEXAS MEDICAL BRANCH HOSPITALS - GALVESTON, TEXAS FORM 5007 - 11/80
AGE (MONTHS)
LENGTH
WEIGHT
PATIENT A: (24 month old female)
NORMAL PATTERN

GIRLS: BIRTH TO 36 MONTHS
PHYSICAL GROWTH
NCHS PERCENTILES*

NAME ____________ RECORD # ____________

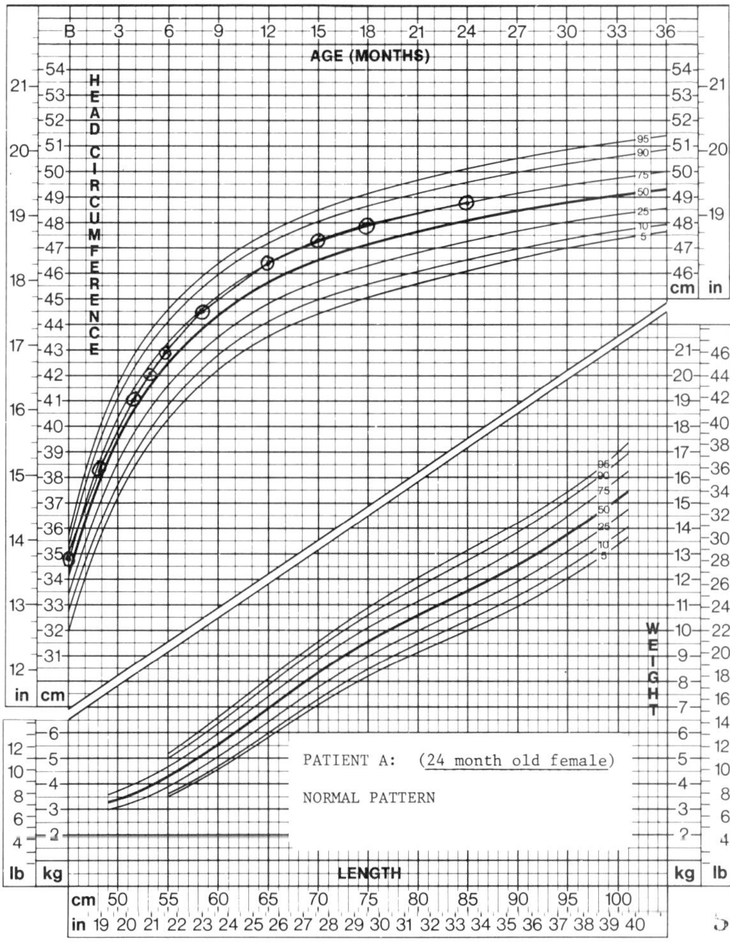

5006

DATE	AGE	LENGTH	WEIGHT	HEAD C.
	BIRTH			

DATE	AGE	LENGTH	WEIGHT	HEAD C.

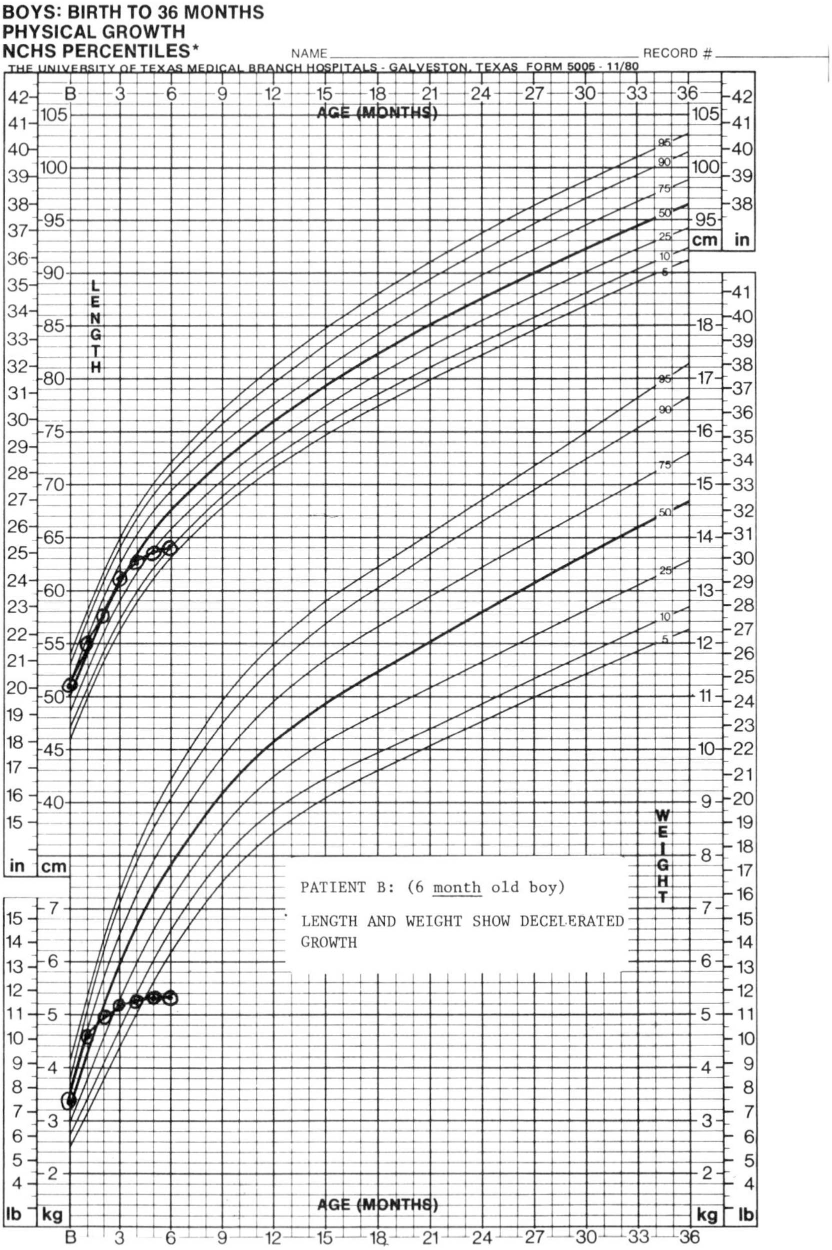
BOYS: BIRTH TO 36 MONTHS
PHYSICAL GROWTH
NCHS PERCENTILES*
NAME
RECORD #
THE UNIVERSITY OF TEXAS MEDICAL BRANCH HOSPITALS - GALVESTON, TEXAS FORM 5005 - 11/80
AGE (MONTHS)
LENGTH
WEIGHT
PATIENT B: (6 month old boy)
LENGTH AND WEIGHT SHOW DECELERATED GROWTH

BOYS: 2 TO 18 YEARS
PHYSICAL GROWTH
NCHS PERCENTILES*

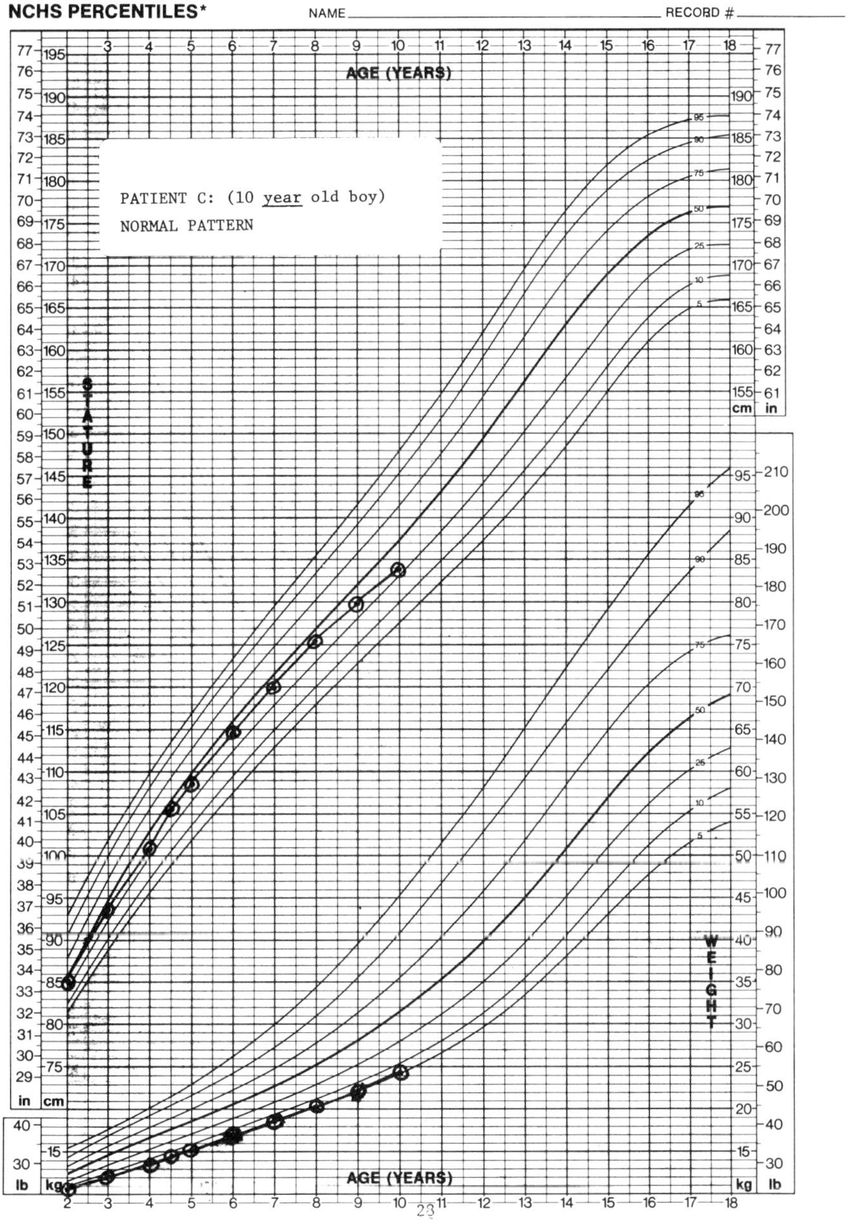

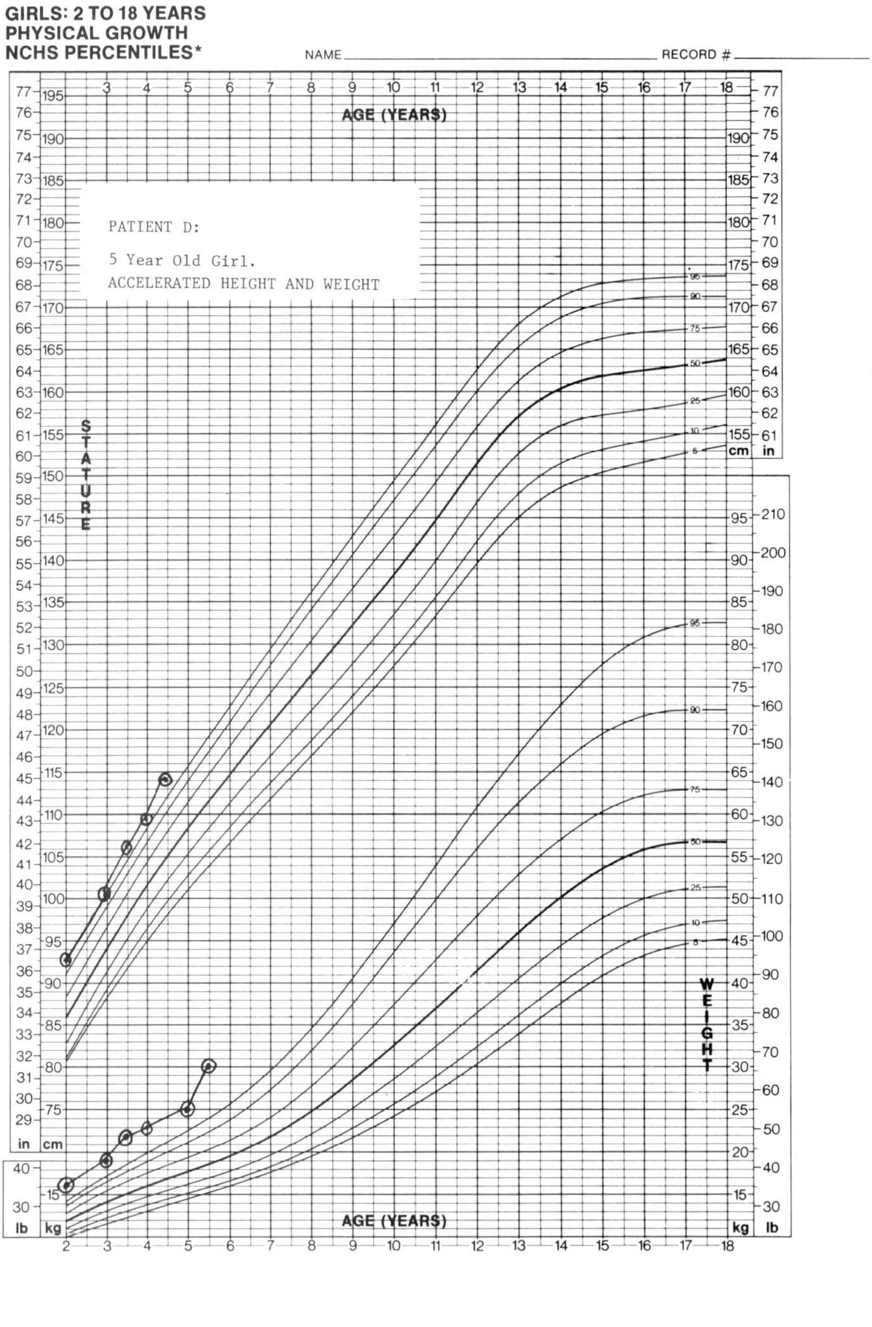
GIRLS: 2 TO 18 YEARS
PHYSICAL GROWTH
NCHS PERCENTILES*
NAME
RECORD #
AGE (YEARS)
PATIENT D:
5 Year Old Girl.
ACCELERATED HEIGHT AND WEIGHT
STATURE
WEIGHT

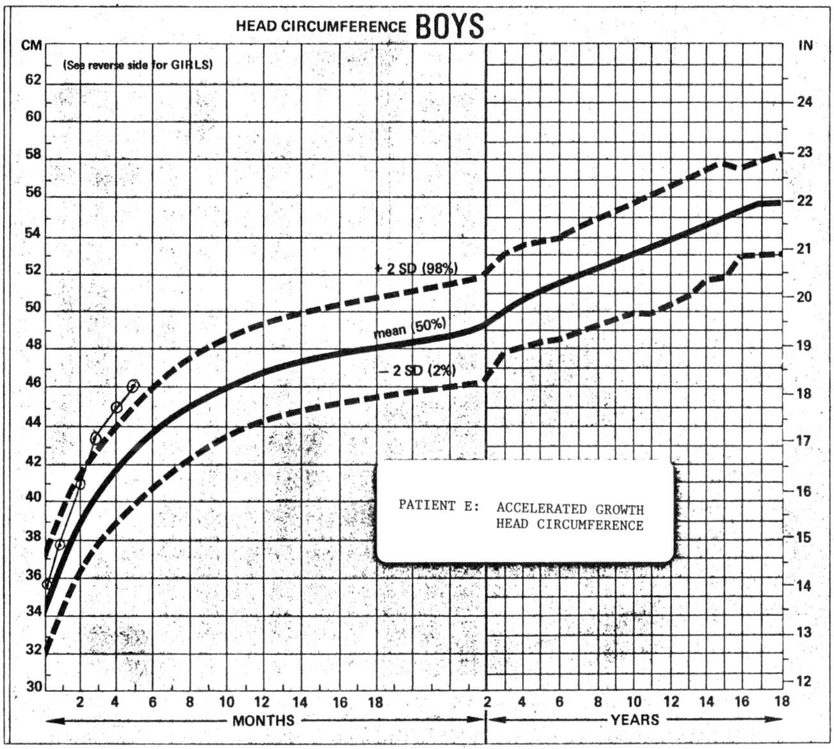
HEAD CIRCUMFERENCE BOYS
(See reverse side for GIRLS)
CM
IN
+2 SD (98%)
mean (50%)
− 2 SD (2%)
PATIENT E: ACCELERATED GROWTH
HEAD CIRCUMFERENCE
MONTHS
YEARS

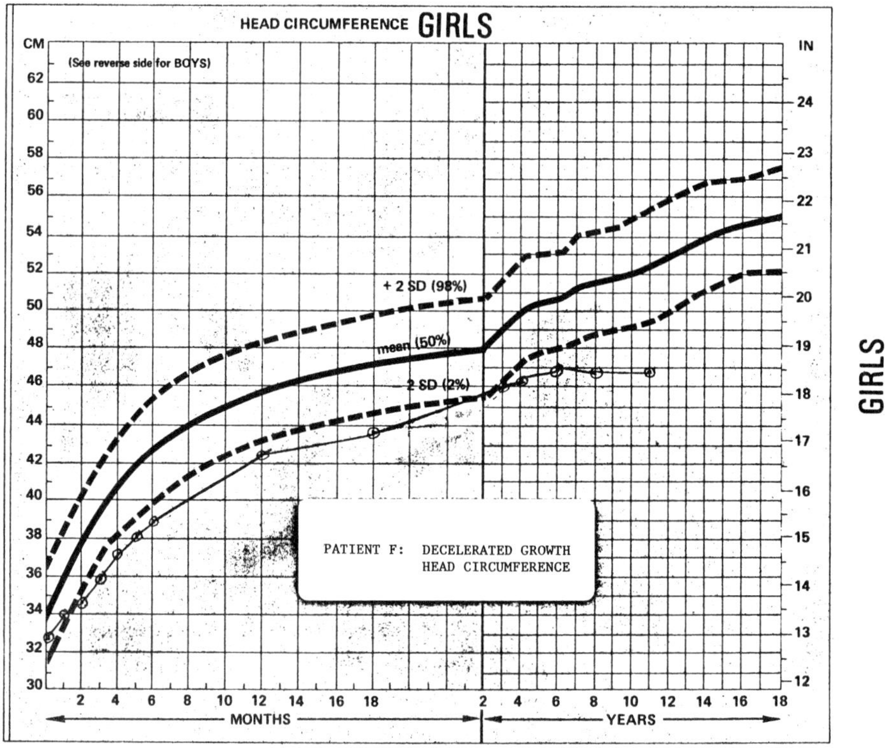
HEAD CIRCUMFERENCE GIRLS
(See reverse side for BOYS)
CM
IN
+ 2 SD (98%)
mean (50%)
– 2 SD (2%)
PATIENT F: DECELERATED GROWTH HEAD CIRCUMFERENCE
MONTHS
YEARS
GIRLS

INDEX

The letter *f* following a page number indicates a figure.